The *Medicina Plinii*

This book presents the first-ever English translation of the *Medicina Plinii*, one of the most influential books of applied medicine and self-medication in Late Antiquity and the Middle Ages.

The work, which predates AD 400, was created as a quick reference work for travellers, and became and remained highly influential, as witnessed by frequent references to it and by various later adaptations. Only the rise of scientific medicine and pharmacology led to its demise and confinement in a small corner of specialist studies. It presents more than 1,150 healing methods and recipes mainly adapted from the encyclopaedic *Natural History of Pliny the Elder*, arranged from the patient's head to foot in order that readers could quickly find treatments for their diseases. The *Medicina Plinii* is of dual interest to present-day scholarship: The book is a monument for the practical application of classical knowledge which has recently found lively interest in the history of science and medicine. At the same time the *Medicina Plinii* provides a fascinating insight into the realities of the world of Late Antiquity, and into the anxieties of the people living in the vast Roman empire.

This book will be of particular interest to scholars and advanced students in the History of Science and Medicine, along with a wider audience interested in medicine, and in life in the Roman world.

Yvette Hunt is Honorary Research Fellow within the School of Historical and Philosophical Inquiry at The University of Queensland. She completed her PhD there in 2013. Among her research interests are ancient medicine and toxicology and their reception in the medieval period, ancient magic, and public entertainment in the Roman period along with the policies which regulated it. In the field of ancient medicine, Yvette has previously published a paper addressing the reception of Dioscorides: "Bang for his buck: Dioscorides as a gift of the tenth-century Byzantine court", in *Byzantine Culture in Translation* (edited by Amelia Brown and Bronwen Neil).

Scientific Writings from the Ancient and Medieval World

Series editor: John Steele, *Brown University, USA*

Scientific texts provide our main source for understanding the history of science in the ancient and medieval world. The aim of this series is to provide clear and accurate English translations of key scientific texts accompanied by up-to-date commentaries dealing with both textual and scientific aspects of the works and accessible contextual introductions setting the works within the broader history of ancient science. In doing so, the series makes these works accessible to scholars and students in a variety of disciplines including history of science, the sciences, and history (including Classics, Assyriology, East Asian Studies, Near Eastern Studies and Indology).

Texts will be included from all branches of early science including astronomy, mathematics, medicine, biology, and physics, and which are written in a range of languages including Akkadian, Arabic, Chinese, Greek, Latin, and Sanskrit.

The Foundations of Celestial Reckoning
Three Ancient Chinese Astronomical Systems
Christopher Cullen

The Babylonian Astronomical Compendium MUL.APIN
Hermann Hunger and John Steele

The Gaṇitatilaka and its Commentary
Two Medieval Sanskrit Mathematical Texts
Alessandra Petrocchi

The *Medicina Plinii*
Latin Text, Translation, and Commentary
Yvette Hunt

www.routledge.com/classicalstudies/series/SWAMW

The *Medicina Plinii*

Latin Text, Translation, and Commentary

Yvette Hunt

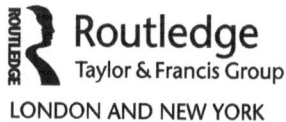
Routledge
Taylor & Francis Group

LONDON AND NEW YORK

First published 2020 by Routledge

2 Park Square, Milton Park, Abingdon, Oxon OX14 4RN
605 Third Avenue, New York, NY 10017

Routledge is an imprint of the Taylor & Francis Group, an informa business

First issued in paperback 2021

Publisher's Note

The publisher has gone to great lengths to ensure the quality of this reprint
but points out that some imperfections in the original copies may be apparent.

British Library Cataloguing-in-Publication Data
A catalogue record for this book is available from the British Library

Library of Congress Cataloging-in-Publication Data
A catalog record has been requested for this book

ISBN: 978-1-138-93482-5 (hbk)
ISBN: 978-1-03-217703-8 (pbk)
DOI: 10.4324/9781315677729

Typeset in Times New Roman
by Apex CoVantage, LLC

For my mother.
For everything.

Contents

Preface

The present translation – the first ever into English – is based on the Latin edition by Önnerfors (1964) and the bilingual Latin/German version of Brodersen (2015). The summaries at the beginning of all three books (which do not always correspond exactly to the equally traditional chapter headings) can already be found in the manuscripts; the division of the text into chapters and sections, however, was only introduced by Rose in 1875.

The text survives because it has been copied repeatedly throughout the Middle Ages. Of course, this process was error-prone, so modern scholars have reconstructed what they consider to be the closest we can get to the lost original. To achieve this, necessary deletions of the text as transmitted are enclosed in square brackets (and are not translated), while necessary insertions appear in angle brackets (and are translated). The commentary first refers to comparanda that are parallel to what the *Medicina Plinii* asserts were found in other ancient literature, and then provides a brief explanation of the text and how it fits within medical knowledge in antiquity. Where it is relevant, I have noted where modern science has investigated this treatment. All dates refer to the Common Era unless otherwise stated.

I have used a very wide array of ancient literature, and where possible have made references to material objects such as papyri and amulets throughout the commentary because I have tried to contextualise the *Medicina Plinii* within its medical, literary, and cultural context, looking at both what influenced its composition, and how these approaches to disease and illness fitted within the broader classical world. Indeed, some of the texts I refer to either cannot be securely dated (e.g. *De morbis acutis et chronicis*) or date as late as the ninth or tenth centuries CE (e.g. *Hippiatrica*, or horse manuals, and *Geoponica*). The reason for including later material is to show how the *Medicina Plinii* appears to have shared (or perhaps influenced) approaches to disease in the centuries following its composition. In addition to this, many later texts preserve material which was originally written centuries earlier, and thus might reflect medical knowledge not just at the time of composition of the *Medicina Plinii*, but even well before it was written. Looking at this text in relation to later literature and material culture helps modern readers to connect not just with the author and his understanding of medicine, but shows why later readers of this text used it and copied it. This approach also illustrates how Latin and Greek medical approaches sometimes overlapped.

This project started with a chance meeting at the University of Queensland in Brisbane while Kai Brodersen (Erfurt) was Margaret Braine Fellow in Classics and Ancient History at the University of Western Australia in Perth. I am grateful to him for advice and for the introduction, to the series editor, John Steele, and the Routledge team, especially Elizabeth Risch, for their patient and efficient support of this project.

Yvette Hunt

Disclaimer

Do not try these at home

The advice outlined in this text was meant for an ancient audience and does not constitute modern medical advice.

Not only was the vast majority of ancient medicine ineffectual, in some cases it was injurious to patient health. Many of the medicaments used are toxic, and even those which are not are dangerous as it is impossible to determine how an individual might react to chemicals they contain. Yes, these remedies can be considered natural, but natural does not mean safe!

This research was conducted for historical purposes only, and the authors are not responsible for the effects on anyone who experiments with these treatments.

Introduction

Kai Brodersen

Euporista – making remedies easily obtainable

> It frequently happened to me during my travels that when, either on account of my illness or that of my companions, I experienced various doctors' frauds; some selling useless remedies at enormous prices, others undertaking those (treatments) which were unable to cure on account of greed. Truly I have learned that some approached illnesses which could be healed in the fewest number of days or even hours in this way; they would prolong them for a long time, so that they could keep their patients for an extended period for profit, and they appear to be crueller than the diseases themselves.
>
> (*Medicina Plinii* Prol. 1)

This complaint opens a little work in which a late-antique author, who called himself "Plinius Secundus Iunior", gave advice on how you could travel through the Roman empire without too much fear of disease, or of doctors. This "Pliny the Younger" continued:

> This is why it seemed necessary to me to gather remedies to illnesses from every source and produce them as a summary; so that whatever place I had come to I might be able to avoid this kind of treachery, and with confidence in this, to engage in travel since then, for I know that should any illness befall me they will neither be making a profit nor assessing an opportunity from me.
>
> (*Medicina Plinii* Prol. 2)

So imagine you fall ill on a journey, but have no access to, or no trust in, medical or pharmaceutical professionals. What can you do? In the ancient world an answer to this potentially vital question was given in books which collected easily obtainable (Greek *euporista*) remedies. These books promised trustworthy advice for patients without access to a trustworthy doctor or apothecary. The *Medicina Plinii* is a prime example for this kind of compilation.

While *euporista* texts had been written centuries prior to the composition of the *Medicina Plinii*, the earliest seems to be the *Euporista* of Apollonius Mys, dating to at least the first century BCE. The earliest extant *euporista* is Dioscorides' *On Simple Drugs* which is now commonly referred to as *Euporista*, probably on account of his use of the term εὐπόριστον in his prologue and the text's approach to disease starting with complaints of the head. This text does not receive the same scholarly attention as Dioscorides' *De Materia Medica*, despite the fact that both were used by Pliny the Elder in his *Naturalis Historia*. These *euporista* must have been reasonably popular during the height of the Roman imperial period. The great doctor and medical writer Galen wrote a *Euporista*, but it was lost within two centuries of its composition (Oribasius *Libra ad Eunapium*, pr. 5). There is a *Euporista* preserved within the Galenic Corpus, now referred to as Pseudo-Galen's *De remediis parabilibus*, which uses the "head-to-toe" approach most commonly used in these works, but it cannot be securely dated.

While the *Medicina Plinii* was written to address the author's mistrust in medical specialists, similar *euporista* were written to address the specific issue of travel by medical specialists. Oribasius, the personal physician to Julian the Apostate, the Roman emperor from 360/1 to 363 CE, wrote a *euporista*, his *Libri ad Eunapium*, as a book for laymen to use while travelling (pr. 1), so health during travel seems to have been an issue of some concern in antiquity.

Another *Euporista* which has survived is that of Theodorus Priscianus whose work, like those of his fellow North African medical writers, bridged the supposed gap between Greek and Latin medical writing. His *Euporista* was originally composed in Greek; he then translated it into Latin. This is extremely interesting as much has been made in modern scholarship about the influence of Pliny the Elder upon his work (e.g. Formisano 2004, 135–40). The nature of this *Euporista* highlights the need for modern scholars to not look at later Latin and Greek medical texts as discrete bodies of literature; cross-pollination was occurring between the two. Theodorus' *Euporista* is considered to have been written as a popular and practical medical manual, and by translating it into Latin he was seeking a broader audience (Theodorus *Euporista*, 1.pr.1); Greek was considered the specialist language of doctors, so like the *Medicina Plinii*, Theodorus' Latin *Euporista* might have sought a lay audience.

Making science accessible

While the science of medicine had a long-standing tradition in the ancient world, a normal patient had no access to, or could not understand, books by the great doctors, or even compendia like the *Compositiones* ("Recipes for Combined Medicaments") of Scribonius Largus, a doctor who served the Roman Emperor Claudius (41–54 CE), or the chapters *De medicina* ("On medicine") of the (otherwise lost) encyclopaedic work by his contemporary Aulus Cornelius Celsus. Another comprehensive work which compiled scientific information available in the first century, the huge *Naturalis Historia* by the great scholar Gaius Plinius Secundus, Pliny the Elder, is preserved.

Pliny the Elder was killed while observing the eruption of Mount Vesuvius in 79 CE which buried Pompeii. His eponymous nephew, often referred to as Pliny the Younger, but not the author of the present book, described the elder Pliny's last hours. Pliny the Elder's encyclopaedia is comprised of 37 books and offers a comprehensive survey of ancient natural history: After an introduction (Book 1) it starts with cosmography, meteorology, hydrology, and general geography (2). This is followed by a detailed geography of the known world (3–6), anthropology (7), zoology (8–11), botany (11–19), medicine and pharmacology (20–32), metallurgy (33–34), theory of colours, painting and sculpture (35), and finally mineralogy (36–37). As for medical and pharmacological information, the *Naturalis Historia* offers an almost overwhelming amount of information, which was sorted by remedies: Books 20–27 deal with herbal medicines, sorted by their environment (garden plants, field crops, wild plants), 28–30 with remedies taken from animals, and 31–32 remedies aquatic creatures. If the reader searched for a cure, such a systematic approach was obviously only of practical use if it was already known which remedy was helpful for a particular affliction. Also, the sheer size of the *Naturalis Historia* made it difficult to use, let alone to have a copy at hand when you needed a remedy.

To make the information in Pliny the Elder's *Naturalis Historia* easier to digest and access, its content was variously excerpted and rearranged in Late Antiquity. Thus a compact collection of the wonders of the world in which the details of the geographical books were combined with those of the natural wonders (especially from zoology, botany, and mineralogy) was created in the early fourth century CE by Gaius Iulius Solinus in his *Collectanea rerum mirabilium* ("Collections of Wondrous Things"), also known as *Polyhistor* ("Know-a-lot"). Solinus condensed Pliny the Elder's *Naturalis Historia*, combined it with details taken from additional documents, and presented the result in a new arrangement. The new *Collectenea* proved to be most successful in Late Antiquity and the Middle Ages: Some 250 copies bear witness to its influence, and several of them comprise further enhancements, including the oldest surviving description of Norway (which neither Pliny nor Solinus could have known, of course).

Similarly, a pharmacological book dating to the late third century CE (it was quoted in the material added to the fourth-century *Euporiston* of Theodorus Priscianus (Rose 1894, 276) and entitled *Herbarius* (*liber*), provided compact excerpts from Pliny the Elder's books on herbal remedies, combined with information taken from other sources, or experience, and rearranged to enhance its practical value. This anonymous work circulated under the name of Apuleius Platonicus, a second-century CE philosopher and author best known today for his novel *Metamorphoses* (also known as "The Golden Ass"); clearly this famous name was chosen to enhance the authority of the information contained in the book. In addition, the *Herbarius* was presented as a work which ultimately originated from the centaur Cheiron (Latin Chiro) who was the wise teacher both of the hero Achilleus (Achilles) and of the healing god Asklepios (Aesculapius).

The *Herbarius* thus claimed to have even more authority than the famous hero and the god of healing. The work presents 129 healing herbs, but begins, after a prologue, with a comprehensive survey presenting nearly 200 diseases and ailments which could be treated with the herbs described in the book, and sorted first from head to toe, and then refers to illnesses affecting the whole body. The *Herbarius* begins with a harsh criticism of professional doctors, presented as a letter by Apuleius to his fellow citizens:

> From many public documents, we have chosen some powers of herbs and treatments for the body and done so in truthfulness because of the verbose stupidity of the professionals. We say that they are guided more by the greed of the medical profession than by real care, and also that we must describe these people mostly because of their deeds and inexperience as addicted to profit, who demand money from the dead! What do they do? Nothing! They wait for an opportunity to make a profit and even extend the time of the treatments! Indeed, I think they are more dangerous than the diseases themselves! As a way out, we want to introduce the names of the diseases, which our time knows of, so that my fellow citizens, both compatriots and foreigners, who are afflicted by a physical ailment, may be helped through our written-down science – against the will of the doctors.
>
> (Herbarius, praefatio)

These attacks on doctors seem to have become so common among such handbooks that even Theodorus Priscianus' *Euporista* includes an attack on doctors for not approaching medicine with the needs of the patient foremost to mind, and he was a doctor (Theodorus *Euporista*, 1.prol.1).

Like the *Herbarius*, the *Medicina Plinii* was based on Pliny the Elder's *Naturalis Historia*, which was the source for about five-sixths of the advice and recipes given. The information from Pliny was supplemented from other sources; this is specifically true for a dozen or so detailed recipes at the end of some sections which present, unlike Pliny the Elder, a lot of information on quantities. Not least, "Pliny the Younger", who referred to himself repeatedly in the first person (prologue, 1.26.5–6; 3.4.1; 3.33 Pr.), claimed that he worked from his own experience and had used some of the remedies himself.

Unlike Pliny the Elder's *Naturalis Historia*, but like the works in the *euporista* tradition, the *Medicina Plinii* sorts the information by complaints from head to toe (Book I and II); followed by whole-body symptoms such as fever, skin diseases, poisons, and bites (Book III). In this last book, the author presented an even more condensed summary of material, "since some materials are beneficial for several conditions" (3.4.1). The aim of presenting a practically useful manual was enhanced by taking apart many of the long and complicated sentences in the *Naturalis Historia* as well. The work thus presents, in quite simple Latin, more than 1,150 healing methods and recipes in a compact format.

The provision of compact texts was also regarded as desirable among Greek readers throughout Late Antiquity and into the Byzantine period. In addition to his *euporista*, *Libri ad Eunapium*, Oribasius wrote a longer work called *Synopsis ad Eustathium*. Like his *euporista*, this work was a longer summary of his medical works written for doctors to use when travelling (*Syn.* 1.pr. 3), providing an accessible, compact format. Similarly, Aëtius provided a synopsis of Galen's *De simplicium medicamentorum temperatmentis ac facultatibus libri xi* in his first two books. Like the author of the *Medicina Plinii*, Aëtius reduced the length of Galen's work to forty per cent (Gowling 2017, 84). He did this by removing much of Galen's introductory discussions as well as some entries, but like the author of the *Medicina Plinii*, he also added material to his text which was procured independently from his primary source, perhaps the result of personal experience, and created a handbook of practical size for practicing physicians (Gowling 2017, 96 & 99).

Much of this move towards the creation of practical condensed volumes was owed to the increased popularity of codices. It therefore should not be surprising that there was a shift among both Greek and Latin medical authors in the manner in which new works were composed, as this change in technology – from scroll to codex – was a perfect medium through which to make scientific literature more accessible (Horden 2013, 5–6; see also Nutton 2013, 12–18 for the influence of the codex on the development of medical handbooks). It should come as no surprise that writers would have adapted their style of composition to also reflect this accessibility to a wider audience. The author of the *Medicina Plinii* was one of the first to draw these two ideas of accessibility together in his work.

The world of the *Medicina Plinii*

The *Medicina Plinii* identifies several historical figures: King Antiochus, either the third who ruled over the Seleucid Empire in Syria from 223–187 BC, or the eighth who ruled from 125 to 96 BCE over parts of that empire (3.37.11), while Mithridates VI held the Kingdom of Pontus on the Black Sea from about 120 BCE, until Gnaeus Pompeius Magnus ("the Great") conquered it for the Romans (3.33.4). Manlius Cornutus (1.18.2) was the governor of the province of Aquitania under the emperors Tiberius or Claudius (14 to 41 CE), and the emperor Nero (54 to 68 CE) were named. We cannot date the doctor Damon (3.3.3; note that Pliny the Elder mentioned a physician named Damion or Dalion in his *Naturalis Historia* 20.40.103) and the athlete Sagares (30.3.11, not mentioned by Pliny the Elder).

However, the language and tradition to which the *Medicina Plinii* belongs show that the work was created later. It can also be shown that the author of the late third century CE *Herbarius* had access to, and used, the *Medicina Plinii* which must therefore predate it. Also, the late fourth century author Marcellus Empiricus appears to have had access to the work, so it is reasonable to date the *Medicina*

Plinii, like the other extract of Pliny the Elder's *Naturalis Historia*, Solinus' *Collectanea*, to the early third century CE.

The late-antique Roman world for which the *Medicina Plinii* appears to have been written, was great and wide. The work mentions not only the Roman people (3.30.14) and the provinces of Aquitania in modern-day France (1.18.2), but also the Aegean island of Cos (Kos) where an inscription was placed (3.37.11), and Egypt as a region which was known for *elephantiasis* (1.19.2). Most importantly, however, the origins of remedies show how large the world had become in Late Antiquity: Italy presented wine from Aminea (also spelled Aminnea) on the Adriatic (2.3.2) and from Falernum in Campania (1.24.2), as well as pitch from Bruttium in southern Italy (1.17.2; 2.27.9; 3.4.16; 3.8.3) and saffron from Sicily (2.4.11). Nuts (3.23.5) and honey came from Greece (1.25.2; 2.4.14; incidentally, fenugreek is *fenum Graecum*, "Greek clover", in Latin: 2.4.3), honey specifically also from Attica (1.12.7; 2.27.15), from where you could also source soda (2.14.6), and parsley from Macedonia (2.4.13). Oak-gall was collected from Asia Minor (2.15.1), especially Commagene (2.10.5), and from Syria (1.12.5), from where sumach was also be obtained (2.4.11). Pontus, the Black Sea region, was not only home to a well-known breed of ducks (3:33:10), but also of wax (2.17.5; 2.27.9). The Aegean island Cimolus (Kimolos) lent its name to the "Cimolian chalk" (1.2.3; 1.7.4; 3.5.5; 3.24.8; 3.27.3), Samos to "Samian earth" (1.2.3), and Cyprus to "Cyprian oil" (1.2.2; 1.4.2; 2.23.3; 3.1.4). Out of Egypt alum (1.4.3; 2.20.4) and behen-nuts (2.5.2) arrived, from Thebes in Egypt, dates (1.25.7), from Alexandria, mustard (3.20.2), and from Cyrene the plant called *laser* (1.15.4), a panacea popular in the ancient world but probably extinct later. From North Africa one used sponges (1.25.4; 3.16.1; 3.22.2) and snails (2.4.7; 2.16.3; 2.19.3), while pomegranates were referred to as "Punic apples" with reference to the world of Carthage (2.1.1; 2.4.11; 2.8.3; 2.8.4; 2.12.4; 3.21.10), which also had "Punic wax" (2.15.5). Similar to pomegranates, quinces were commonly called "Cydonian apples", referring to the city Cydonia in western Crete (the modern city of Chania) where they were grown in huge numbers, and were commonly recommended by the author (1.4.2; 1.8.4; 1.25.3,7; 2.4.4,11; 2.5.3; 2.7.2; 2.10.4; 3.4.10).

Travellers in the Mediterranean world obviously did not need much advice on problems of too much exposure to sunlight (only 1.1.4), but felt threatened by chilblains (2.25) and frostbite (3.13); even a walk through snow – clearly a rare event – needed to be prepared for (3.13.1).

Who travelled in this world? What were the typical travel afflictions? And what were the remedies suggested in the text? Travellers were identified mainly as men (the *Medicina Plinii* does not adopt remedies for women from Pliny the Elder), but apparently also for families, as there were recipes for teething infants (1.13) and for ulcers in children (1.3.1).

The journeys were conducted on foot, on horseback, or by horse-drawn carriage: ancient footwear was made – like simple sandals today – mostly from soles which were fastened to the foot with straps. If you walked a lot, this could lead to foot wounds: the straps rubbed and created sore points on the foot or even caused ulceration. The toenails could hurt, the soles could become rubbed, tearing the skin on the heel could cause fissures, and there might be corns and calluses. What to do? Foot wounds were treated by applying ashes of earthworms in old oil or burning slugs alive, and ulceration by the ashes of chicken or pigeon droppings in oil (2.25.4). Sores were removed by the ashes of an old sandal sole or goat horn, each in oil, or a layer of lamb or ram lung (2.25.5–6). For abscessed toenails (foot-rot or whitlows) one used the dust of a ground horse's tooth, and for abraded feet the blood of a green lizard as a healing ointment, while fissures were treated with the ashes of a tortoise shell, mixed with wine and oil, or bear grease with the addition of alum (2.25.6). For corns and calluses on the feet it was useful to rub the urine of mules with the mud it created or apply sheep excrement or the liver or blood of a green lizard in a tuft of wool. Also, you could boil earthworms in oil or pigeon droppings in vinegar and apply them – or put fresh boar excrement on and leave it for three days. Also useful were beans with *laser* (see above), placed in vinegar (2.26.2–4). Similarly, travelling on horseback could lead to discomfort. Thighs chafed by riding can be brushed with foam from the horse's mouth (2.22.3).

Most frequently, however, people travelled by horse-drawn carriages, which left tracks in the ground (3.35.1–2). A traffic accident could lead to the patient being pushed or knocked down, dragged or be hurt by the wheels. To remedy this, boar excrement cooked in vinegar was useful; for other injuries dry dust from boar excrement or pig manure in a drink or in water (3.30.7–9). Incidentally, axle-grease (Latin *axungia*), which was mostly made of lard (as 3.13.2 states), was repeatedly recommended (1.7.3,5; 1.22.3; 2.21.4,5; 2.27.3.6, 7; 3.1.1; 3.4.11,15 and 16; 3.5.3; 3.8.3; 3.1.1,2; 3.13.2; 3.29.2) – obviously this was always easily available, as was the paste used to wash your hands, made from bean flour (1.18.6; 2.21.4; 2.26.5; 3.6.2). Occasionally the journey was made by boat: a recipe recommended the use of ship-biscuit (2.6.2); repeatedly, sea water was recommended – if this was unavailable when travelling over land you could mix it yourself using water and salt (Prol. 4).

Drink and food – *Passum, Mulsum, Pusca, Garum,* and *Moretum*

A number of drinks were common throughout the empire. Wine was usually taken mixed with water; undiluted wine appears in the *Medicina Plinii* repeatedly as a remedy. *Passum* was a type of sweet raisin wine; it is still made today and called "Passito de Pantelleria". This is also commonly recommended throughout the text. *Mulsum* (also called *mulsum vinum*) was made either from wine or must with honey and was sometimes mixed with water or vinegar. *Mulsa aqua* (also called *mulsa*) was a type of mead made of fermented honey and water. Vinegar itself was drunk, as was *pusca*, a simple non-alcoholic drink that consisted of water, a little vinegar, and possibly spices. *Pusca* was the refreshment offered to Jesus Christ on the cross. *Moretum* was a cheese dish produced in a mortar with herbs. *Garum* was a spicy sauce based on fermented fish guts; it was very similar to and sometimes confused with *liquamen* which was made using the whole fish. *Garum*'s sediment was called *allex*.

Of course, some food and drink may well be too hot or cause constipation or diarrhoea:

> If something extremely hot scalded the inside of the mouth, it is promptly healed by a gargle of dog milk.
>
> (*Medicina Plinii* 1.12.4)

For constipation, the *Medicina Plinii* recommends cooking an old snake skin with rose oil in a silver-lead alloy vessel and spreading it on the body; alternatively oysters cooked in *mulsum*, cow's milk, or a soup of pan-braised sea fish, taken with lettuce or with bread. For intestinal cramps, it helped to eat overcooked vegetables with salt or to drink sea water taken from the high seas or stagnant sea water with wine or vinegar or, if you drink the pure sea water, chew radish in vinegar to promote vomiting. The effect could also be achieved by eating wheat-meal gruel without oil (2.9.1–4).

For the opposite complaint, diarrhoea, several remedies and methods are presented: one could drink crushed riverine crabs in water or skirret juice in goat milk, rub ground basil on the body or cook Italian millet in goat milk and take it daily as a soup. One could pound old ship-biscuit, cook and drink water, possibly with boiled beans, or you could eat lentils boiled in rain water as a soup or drink undiluted vinegar – and much more; the number of recipes for diarrhoea is indeed very large (2.6.1–8).

From toothache to poisoning

Toothache can affect travellers everywhere. To maintain dental health they were advised to start the day with putting a grain of salt under the tongue until it dissolved (1.13.20) – the toothbrush had not been invented yet. The work presents detailed advice on what to do in case of dental problems – particularly loose, aching or hollow teeth, but does not even mention the usual radical method applied in antiquity: pulling bad teeth (1.13). A remedy against bad breath was rubbing the teeth with mice ash and honey, possibly with the addition of roots from a tamarisk growing near the sea; also useful was rinsing the mouth with pure wine in the evening or with cold water in the morning (1.12.1).

It is also noteworthy that the *Medicina Plinii* includes hair dyes: "It is worthwhile to assist those who are embarrassed to be old, even if they want to dye their grey hair, as if they could strip years away from their true age." They should anoint their scalp with "earthworms' ash in oil" (1.5.5) – a tincture, incidentally which, provided you used old oil, also healed foot wounds (2.25.4).

A special risk for travellers in Late Antiquity, however, were poisons and bites which are discussed only in the last chapters of the *Medicina Plinii*, with the exception of dog-bites which were addressed a little earlier in Book Three. Not only could mad dogs bite and cause "hydrophobia" (a typical symptom of rabies), but even non-rabid bites posed a danger (3.10–11). There were also poisonous spiders (3.36), snakes (3.37) and shrew-mice (3.35) – it was unknown in antiquity that their bite is actually not poisonous. Not least, the traveller could also encounter villains who intentionally administered a poison (3:33) – and could be bitten not only by animals, but also by humans (3.37.14)!

Insights into a distant world

While we often think that we are somehow familiar with the world of travellers in history, the *Medicina Plinii* presents us in many ways with a rather distant world. One wrote on papyrus, one could buy breast milk on the road, slavery was an undisputed fact of life, crucifixion was a method used for the death penalty, and vultures could be seen to pick at corpses.

Papyrus was ubiquitous as writing material; the individual strips were glued together with special flour – flour which was also a remedy (1.25.4). Breast milk was required for three herbal remedies (1.6.11; 1.8.1; 3.30.10); apparently it could be bought from wet-nurses, whose job it is to breast-feed infants. Slaves were part of the groups which travelled; they also accompanied their master to the public baths (3.32.1). They were regarded as property, so to avoid the risk of their devaluation one could treat their impending baldness (1.4.1). The traveller had fun with boys and men – which was why some travellers used hair dye because men prefer red hair on boys, but not on men (1.5.1).

The world was cruel: as a remedy for quartan fever (a symptom of malaria), the head of a nail or rope taken from a recent crucifixion was recommended (3.15.1). Vultures fed on human corpses (3.21.9), and a knife or dagger used to wound or kill a man could also be obtained while travelling (1.22.4; 3.21.2).

Weights and measures

Although most recipes in the *Medicina Plinii* do not refer to quantitative data, some do state lengths, capacities or weights, which the work partially explains itself (Prol. 9).

The standard length was the foot (*pes*, almost 30 centimetres), 1/12 of a foot was an inch (*uncia*). For capacities the standard size was one bucket (*congius*, about 3 litres), a sixth of the pitcher (*sextarius*), which in turn consisted of 2 pints (*hemina*), 8 pans (*acetabulum*), 10 ounces (*uncia*), 12 ladles (*cyathus*), or 48 spoons (*cochlear*); 1 small spoon (*lingula/ligula*) was a somewhat smaller unit. A "pinch" referred to the amount of material one could lift with three fingers. For weights, the standard measurement was the pound (*libra*, about 330 grams) consisting of 12 ounces (*uncia*) or 24 asses (*as*). So depending on context, *uncia* could refer to length or capacity or weight. Sixteen *as* (or 2/3 pounds) corresponded to a *drachma*; this Greek unit was considered to be equal to the Roman (silver) *denarius*; a *victoriatus* was originally 3/4 of a *denarius*, but was worth 1/2 by the mid-first century BCE. A *drachma* consisted of 2 spoons (*cochlear*), 3 scruples (*scripulus*), 4 sesterces (*sestertius*), or 6 obols. A hundred *drachmae* formed a *mina*. A *sestertius* was understood not only as a unit of weight, but also as a coin. Finally, for consistency of materials, the author drew comparisons taken from everyday life, using honey (1.12.6; 1.16.5; 1.25.8; 1.26.7; 2.4.12; 2.8.4; 2.20.4) or carpenter's glue (3.30.12) as a reference.

A travel health kit

While doctors were not always available, or mistrusted, and while the earlier scholarly or encyclopaedic works on medicine and pharmacology appeared to be too bulky or not well enough organised for practical use, compilations of easily obtainable (*euporista*) remedies promised healing without having to ask, trust, and pay doctors.

> We proffer many remedies so that it is possible to use them when required, when any of these present themselves.
>
> (*Medicina Plinii* 1.6.1)

Overall, about two-thirds of the procedures and remedies referred to in the *Medicina Plinii* made use of plant, animal, and mineral substances which belong to what is now called "folk medicine". They partly coincide with "natural healing advice" today, but partly also correspond to the so-called "rational" medicine and thus, according to the author's contemporary conventional medical opinion, to effective remedies. The remaining third of substances are taken from what scholars refer to as "dirt pharmacy" (like ear wax or animal droppings) and some include elements of magic (e.g. 2.19.1; 2.22.2). Thus, a recommended remedy against quartan fever (a symptom of malaria) reads as follows:

> If a prepubescent boy removes the swollen bark of the wild fig from a broken branch with his teeth and the inside itself is attached before the rising of the sun, it is known to prevent *strumae*. Beaten sea-urchins' shells with alum in old oil and porridge.
>
> (*Medicina Plinii* 3.6.1)

> You write on a clean piece of paper which he who suffers should carry tied on the right arm: "Withdraw from him, Gaius Seius, tertian. Solomon follows you!" Likewise, he should bind bread and salt in a cloth with thread and with the thread he should tie it around a tree and he should swear three times by bread and salt: "Tomorrow guests are going to come to me; receive these!" He should say this three times.
>
> (*Medicina Plinii* 3.15.7–8)

Obviously, the *Medicina Plinii* cannot be used as a good guide to symptom-free journeys throughout the world of today. But who knows – maybe it will help even today for grey hair when you rubbed your head with the ashes from earthworms in oil?

The *Medicina Plinii*

Text

Liber I

capitula libri I

Prologus

The *Medicina Plinii*
Translation

Book One

Chapters of Book One

Prologue

Prologus plinii secundi iunioris

1   Frequenter mihi in peregrinationibus accidit ut aut propter meam aut propter meorum infirmitatem varias fraudes medicorum experiscerer, quibusdam vilissima remedia ingentibus pretiis vendentibus, aliis ea quae curare nesciebant cupiditatis causa suscipientibus. quosdam vero comperi hoc genere grassari ut languores, qui paucissimis diebus vel etiam horis possint repelli, in longum tempus extraherent, <ut> et aegros suos diu in reditu haberent saevioresque ipsis morbis existerent.

2   quapropter necessarium mihi visum est ut undique valitudinis auxilia contraherem et velut breviario colligerem, ut quocumque venissem possem eiusmodi insidias vitare et hac fiducia ex hoc tempore <iter> ingredi, ut sciam, si quis mihi languor inciderit, non facturos illos ex me reditum nec taxaturos occasionem.

3   Ante omnia autem puto in promptu habenda quae subito desiderata difficillima videntur <inventu>, sicut oleum vetus. quod si ad manum non fuerit, celerrime fieri potest. defervefactum enim vel recentissimum et odorem et vires vetustissimi praestat.

4   et si forte curatio exegerit aquam marinam quae<ri> in mediterraneo, sol<licitudini> loc<us> non erit. bessis sextarii salis marini in quattuor sextarios aquae coniectus temperatum mare repraesentat, sextarius vero salsissimum. si vero plus adiciatur, exsuperat sal aquam nec liquari potest.

5   Oxymeli faciemus duobus cyathis mellis in sextario aceti resolutis.
Thalassomeli quemadmodum conficiatur dicemus cum ad usum eius venerimus.

6   Opus erit aliquando et polenta, quam sic comparari oportet. perfusum aqua hordeum nocte una siccatur. deinde in XX libris hordei adiciuntur tres librae lini seminis et coriandri selibra, salis acetabulum unum. tunc mane torretur et mola frangitur.

7   In omnibus curationibus meminerimus utillimum esse mel in quo apes mortuae sunt. quo uti si continget, affectandum erit.
Lanam sucidam aeque meminerimus optimam esse e collo.

8   Iubemur in quibusdam remediis uti cinere vel avium vel animalium aliarumque rerum. omnia huius generis debebunt cremari in olla nova, addito operculo circumlitoque argilla, in furno ferventi.

9   Omnibus gargarizationibus calidis utemur.
Oportet et pondera medicinalia mensurasque nosse. drachma tres scripulos habet. drachma pondus est denarii argentei, obolus drachmae pars sexta. cyathus drachmae decem, acetabulum drachmae quindecim, cochleare drachma dimidia, mina drachmae C. sextarius medicinalis habet uncias X.

10 Haec sunt fere quae in universitatem observanda sunt. nunc singulis membris sua remedia applicabimus. procedente opusculo tertianis quartanis et huiusmodi malis quemadmodum occurratur, sicut in notitiam nostram venit, tractabimus. incipiemus ergo a capite.

Prologue of the second Pliny the Younger

1   It frequently happened to me during my travels that when, either on account of my illness or that of my companions, I experienced various doctors' frauds; some selling useless remedies at enormous prices, others undertaking those (treatments) which were unable to cure on account of greed. Truly I have learned that some approached illnesses which could be healed in the fewest number of days or even hours in this way; they would prolong them for a long time, so that they could keep their patients for an extended period for profit, and they appear to be crueller than the diseases themselves.

2   This is why it seemed necessary to me to gather remedies to illnesses from every source and produce them as a summary; so that whatever place I had come to I might be able to avoid this kind of treachery, and with confidence in this, to engage in travel since then, for I know that should any illness befall me they will neither be making a profit nor assessing an opportunity from me.

3   First, however, I think it is necessary to have everything in readiness which seems most difficult to find at short notice, like old oil. But if it is not at hand, it can be made extremely quickly. In fact, even the freshest boiled thoroughly exceeds the smell and strength of the oldest.

4   And if by chance a treatment requires that sea water be obtained when inland, there will be no place for anxiety. Two-thirds of a *sextarius* of sea salt thrown into four *sextarii* of water creates mild sea water. Indeed, a *sextarius* is much too salty. In fact, if more is added, the salt overcomes the water and it cannot be dissolved.

5   We will make *oxymel* by dissolving two *cyathi* of honey in a *sextarius* of vinegar. I will say how *thalassomeli* is made when we come to its use.

6   Sometimes *polenta* will be useful, which ought to be prepared thus. Barley wet with water, is dried for one night. Afterwards, three *librae* of linseed, half a *libra* of coriander, and one *acetabulum* of salt is added to 20 *librae* of barley. Then it is roasted in the morning and crushed with a mill.

7   We should keep in mind that in all treatments the most useful honey is that in which bees have died. It should be planned to use this if it can be arranged. We should equally keep in mind that the best greasy wool is from the neck.

8   We are directed in some remedies to use the ash of either birds or animals and other things. Everything of this type ought to be burnt in a new pot, with the lid inserted and smeared over with potters' clay, in a hot oven.

9   We will employ every gargle hot.
    And it is necessary to know the medicinal weights and measures. The *drachma* has three *scripuli*. The *drachma* is the weight of a silver *denarius*, an *obolus* is the sixth part of a *drachma*. A *cyathus* is ten *drachmae*, an *acetabulum* is fifteen *drachmae*, a *cochlear* is a half *drachma*, a *mina* 100 *drachmae*. A medicinal *sextarius* has 10 *uncia*.

10 These things are generally what ought to be heeded on the whole. Now we will assign their remedies to each part. As our little work is proceeding, we will discuss how tertian fever, quartan fever, and maladies of this kind are remedied as it comes to our attention. Therefore we will start from the head.

1   capitis dolori

1   Capitis dolor levatur si de porri sectivi suco cochlearia duo et unum mellis permixta infundantur vel in nares vel in auriculas. veteres dolores et vertigines betae nigrae suco temporibus inlinito emendantur. in dolore utilissimum est caput ungui suco intibi <cum rosaceo et aceto. ocimum> cum rosaceo aut myrtino aut aceto fronti imponitur.

2   ruta ex vino bibitur; et tritae sucus instillatur capiti cum aceto aut rosaceo. corona de puleio prodest imposita. pollinem siliginis admixto ovi albo, simul et quiddam salis [albi] conspargi oportet frontique inlini, et super fascia pedalis alligetur. anethum ita uti de horto sublatum est decoquitur ex oleo, et suco eius dolor unguitur.

3   serpullum decoctum in aceto inlinitur fronti et temporibus. et si difficilis somnus sit, amigdalino oleo caput perungui oportet. tempora in dolore alio elixo inlinuntur. nucleorum persici farina cum melle et aceto capiti inlinitur. nuclei amigdalini triti fronti utiliter imponuntur, etiam in febre. bacae lauri impari numero in oleo contritae capiti instillantur.

4   si a sole doleat, cupressi folia contrita cum polenta imponuntur. hederae folia mollissima quaeque trita cum aceto et rosaceo adversum omnem dolorem fronti inlinuntur. herba quae in capite statuae nascitur collecta in alicuius vestis panno et lino rufo inligata confestim dolorem sedat. panacis radix in oleo conteritur et caput perunguitur.

5   veratrum in rosaceo decoctum et contritum capiti instillatur. peucedano ex oleo et aceto trito hemicrania unguntur. ossa de capite vulturis sub collo alligari prodest. gallinaceus pullus inclusus abstinetur nocte et die, sed et is qui languet, deinde eius gallinacei vel plumae vel crista alligatur collo dolentis.

6   surculus ex nido milvi pulvino subditur nescienti aegro. murinarum pellium cinis ex aceto fronti inlinitur. cochleae matutino se pascenti caput harundine praeciditur et in linteolo licio alligatur colloque suspenditur. fracto capiti tela araneae imposita ex oleo et aceto; non recedit nisi sanet dolorem.

7   aqua pota quae superfuit de bovis aut asini potione remediat si ter potetur. cervini cornus cinis inlitus ex aceto et rosaceo prodest.

1 *For pain of the head*

1   Pain of the head is relieved if two *cochlearia* of chive's juice and one of honey, mixed together, are poured into either the nostrils or the ears. Long-standing pains and dizziness are improved by smearing dark beet's juice on the temples. It is most useful for pain to anoint the head with endive juice, with rose oil and vinegar. Basil is applied to the forehead with rose oil or myrtle oil or vinegar.

2   Rue is drunk in wine; ground rue juice is trickled onto the head with vinegar or rose oil. Wearing a pennyroyal wreath is useful. Fine wheaten flour with added egg white ought to be smeared on the forehead, and at the same time be sprinkled with some salt, and a foot-wide bandage is bound over it. Dill is decocted with oil when it was taken from the garden, and the pain is anointed with its juice.

3   Tufted thyme decocted in vinegar is smeared on the forehead and temples. And if sleep is difficult, the head ought to be anointed with almond oil. Temples are smeared with thoroughly boiled garlic for pain. Meal of peach kernels is smeared on the head with honey and vinegar. Ground almond kernels are usefully applied to the forehead, even with a fever. An odd number of laurel berries crushed in oil are trickled onto the head.

4   Cypress leaves crushed with *polenta* are applied if one feels pain from the sun. The most tender ivy leaves, ground with vinegar and rose oil, are smeared on the forehead against every pain. A plant which grows on a statue's head, collected in a rag from any garment and tied on with a red thread, immediately allays pain. All-heal's root is crushed in oil and the head is thoroughly anointed.

5   Hellebore, crushed and decocted in rose oil, is trickled onto the head. Pains on one side of the head are anointed with ground sulphurwort in oil and vinegar. It is useful for bones from a vulture's head to be tied under the neck. A chicken penned up is starved for a night and a day, as is he who is ill, then either the feathers or the comb of that bird is tied around the neck of the sufferer.

6   A twig from a kite's nest is placed without the patient's knowledge under the pillow. The ash of the skins of mice is smeared on the forehead with vinegar. A snail's head is cut off with a reed while it is grazing early in the morning and is tied and suspended from the neck on a linen thread. A spider's web applied with oil and vinegar to a fractured skull does not come off until it heals the pain.

7   The drinking water which is left over from a cow's or ass' draught cures if it is drunk three times. The ash of deer horn smeared on with vinegar and rose oil is beneficial.

2   *pthiriasi et prurigini [id est pediculos in capite]*

1   Pthiriasis pruriginesque plerumque in perniciem solent convertere. quibus succurrendum est. perunguntur itaque bulbis tritis ex vino, item sulphure ex vino. item per se ex cedro inlinuntur. alium cum aceto et nitro tritum infricatur.

2   farina feniculi cum vino et nitro pruriginem purgat, et furfures ex aceto. idem praestat radix veratri in oleo decocta trita suffusaque. hyssopum ex oleo tritum et instillatum capiti pthiriasi medetur et pruritibus. ova ex vino et oleo cyprino et cedro pruritus scabiemque tollunt.

3   prurigines discutiuntur felle ovillo inlito cum creta Cimolia donec inarescat. lendes et alia capitis taetra animalia quae nocent lotione aquae marinae necantur. item si inlinatur Samia terra cum nitro et oleo. nitrum alumini mixtum capiti infrictum prurigines tollit.

3   *ulceribus in capite manantibus*

1   Ulcera in capite manantia tamquam proprio morbo praecipue infantibus nascuntur, sed et viros et mulieres cum ceperint graviter infestant. quae fota urina tauri efficacissime sanantur. vitulino felle cum aceto tepefacto inlinuntur.

2   sevum vituli cum sale utilissimum est. testarum muricum purpurarumve cinere ex melle inlinuntur. alium cum sua reste comburitur cinisque eius ex oleo imponitur. menta trita et apposita siccat.

3   oleum amigdalinum cum vino expurgat. galbanum inlinitur ex melle. folia rubi in quo mora nascuntur contrita imponuntur. misy tritum cum vino in lana superponitur. malva macerata in urina humana et trita imposita valde desiccat.

4   Omnia autem capitis ulcera cum purgata sunt iucundissime ad cicatricem perducuntur hoc ceroto. spumae argenti tunsae et cribratae libra, cerussae libra una teruntur, et cerae albae libra <ex> olei rosacei libra remittitur et refrigera[n]tur; deinde raditur et miscetur cum spuma et cerussa.

5   adiciuntur ovorum quattuor lutea cruda. prodest et resinae pituinae libra mixta cum cerae albae selibra et in oleo decocta, ita ut in acopi modo perunguatur pistillo mixtum.

4   *alopeciis*

1   Alopeciae magnam foeditatem afferunt et propter hoc servorum pretia diminuuntur. itaque necessarium est eas quoque emendare. quae celerrime complentur pellium viperarum cinere sparso. nasturcium cum sinape tritum impositum emendat.

2   cydonia cocta ex vino et cum cera trita inlita capillos restituunt. roboris pilulae cum adipe ursina tritae emendant. glandis faginae cinis cum melle et oleo Cyprio inlinitur. cinis ungularum mulae vel muli ex oleo myrteo, cinis murium impressus, cinis erinacei recens cum pice liquida.

2   *For the louse-disease and itch*

1   *Phthiriasis* and itch commonly turn to ruin. Therefore they are thoroughly anointed with ground bulbs in wine, and the same manner with sulphur in wine. Likewise they are smeared with cedar oil by itself. Ground garlic with vinegar and soda is rubbed in.

2   Fennel meal with wine and soda, and bran in vinegar, cleanses itch. Also ground decocted hellebore root poured over in oil is excellent. Ground hyssop trickled onto the head in oil is good for *phthiriasis* and itches. Eggs with wine, Cyprian oil, and cedar oil remove itch and *scabies*.

3   Itches are dissipated by sheep bile smeared on with Cimolian chalk until it dries. Nits and other loathsome creatures of the head which cause harm are killed by washing in sea water. Likewise, if Samian earth is smeared on with soda and oil. Soda mixed with alum and rubbed onto the head removes itches.

3   *For weeping sores on the head*

1   Weeping sores on the head arise, as it were, as a specific disease principally among children, but they also severely injure men and women when they beset them. They are most affectively cured by fomentation with bull's urine. They are smeared with calf bile with warmed vinegar.

2   Calf's tallow with salt is most useful. They are smeared with murex or purple-fish shells' ash in honey. Garlic is burnt with its own leaf and its ash is applied with oil. Ground mint applied dries it.

3   Almond oil cleanses with wine. *Galbanum* is smeared on with honey. Crushed leaves of the bramble on which berries grow are applied. Ground *misy* is applied over it with wine on wool. Mallow steeped in human urine, ground, and applied, strongly desiccates.

4   However, all sores of the head, after they were cleansed, are made to scar over most pleasantly by this cerate. A *libra* of crushed and sifted litharge; one *libra* of ground white lead; a *libra* of white wax is melted in a *libra* of rose oil and cooled; then it is smoothed and mixed with the litharge and white lead.

5   Four raw egg yolks are added. It is also useful for a *libra* of pine resin mixed with half a *libra* of white wax and decocted in oil, so that it might be thoroughly rubbed on in the manner of a salve that was mixed with a pestle.

4   *For* alopeciae

1   *Alopeciae* cause great shame, and because of it the value of slaves is reduced; therefore it is necessary to cure it. This is quickly accomplished by a sprinkling of the ash of vipers' skins. Ground cress applied with mustard improves it.

2   Quinces cooked in wine, ground, and smeared on with wax restore hair. Ground oak's catkins improve it with bear grease. Beech-nut ash is smeared on with honey and cypress oil. Ash of a molly- or john-mule's hooves in myrtle oil, pressed mice ash, or fresh hedgehog ash with liquid pitch.

3   gallinacei recens fimus inlinitur. sandaraca ex aceto. fluentem capillum
    continet leporis cinis cum oleo myrteo. fel taurinum cum Aegyptio alumine
    tepefactum inlinitur.

5   *capillis denigrandis*

1   Potest videri supervacuum inter remedia corporis ponere ea, quae ad decorem
    pertinent. sed quosdam pudet aut ipsos rubeos esse, aut in tantum luxuriae
    indulgent ut deliciae eorum inter se dissentiant volentium in pueris rufos
    capillos, in viris recusantium.
2   Quemadmodum denigrentur monstrabimus. ovum corvinum in aeneo vase
    permiscetur, deinde raso capiti in umbra inlinitur. habere debet in ore oleum
    is qui curabitur donec siccescat ovum, ne ei dentes denigrescant. quarto die
    abluitur.
3   sextarius sanguisugarum in duobus sextariis aceti diebus XL maceratur; ex
    oleo tritus deraso capiti in umbra inlinitur. dum siccescat, sicut superius
    praediximus, in ore oleum tenendum est.
4   siliquae ervi prius quam exarescant numero L cum suis foliis et caulibus
    conteruntur et capiti raso inlinuntur. folia cupressi trita ex aceto efficiunt ut
    capilli nigri renascantur. spondilio peruncti crispi fiunt.
5   Operae pretium est his qui erubescunt senes esse succurrere, et si canos suos
    inficere volunt, tamquam annos detracturi sint hoc nomine aetati, vermium
    terrenorum cinerem adiciant in oleo quo caput perunguant.

6   *auriculis*

1   Proxima mihi videtur cura aurium, quae acutissimum dolorem inferunt simul
    ut passae sunt vel minimam offensam. scio certe quosdam medicos huius
    curationis sibi summam scientiam vindicasse et magnas mercedes poposcisse,
    cum adversus morbos aurium unum aut alterum nossent remedium. nos multa
    proferimus, ut cum res exegerit possimus uti, cum ex his aliqua occurrerint.
2   Gari excellentis cyathus, aceti cyathus unus, mellis cyathus et dimidius: in
    calice novo sensim decoquitur, spuma subinde penna tollitur, et cum spuma
    resederit, removetur et ex eo tepidum infunditur.
3   ad omnes infusiones auriculae conchiliata lana obturandae sunt. ranarum
    adeps remissus instillatus dolorem statim tollit. si tument aures, suco corian-
    dri mitigandae sunt prius. sucus hederae tepidus cum vino instillatur.
4   [mel cum rosaceo inditur] mel cum rosaceo et manna turis ad instar cochlearii
    adiciuntur. hoc et vulnera sanat et umores exsiccat. parum audientes utiliter
    acetum gargarizant. auricularum fracturis medentur bulbi triti et appositi et
    quinto die soluti.

3   Fresh chicken's dung is smeared on. Red arsenic sulphide with vinegar. Hare's ash with myrtle oil. Warmed bull bile is smeared on with Egyptian alum.

5   *For blackening hair*

1   It may seem unnecessary to place among these remedies for the body those which relate to beauty, yet it either shames some that they themselves are a redhead, or they indulge in such extravagance that their favourites differ from each other, thus: wanting red hair on boys, and rejecting it on men.

2   We will instruct how it is blackened. A raven egg is beaten in a bronze vessel, and then is smeared onto a shaved head in the shade. He who will be treated thus ought to hold oil in the mouth until the egg becomes dry, lest they blacken the teeth. It is washed off on the fourth day.

3   A *sextarius* of leeches is steeped in two *sextarii* of vinegar for 40 days; ground, it is smeared onto a shaved head in the shade with oil. While it dries, oil ought to be kept in the mouth just as we recommended above.

4   Bitter vetch pods, 50 in number, are crushed with their leaves and stems, and smeared on a shaved head. Ground cypress leaves with vinegar cause hair to regrow black. Anointed with *spondylium*, hair becomes curly.

5   It is worthwhile to assist those who are embarrassed to be old, even if they want to dye their grey hair, as if they could strip years away from their true age; they add earthworms' ash to oil with which they may anoint the head.

6   *For ears*

1   Next appears to me to be the treatment of ears, which inflict the most severe pain, while at the same time are afflicted by the smallest problem. I know without a doubt that some doctors claimed the greatest knowledge in their treatments and demanded immense prices, while they only knew one or two remedies for ear diseases. We proffer many so that it is possible to use them when required, when any of these present themselves.

2   A *cyathus* of excellent *garum*, one *cyathus* of vinegar, and a *cyathus* and a half of honey: it is decocted slowly in a new cup; foam is constantly removed with a feather, and when the foam subsided, it is removed and is poured in from it warm.

3   Ears need to be stoppered with purple wool for all infusions. Melted frog's grease trickled in immediately removes pain. If ears swell they first need to be reduced with coriander's juice. Warm ivy juice is trickled in with wine.

4   Honey with rose oil and grains of frankincense, about equal to a *cochlear*, are added. This heals wounds and dries up humours. For insufficient hearing they usefully gargle vinegar. Applied ground bulbs removed on the fifth day heal fractures of the outer ears.

5   foliorum rubi in quo mora nascuntur sucus tepidus instillatur. fel pecudis cum
melle aures purgat. canini lactis instillatio sedat dolorem, gravitatem aurium
adeps remissus cum absinthio trito. cum oleo infusus emendat. murium cinis
cum melle instillatus inhibet dolorem. si aliquod animal intravit, praecipoum
est remedium murium fel aceto dilutum instillare.

6   si aqua <ingrediatur et non statim> fugiat, [et] adeps anserinus cum cepae suco
inlinitur. deplorata autem vitia aurium sic sanantur. gliri detrahetur pellis et
intestina eiusdem decoquuntur in vase novo cum mellis heminis tribus usque ad
tertias atque ita adservatur, et cum opus est, strigle medicamentum tepefactum
infunditur. valde laudantur et terreni vermes cum anseris adipe cocti et instillati.

7   verberatis auribus cochleae, quae in usu sunt cibi, apponuntur tritae cum myrrha et ture. cochleae minutae latae tritae fracturis aurium inlinuntur.

8   senectus serpentis ferventi testa usta et contrita instillatur ex oleo rosaceo
contra vitia omnia sed praecipue graveolentia<m>, et si purulentae sint aures
melius ex aceto et felle caprino et bubulo.

9   haec senectus post annum vires non habet. membrana ex ventre gallinaceo quae
proicitur ex vino trita et adipe<s> gallinarum tepefacta infunduntur. blattae sine
capite et pedibus et alis tritae inlitae in linteolo contusis auribus imponuntur.

10   nitrum ex vino liquatum purulentis auribus medetur. sonitus et tinnitus discutit nitrum tritum et siccum insparsum <vel> ex rosaceo tepido [et] in auribus
inmissum. purulentis auribus infunditur fel tauri cum porri sectivi suco.

11   si gravitas sit aurium, eodem felle cum lacte muliebri perluendae sunt. equini
fimi cinis cum rosaceo instillatur. sevum vituli cum adipe anseris et ocimi
suco, fel taurinum vel caprinum cum rosaceo tepido auribus inditur.

12   omnibus quae inmittuntur tepidis utendum est. urina apri tepida infunditur: ad
hos usus servatur in vitreo vase. si aqua intraverit in auriculam dextram, sin-
istro pede desultare oportet capite in dextro umero inclinato, si in sinistram,
ex diverso. si quod animal intraverit et inspuatur in aurem, exire creditur.

7   *parotidibus [id est farcimina quae sub auribus nascuntur]*

1   Raro medici parotidibus curationem non devocant ad scalpellum, cum et
reprimi possint et si res exegerit aperiri molliore curatione. reprimit eas
radicis brassicae cinis cum melle inlitus.

2   lupini ex aceto cocti tritique discutiunt. vitium cinis cum cera et resina paribus
ponderibus imposita desiccant. apponitur muricum testarum cinis cum melle
vel conchyliorum ex mulso.

5 Warm juice of the leaves of the bramble on which berries grow is trickled in. Livestock's bile cleanses the ears with honey. An infusion of dog milk moderates pain, melted grease for hardness of hearing with ground wormwood. Poured in with oil, it improves them. Mice ash trickled in with honey checks pain. If any insect entered, a specific remedy is to trickle in the bile of mice, diluted with vinegar.

6 If water enters and does not immediately escape, goose grease with onion juice is smeared on. However, desperate complaints of the ears are healed thus: the skin will be removed from a dormouse and the intestines of the same are continuously decocted with three *heminae* of honey in a new vessel to one-third, and is thus preserved. And when it is beneficial the warmed medicament is poured in with a *strigilis*. Earthworms cooked with goose grease and poured in are highly praised.

7 Snails which are enjoyed at meals are applied, ground with myrrh and frankincense, to beaten ears. Ground tiny, broad snails are smeared onto fractures of the ears.

8 A snake's slough, burnt in a very hot pot and crushed, is trickled in with rose oil treats all complaints, but especially a foul smell, and if the ears are purulent with vinegar and goat and ox bile is better.

9 This slough has no strength after a year. The membrane which is thrown away from a chicken's belly ground in wine and hens' grease are poured in warm. Cockroaches without head, feet, and wings, ground and smeared on a little linen cloth, are applied to bruised ears.

10 Dissolved soda with wine heals festering ears. Soda, dried, ground, and sprinkled, or inserted in the ears with warm rose oil, dispels noises and ringing. Bull's bile is poured in festering ears with chive's juice.

11 If there is fetidness of the ears, they need to be washed with the same bile with breast milk. Horse dung ash with rose oil is trickled in. Calf's tallow with goose grease and basil juice; bull or goat bile put in the ears with warm rose oil.

12 All things which are inserted need to be used warm. Warm wild boar's urine is poured in; for this use it is kept in a glass vessel. If water entered the right ear, one ought to hop with the left foot with the head bent onto the right shoulder; if into the left, the opposite. If any insect has entered, the ear is spat into and it is believed to exit.

7 *For inflammation of the parotid glands*

1 Rarely do doctors not call upon the scalpel to treat swellings of the parotid glands, even though they can be repressed and – if the condition required it – opened with a softening treatment. Cabbage root's ash smeared on with honey represses them.

2 Lupines boiled in vinegar and ground dissipate them. Vines' ash applied with wax and resin in equal weights dries them up. Murex shells ash is applied with honey or that of cockles in honeyed wine.

3   sepiae ossa cum axungia vetere tusa medentur. lini semen tusum eum melle mixtum mitigat. ficus siccae decoctae ex vino tritae adhibentur. comprimit eas fimus columbinus cum farina hordeacea ex melle.

4   noctuae cerebrum vel iecur cum oleo tepido infunditur auriculae. parotidi multipedae cum resinae parte tertia inlinuntur. creta Cimolia ex aceto siccat.

5   plantago cum axungia vetere persanat. ursinus adeps conteritur cum sevi taurini pari pondere et cerae. fimo caprae cum axungia inlinuntur. caput viperae in linteolo involutum et faucibus alligatum sanat.

8   *epiphoris [hoc est oculorum umoribus]*

1   Cochleae sine putamine tritae inlitae fronti cum turis polline validissime prosunt. tumores oculorum sedat mulsum tepidum in penicillo super impositum. corticis sepiae farina in epiphora ex lacte mulieris circumlinitur.

2   caro peponis mirifice refrigerat. alba beta trita fronti imponitur. eundem effectum habent bulbi triti oculis impositi. apio viridi trito cum pane oculi teguntur. ocimo ex vino optimo trito oculi circumlinuntur.

3   ruta cum polenta contrita et imposita lenit dolorem. anethi radix in vino trita inlinitur. papaveris cauliculus vel siccus vel viridis cum suo fructu tritus imponitur. lini semen cum ture ex aqua tusum circumlinitur. siliginis grana in ferro tostata ex vino trita circumlinuntur.

4   item lenticula cum cydoneis cocta et una trita adhibetur. lentisci teneri folia contrita et fronti imposita epiphoram suspendunt. mandragorae radices tusae cum rosaceo ex vino tritae circumligatae et epiphoram sanant et dolorem statim sedant.

5   folia cicutae trita et ita fronti imposita epiphoram et tumores et dolorem tollunt. anacollima hoc modo fieri solet: lana non curata cum albo ovi et turis polline fronti applicatur. ovi album oculis infusum epiphoras sedat et uredines mitigat et refrigerationem praestat. lutea ovorum ex rosaceo et mulso in lana super oculos imponuntur.

6   caseo molli caprino ex aqua ferventi imposito epiforae sedantur. fimus caprinus ex melle oculis inlinitur. vulpinam linguam habentem in armilla lippiturum negant.

3   Pounded cuttlefish bones heal with old axle-grease. Pounded linseed mixed with honey alleviates them. Dried figs decocted in wine and ground are applied. Pigeon dung with barley meal in honey compresses them.

4   A little owl's brain or liver is poured in the ear with warm oil. *Multipedae* are smeared on the inflammation with a third part of resin. Cimolian chalk dries with vinegar.

5   Plantain with old axle-grease completely heals. Bear grease rubbed in with an equal weight of bull tallow and wax. They are smeared with a nanny-goat's dung and axle-grease. A viper's head wrapped in a little cloth and tied around the throat cures it.

8   *For* epiphorae

1   Snails ground without a shell and smeared on the forehead with frankincense dust are extremely beneficial. Warmed honeyed wine applied in a soft sponge soothes swellings of the eyes. Cuttlefish shell's dust is smeared all over *epiphora* in breast milk.

2   *Pepon*'s flesh cools marvellously. Ground white beet is applied to the forehead. Ground bulbs applied to the eyes have the same effect. Eyes are covered with ground, fresh *apium* with bread. The eyes are smeared all over with ground basil with top quality wine.

3   Rue applied with crushed *polenta* alleviates pain. Ground dill's root is smeared on with wine. A poppy's stem, either dried or fresh, ground with its fruit is applied. Pounded linseed with frankincense is smeared all over with water.

4   Grains of wheat roasted on iron and ground in wine are smeared all over. Likewise, cooked little lentils ground together with quinces are used. Tender mastic leaves ground together and applied to the forehead suspend *epiphora*. Mandrake's roots pounded with rose oil, ground in wine, and smeared all over heal *epiphora*, and immediately allay pain.

5   Ground hemlock's leaves applied in this manner to the forehead remove *epiphora*, swellings, and pain. An adhesive plaster ought to be made in this way: unprocessed wool is applied with egg white and frankincense flour to the forehead. Egg white poured into the eyes stays *epiphora*, soothes the burning sensation, and promotes cooling. Egg yolks with rose oil and honeyed wine are applied on wool over the eyes.

6   *Epiphora* is stayed by soft goat cheese applied in very hot water. Goat dung in honey is smeared on the eyes. They say that keeping a fox tongue in a bracelet will prevent *lippus*.

9   *oculis suffusis sanguine*

1   Sanguis instillatur columbae vel palumbi vel perdicis vel turturis. superimponi debet splen<ium> ex melle coctum lanaque sucida ex oleo aut vino. et radix rutae inlita emendat.

10   *naribus*

1   Plerumque evenit ut ex naribus is modus sanguinis profluat qui nisi reprimatur afferat mortem, neque aliter exiliat quam solet e vena percussa erumpere. occurrendum est itaque velocissimo periculo et magno impetu et subito saevienti.

2   in hoc itaque casu porro sectivo trito nares obturantur. ruta trita aeque reprimit in naribus indita. eodem modo et radice urticae utendum est.

3   semen urticae cum lana sucida coicitur in nares cum oleo rosaceo et auriculae lana sucida spisse obturantur, et ita sanguis continetur.

4   coagulum agninum mirifice facit ex aqua subactum et infusum. adeps anserinus cum butyri pari pondere ingeritur pastillis. prosunt cochleae contritae et fronti inlitae.

5   Graveolentiae narium sic subvenitur. sucus hederae infunditur, aristolochiae cum cypero. dracontei semen cum melle pari pondere naribus inditur. hoc etiam si carcinomata sint emendat. dicitur prodesse qui hoc malo vexabitur ut osculetur nares mularum.

11   *destillationi*

1   Cinis testarum ostreorum in cibo; pane colligitur in modum salis. porri capitati folia cruda sine pane eduntur.

2   caninum corrigium numquam unctum cuilibet digito in manu circumligatur. ostrea cum sua testa ita ut electa sunt in carbonibus coquuntur et in cibo dantur.

3   oleum calidum eunti dormitum in cerebrum infunditur et in nares coicitur. in manu dextera duo digiti medii lino alligati inter se destillationem compescunt.

12   *oris vitiis*

1   Oris saporem commendari affirmant murino cinere cum melle si fricentur dentes. admiscent quidam tamaricae maritimae radices. mero ante somnos colluere ora propter halitus, frigida <matutinis> utile dicitur.

2   folia fagina commanducantur adversus gingivarum et labiorum vitia. aeque folia rubi in quo mora nascuntur. eiusdem generis rubi teneri pampini decoquuntur ex vino ad tertias idque vinum in ore continetur.

9   *For eyes suffused with blood*

1   Pigeon's, wood-pigeon's, partridge's, or turtledove's blood is trickled in. A patch boiled in honey and greasy wool boiled in oil or wine ought to be placed over. And rue's root smeared on improves it.

10   *For noses*

1   It frequently happens that so much blood flows from the nose that unless it is repressed it causes death, and does not burst forth other than as it is accustomed to erupt from a struck vein. Therefore one must address the sudden raging and swiftest danger with great vigour.

2   Therefore in this case the nostrils are stoppered with ground chive. Equally, ground rue put in the nostrils represses it. Nettle's root ought to be used in same way.

3   Nettle's seed with greasy wool is set in the nostrils with rose oil and the ears are closely stoppered with greasy wool; thus the blood is contained.

4   Lamb rennet worked with water and poured in acts marvellously. Goose grease with an equal weight of butter is formed into pastilles. Pounded snails smeared on the forehead are useful.

5   Foul smells of the nose are assisted thus. Ivy's juice or *aristolochia*'s juice with galingal is poured in. Dragon arum's seed is set in the nostrils with an equal amount of honey. This improves it even if there are *carcinomata*. It is said that it is useful for the person tormented by this complaint to kiss the nose of a molly-mule.

11   *For a runny nose*

1   Oyster shells' ash in food; it is gathered in bread in the manner of salt. Raw headed-leek's leaves are eaten without bread.

2   A thong of dog-leather that has never been oiled is tied around any finger on a hand. Oysters are cooked, as they were extracted with their shell, on coals and given in food.

3   When going to sleep, hot oil is poured onto the top of the head and put in the nostrils. Two middle fingers of the right hand tied to each other with thread restrain a runny nose.

12   *For complaints of the mouth*

1   They assert that the mouth's taste is made agreeable if the teeth are rubbed with mouse ash and honey. Some mix in the marine tamarisk's roots. It is said that it is useful for the breath to rinse with unmixed wine before sleep and with cold water in the morning.

2   Beech leaves are chewed for complaints of the gums and lips. Likewise, so do the leaves of the bramble on which berries grow. The tender shoots of the same type of bramble are decocted to one-third, and that wine is held in the mouth.

3   ulcera plantaginis sucus emendat, et folia eius cocta radicesque eius commanducatae. membrana ex ovo cocto vel crudo detracta labiorum fissuris medetur. oris halitum emendat murinus cinis cum melle dentibus infricatus.

4   linguae ulcera et labiorum hirundines ex mulso coctae sanant. adeps anserinus aut gallinae rimas emendat. si ferventia os intus exusserint, continuo sanatur gargarizatione lactis canini.

5   adversus foetorem oris folia myrti et lentisci pari pondere et gallae Syriacae dimidium pondus una teri oportet et aspersa vino vetusto matutino mandere vel hederae bacas cum casia et myrrha pari pondere aspersa vino.

6   eadem ratione ulcera oris emendantur. hoc et ad stomachum optime, sed melius mororum domesticorum [sed melius eorum quae in rubis nascuntur] sextarii tres leni vapore decoquuntur, ut ad spissitudinem mellis veniat:

7   tum additur de myrrha pondus denarii et tantundem croci et in unum totum teritur, et inde prout visum fuerit aeger accipit. item suci mororum sextarii duo cum uno Attici mellis decoquuntur, et inde stomachicus prout visum fuerit accipiet.

8   capitis leporini cinis adiecto nardo mulcet graveolentiam. ulcera et rimas sevum bovis vel vituli cum adipe anseris emendat. amurca ex oliva nigra oris vitiis subvenit.

13 *dentibus*

1   Cucurbitae sativae decoctae sucus inhibet dolorem et mobilitatem stabilit in ore compressus. inula ab ieiunis commanducata dentes confirmat.

2   aqua in qua alium decoctum est gargarizatur, et idem alium cavis dentibus inditur. asparagi erratici sucum in ore contineri oportet adversum mobilitatem.

3   acetum si in ore contineatur gingivas stringit et dentes continet. olivae nigrae amurcae muria eosdem stabilit. caprifici radix ex vino decoquitur, vinum in ore continetur, radix trita maxillae imponitur adversus dolorem.

4   mori radix per messes inciditur, et haec mittit sucum aptissimum dolori. nucleus gallae commanducatus dolori medetur. taedae pingues in astulas conciduntur et in aceto coquuntur, idque acetum in ore continetur.

5   aqua in qua lentiscus decocta est mobiles confirmat. ruborum in quibus mora nascuntur pampini decoquuntur in vino austeri et commanducantur adversum mobilitatem, idque vinum in ore tenetur.

6   millefolium in dolore manditur tritumque maxillae imponitur. radix hyoscyami ex aceto commanducatur. plantaginis radix manditur et eiusdem suco in aceto decoctae tepefacto dentes conluuntur.

7   quinquefolium in quo fraga nascuntur eluitur aceto sive aqua marina, deinde coquitur ad tertias ex vino et aceto, idque in ore diu continetur. quidam malunt cinere eius dentes fricare. hysopo utiliter conluuntur.

3   Plantain's juice improves ulcers, and its cooked leaves and roots chewed. The membrane stripped from cooked or raw eggs heals chapped lips. Mouse ash with honey rubbed on teeth improves the mouth's breath.

4   Swallows cooked in honeyed wine heal ulcers of the tongue and lips. Goose or hen's grease improves cracks. If something extremely hot scalded the inside of the mouth, it is promptly healed by a gargle of dog milk.

5   An equal weight of myrtle and mastic leaves and a half weight of Syrian oak-gall ought to be ground into one, sprinkled with old wine, and chewed in the morning to address a foul smell in the mouth. Or ivy's berries with an equal weight of cassia and myrrh sprinkled with wine.

6   Mouth ulcers are improved by the same reckoning. This is best for the stomach, but better are three *sextarii* of cultivated mulberries decocted over a gentle heat, so it reaches the thickness of honey:

7   Then a *denarius* weight of myrrh and just as much of saffron are added, and they are ground together into one, and the patient takes from this as seems suitable. Likewise, two *sextarii* of mulberry juice are decocted with one of Attic honey, and the stomach patient will take from this as seems suitable.

8   Ash of a hare's head with added nard sweetens fetidness. The tallow of cattle or a calf with goose grease improves ulcers and fissures. *Amurca* from the black olive assists complaints of the mouth.

13   For teeth

1   Decocted cultivated gourd's juice curbs pain, and held in the mouth stabilises looseness. Elecampane chewed while fasting secures teeth.

2   Water in which garlic was decocted is gargled, and the same garlic is put in the cavities in the teeth. Wild asparagus' juice ought to be held in the mouth against looseness.

3   Vinegar, if it is held in the mouth, strengthens gums and secures teeth. The brine of black olive's *amurca* stabilises them. Wild fig's root is decocted in wine, the wine is held in the mouth, and the ground root is applied to the jaw to address pain.

4   The mulberry tree's root is incised during harvest time, and this releases juice most suitable for pain. The chewed inside of an oak-gall remedies pain. Resinous pitch-pines are cut into chips and cooked in vinegar, and that vinegar is held in the mouth.

5   The water in which mastic was decocted secures loose teeth. The shoots of the brambles on which berries grow are decocted in dry wine and chewed against looseness, and that wine is held in the mouth.

6   *Millefolium* is gnawed for pain, and is applied ground to the jaw. Henbane's root in vinegar is chewed. Plantain's root is gnawed and teeth are rinsed with the warm juice of the same, having been decocted in vinegar.

7   Cinquefoil on which strawberries grow is washed with vinegar or sea water, then is boiled to one-third in vinegar and wine, and it is held in the mouth for a long time. Some prefer to rub teeth with its ash. They are usefully rinsed with hyssop.

8   Cavis dentibus cinis murini fimi inditur. vermes terreni decocti in oleo et triti infunduntur auriculae ab ea parte qua dentes dolent. eorundem vermium cinis exesis dentibus coniectus et cera obturatus perfacile eos cadere cogit.

9   idem vermium cinis inlitus dolentibus iuvat: comburi debent in testa. harenulae quae in cornibus cochlearum inveniuntur cavis dentibus inditae continuo finiunt dolorem.

10   idem praestat fimus corvi in lana alligatus. inviolati praestantur dentes si quis cottidie mane ieiunus sub lingua habeat granum salis donec liquescat. cervini cornus farina in dolore vel colluuntur vel fricantur.

11   tali bubuli cinis dentifricium est. ossa ex ungulis suum combusta eundem usum praestant. caprino lacte utiliter dentes colluuntur.

12   ebuli radicem ex aceto decoque, et diu in ore teneatur. folia de buxo et ramusculos anethi tres in olla mittis et cum aceto ad tertias decoques: tepefactum in ore teneat.

14   *dentioni infantium*

1   Dentes equis qui primi cadunt alligati facilem dentionem praestant: melius si terram non tangant. lacte caprino aut leporino cerbello gingivae perfricantur.

2   delphini dentium cinis cum melle gingivis inlinitur, et eius dente gingivae tanguntur. eundem effectum habent dentes caniculae. cerebrum pecudis in cibo datur.

15   *uvae*

1   Cinis testarum ostreorum addito melle inlinitur. garum optimum cochleari subicitur. radicum brassicae cinis tactu reprimit. cinis anethi uvam levat.

2   sinape gargarizatur cum aceto et melle. sucus urticae gargarizatur. rubi in quo mora nascuntur cauliculi decoquuntur ex vino idque vinum gargarizatur praesentaneo remedio.

3   eorundem ruborum folia arefiunt in umbra crematorumque cinere cochleari tacta resilit. hirundininus cinis cum melle inlinitur.

4   laseris Cyrenaici granum carbone sicca et subice cochleario. si iacet uva, verticem morsu alterius hominis suspendi utile est. caseus recens cum melle suggillati[m] uvam emendat.

8 Mouse dung's ash is put in cavities in teeth. Earthworms decocted in oil and ground are poured into the ear on that side on which teeth hurt. The ash of the same worms forced into hollowed teeth and stoppered with wax forces them to easily fall out.

9 The same ash of worms smeared on helps with pain: they ought to be burnt in a pot. The grains of sand which are found on snails' horns put in cavities in teeth immediately stops pain.

10 Likewise, raven's dung in wool tied around is excellent. Uninjured teeth are preserved if someone while fasting in the morning holds a grain of salt under the tongue until it melts each day. For pain they are either rinsed or rubbed with the powder of deer horn.

11 Ash of an ox's anklebone is a tooth powder. The burnt bones from pigs' trotters used the same way are excellent. Teeth are usefully rinsed with goat milk.

12 Decocted dwarf elder's root in vinegar, and it should be held in the mouth for a long time. You throw leaves from boxwood and three twigs of dill into a pot and decoct them in vinegar to one-third; one should hold it while warm in the mouth.

14 For cutting babies' teeth

1 The first teeth which fall from horses tied around are excellent for easy teething; it is better if they do not touch the ground. Gums are rubbed with goat milk or hare brain.

2 Ash of a dolphin's teeth is smeared on the gums with honey and the gums are touched with its tooth. The teeth of a *canicula* have the same effect. The brain of livestock is given in food.

15 For the uvula

1 Oyster shells' ash is smeared on with added honey. Top quality *garum* is held under it in a spoon. Cabbage roots' ash represses it by touch. Dill's ash lifts the uvula.

2 Mustard is gargled with vinegar and honey. Nettle's juice is gargled. Shoots of bramble on which berries grow are decocted in wine, and that wine is gargled as an instantaneous remedy.

3 They dry the same bramble's leaves in the shade, and having been burnt, with a touch of this ash in a spoon, it shrinks. Swallow ash is smeared on with honey.

4 Hold under it, in a spoon, a grain of Cyrenaic *laser* that was dried on coals. If the uvula is relaxed, it is useful for the top of the head to be held up by the bite of a person. Fresh cheese with honey improves a bruised uvula.

16 *tonsillis*

1   Quas tonsillas appellant ex utraque gutturis parte et faucibus lactis ovilli calidi gargarizatio prodest. fimus columbinus tritus ex passo gargarizatur.

2   ficus arida et nitrum una teruntur, deinde faucibus adlinuntur: asperitatem faucibus emendat et destillationem. alium tritum ex pusca gargarizatum. cochleae dempta tantum terra coqui debent inlotae, deinde conteri et in passo dari potui.

3   si quis grillum contriverit manu, suas tonsillas vel alienas tetigerit, levabit. lacte caprino cum myrrha decocto ex sale exiguo gargarizabitur.

4   tonsillis privatim medentur renes vulpis aridi cum melle triti et inliti. hirundi-nus cinis ex melle ab interior parte tonsillis inlinitur.

5   Lini semen et anethum in oleo et aqua decoctum inponitur et acetum garga-rizatur. rubi in quo mora nascuntur caules teneri tunduntur; exprimitur sucus ex his, qui in sole ad crassitudinem mellis cogitur:

6   hic inlinitus ab interiore parte mire prodest. herba quae nascitur super fimeta rustica efficacissime bibitur in aqua ubi mus decoxerit.

7   et verminaca imposita prodest. caninum corr<ig>ium ter collo circumdatur. fimus columbinus, vinum, oleum in unum trita inlinuntur.

17 *anginae [id est intra fauces farcimina quae nascuntur]*

1   Menarum salsarum cinis de capite [id est salsorum piscium] ex melle inlinitur. alium tritum ex pusca gargarizatur. lini semen et anethum in oleo ex aqua decoctum ad tertias imponitur. acetum et sal gargarizatur.

2   nucis nuclei iuglandis triti cum ruta et oleo imponuntur. pix Bruttia cum melle inlinitur. fel taurinum vel anserinum cum melle, ex quo inlitis anginis celeriter succurritur.

3   pullus hirundininus, si fieri potest ripariae, si minus silvestris, si neutrum eius quae in domibus nidificat devoratus totum annum securum ab angina facit.

4   eosdem pullos quidam strangulant et comburunt cineremque eorum in cibo dant aut in potione. milipedae numero XX in unum tritae in aquae mulsae hemina aut aceti melle addito decoquuntur donec lentescat totum quod coquitur, et sic imponitur.

5   hyssopum cum vino decoctum gargarizatur. peucedanum cum coagulo vituli marini aequis ponderibus inlinitur. suci de quinquefolio pondus denarii ex aquae cyathis tribus potui datur.

6   fel caprinum vel taurinum aut ursinum cum melle inlinitur. ipsius hominis quacumque ex parte sanguis missus inlinitur efficacissime prodest.

16 *For tonsils*

1   A gargle of hot sheep's milk is useful for what is on either side of the gullet which they call tonsils, and the throat. Ground pigeon dung is gargled in raisin wine.

2   Dried fig and soda are ground into one and then smeared on the throat: it improves roughness of the throat and catarrh. Ground garlic is gargled in *posca*. Snails with only the earth removed ought to be cooked unwashed, then crushed and given in a draught of raisin wine.

3   If someone crushed a cricket by hand and he touched his or another's tonsils, he will relieve it. When decocted with myrrh, goat milk will be gargled with a little salt.

4   Dried fox's kidneys, ground and smeared on with honey, are a specific remedy for tonsils. Swallow ash is smeared on the inner side for the tonsils with honey.

5   Linseed and dill boiled down in oil and water are applied and vinegar is gargled. Tender stems of the bramble on which berries grow are crushed; the juice from these is squeezed out, and is congealed in the sun until the consistency of honey.

6   This is usefully smeared on the insides. A plant which grows atop a rural dung-heap is drunk most effectively in water in which a mouse was decocted.

7   Applied vervain is useful. A thong of dog-leather is wrapped around the neck three times. Pigeon dung, wine, and oil ground into one are smeared on.

17 *For* angina

1   The ash from salted *mena*'s head is smeared on with honey. Ground garlic is gargled in *posca*. Linseed and dill, decocted in oil with water to one-third, are applied. Vinegar and salt are gargled.

2   Ground walnut's kernels are applied with rue and oil. Bruttian pitch is smeared on with honey. Bull or goose bile with honey; quick relief is brought to *anginae* smeared with this.

3   A devoured chick of a swallow, if it is possible of a sand martin, if not, of a wood-swallow, and if neither, of that which nests in homes, makes one safe from *angina* for a whole year.

4   Some strangle and burn the same chicks and give their ash in food or in a potion. Millipedes, 20 in number, ground into one in a *hemina* of mead or of vinegar with added honey are decocted until the whole thing becomes sticky because it is cooked, and is applied thus.

5   Hyssop decocted with wine is gargled. Sulphurwort with an equal weight of seal's rennet is smeared on. A *denarius* weight of cinquefoil juice is given as a draught in three *cyathi* of water.

6   Goat, bull, or bear bile is smeared on with honey. Blood let from any part of the person himself is smeared on: it is extremely beneficial.

18 *lichenis [id est inpetigines]*

1   Graeco nomine lichenes appellantur, quod vulgo mentagram appellant vitium, quod acerrime per totam faciem solet serpere oculis tantum inmunibus.

2   descendit et in collum et in pectus manusque; foedat et cutem furfure. Manlius Cornutus praetor provinciae Aquitanicae legatus <HS> CC in hoc morbo locavit se curandum.

3   Huic ergo vitio sic conantur mederi. cantharidas inlinunt cum suco uvae tamineae et sevo ovis vel caprae. murinus fimus ex aceto. cinis erinacei ex oleo. in hac curatione prius faciem ex nitro et aceto foveri praecipiunt.

4   inlinunt et adipem vituli marini. delphini iocineris cinerem ex aqua inlinunt. eos qui sic vexabuntur osculari non oportet, quoniam contactus perniciosus est. ficulni caules ex aceto cocti tritique inlinuntur.

5   hibisci radix cum glutine lupino ex aceto decocta ad quartas. flos visci cum calce subactus laudatur. tithymalli flos cum resina decoctus adhibetur.

6   thapsiae radix trita cum melle imponitur. glutinum factum ex genitalibus vitulorum liquatur ex aceto cum sulphure vivo ramo ficulneo permixto, ita ut recens bis in die imponatur. lomentum aequis partibus cum turis polline imponitur ex aqua.

19 *elephantiasi*

1   A facie hoc malum plerumque incipit et nare prima surgit veluti lenticula; quae celerrime per totum corpus serpit, maculosa variis coloribus et inaequali cute, alibi crassa, alibi tenvi, dura <aliis> locis et quasi sub scabie aspera, postremo nigrescente <et ad ossa carnes apprimente>, tumentibus digitis in pedibus manibusque.

2   hic morbus peculiaris est Aegyptiorum populis. totus exitiosus est, cum in reges incidit, quoniam his solia in balneis humano sanguine temperantur.

3   his qui hoc malo afficiuntur cinis mustelae et eiusdem sanguis mixtus inlinitur. radix asparagi decocta in aceto trita apponitur. mentastri folia commanducata adhibentur; cedro inlinuntur.

20 *ulceribus in facie manantibus*

1   Bulbi triti ex aceto et sulphure medentur. nitrum ex melle et lacte bubulo succurrit. faciem purgat atque erugat adeps cygni.

18   *For lichen*

1   Called by the Greek name "lichens", that complaint is generally called *mentagra* because it is in the habit of creeping most severely over the whole face, leaving only the eyes free.

2   It descends down the neck onto the breast and hands; it disfigures the skin with *furfur*. The praetor Manlius Cornutus, the legate of Aquitaine, invested 200,000 *sesterces* in curing himself of this disease.

3   Thus they try to treat this complaint. They smear blister beetles with a taminian grape's juice and sheep's or nanny-goat's tallow. Mouse dung in vinegar. Hedgehog's ash in oil. For this treatment they advise that the face be fomented first with soda and vinegar.

4   And they smear on seal's grease. They smear on a dolphin's liver's ash with water. Those who will be plagued should not be kissed because contact is dangerous. Cooked and ground in vinegar, fig tree shoots are smeared on.

5   Marshmallow's root with lupine-glue decocted to one-quarter in vinegar. Mistletoe's juice kneaded with lime is praised. Spurge's juice decocted with resin is employed.

6   Ground *thapsia's* root is applied with honey. Glue made from calves' genitals is melted in vinegar with native sulphur and mixed through with a fig bough so that it might be applied fresh twice a day. *Lomentum* is applied in equal parts with frankincense dust in water.

19   *For* elephantiasis

1   This complaint generally starts on the face and it grows like a freckle from the tip of the nose, which quickly creeps over the whole body: with speckles in various colours and uneven appearance, in one spot thick, in another thin; in another place hard and rough like under *scabies*; finally growing dark and pressing flesh into the bones, with the digits of the hands and feet swelling.

2   This disease is specific to the people of Egypt. It is totally pernicious when it assails the kings, because the tubs in the baths are prepared with human blood.

3   Weasel's ash mixed together with its blood is smeared on for those who are afflicted with this complaint. Asparagus' root decocted in vinegar and ground is applied. Chewed catmint's leaves are employed; they are smeared on with cedar oil.

20   *For weeping sores on the face*

1   Ground bulbs in vinegar and sulphur heal them. Soda with honey and ox milk helps them. Swan's grease cleanses and removes wrinkles from the face.

21   *cervicibus et his quae mollienda sunt*

1   Adipis anserini perunctio remollit. eodem modo adeps gruis. farina lini seminis nitro adhibito ex vino calido in modum malagmatis temperatur.

2   farina hordeacea cum fico tusa. lenticula in aceto discocta. fici folia et ipsa
poma inmatura contrita. hammoniacum cum melle impositum. iuniperi
semen ex oleo inlinitur.

3   folia alni [vel alei] ex aqua ferventi remedio sunt tumori. ovorum lutea cum
adipe anserino et rosaceo. fel taurinum vel caprinum inlinitur.

4   butyro aut adipe ursino perfricantur. opisthotoniam levat urina caprae auribus
infusa. fimus caprinus cum bulbis inlinitur. opisthotonicis ex milvi iocinere
arido tres oboli in tribus cyathis aquae mulsae bibendi dantur.

5   adeps lupinus utiliter inlinitur. in cervicum dolore poplites utiliter fricantur, et
e diverso in poplitum dolore cervicem fricari remedium est.

22   *umeris et lateribus*

1   Doloribus umerorum mustelae cinis cum ovo inlinitur. sal in sacco ex aqua
ferventi calefactus adicitur.

2   Haec quae supra scripta sunt eodem modo et ad dolorem laterum faciunt,
peculiariter vero quae sequuntur. galbanum impositum. cochleae in tisana
coctae et resina terebintina in cibo prosunt.

3   cochleae lateri impositae. upupae caro in cibo laudatur. lanae sucidae ex oleo
calido imponuntur, melius <ex> axungia vetere.

4   [vel] vellera sulphure vivo suffita efficaciter excalefaciunt. pugionis mucrone
quo homo percussus est leviter pungi prodest.

23   *pectori*

1   Plurimis morbis obnoxium pectus est et impatientissimum frigoris. quod
cum vexatum est, non uno genere saevit sed infert tussim, purulentas excrea-
tiones, sanguinis vomitus, pthisin, synanchen. quibus singulis quemadmodum placeat succurri explicare conabimur.

24   *tussi*

1   Sedatur tussis alio in faba fricta discocto eaque faba in cibo sumpta, vel ex
melle in cibo sumpta. et tussi et purulentis excreationibus medetur.

2   adversum diuturnam tussim Falernum vinum utiliter sorbetur merum ab ieiunis. ficus aridae coquuntur cum hysopo ex aqua eaque aqua tussientibus
propinatur.

21 *For the neck and those things which need to be softened*

1   An anointment of goose grease softens again. Crane's grease does so in the same way. Linseed meal with added soda is combined in hot wine in the manner of an emollient.

2   Barley meal with crushed fig. Little lentils decocted in vinegar. Fig's leaves and its crushed unripe fruit. *Ammoniacum* gum applied with honey. Juniper's seed is smeared on with oil.

3   Leaves of alder in boiling water are a remedy for swelling. Egg yolks with goose grease and rose oil. Bull or goat bile is smeared on.

4   They are rubbed all over with butter or bear grease. Nanny-goat's urine poured into ears relieves *opisthotonia*. Goat dung is smeared on with bulbs. For sufferers of *opisthotonia*, three *oboli* of dried kite's liver is given to drink in three *cyathi* of mead.

5   Wolf grease is smeared on usefully. For pain in the neck, the knee is usefully rubbed, and the remedy for pain of the knees is to rub the neck in reverse.

22 *For the shoulders and sides*

1   Weasel's ash with egg is smeared on for pains of the shoulders. Salt warmed by boiling water is applied in a bag.

2   Those remedies which were written above work in the same way for pains of the sides, but indeed specific are those which follow. Applied *galbanum*. Snails cooked in barley gruel and turpentine resin are beneficial in food.

3   Snails applied to the side. Hoopoe flesh in food is recommended. Greasy wool is applied with hot oil, or better with old axle-grease.

4   Fleece fumigated with native sulphur actually warms effectively. It is useful to be lightly pricked with the point of a dagger with which a person was struck.

23 *For the breast*

1   The breast is subject to many diseases and is most intolerant of the cold. Because when it was troubled, it rages not with one type, but it inflicts a cough, purulent expectorations, the vomiting of blood, tuberculosis, and *angina*. We will try to explain how it is believed that each is to be treated.

24 *For a cough*

1   A cough is soothed by garlic decocted in rubbed beans and those beans eaten in food, or with honey and eaten with food. It is a remedy for a cough and the expectoration of purulent matter.

2   Unmixed Falernian wine is usefully drunk while fasting for a long-standing cough. Dried figs are boiled with hyssop in water, and that water is drunk for coughing.

3   sunt membranae in ventribus gallinaceorum quae proiciuntur: harum cinis potionibus inspersus destillationes pectoris et umidas tusses siccat.

4   testae cochleae crudae tritae cum aquae tepidae cyathis tribus sorbentur. ad tussim sedandam cochleae cum testis suis tritae adiecto croco eduntur.

5   sevum ovium decoctum cum vino austeri tussi medetur. ova cocta cum melle trita in cibo dantur. ova cruda permixta cum pari modo passi bibuntur.

6   sandaraca cum resina terebintina ovo sorbili indita editur. ursinum fel permixtum cum melle. salivae equi triduo potatae ternis potionibus ex aqua calida sanant: equum morti tradunt, hominem sanant.

7   pulmo cervinus cum gula arefactus in fumo, deinde tusus ex melle cottidie sumendus. sorbitiunculam ex alica sevo caprino peruncta[m] dabis, picem liquidam in ovo. iecur lupi coctum esui datur.

25   *sanguinem reicientibus*

1   Si <qui> ex alto praecipitati sunt, millefolium bibendum datur ex aceto. cruenta excreantibus quinque ovorum mediola cruda in vini hemina propinantur.

2   si et purulenta sint eodem tempore, ovum crudum cum pari mensura porri sectivi suci itemque Graeci mellis calefactum hauritur. ad excreationem cruentam cochleae elixae teruntur et ex aqua bibuntur.

3   prodest aqua pota in qua cydonia decocta sunt. cochleae inlotae ex aqua marina coquuntur et ita devorantur. cochleae cum testis suis tritae addito croco eduntur.

4   spongiae Afrae cinis cum porri sectivi suco sorbetur. porri capitati sucus cum farina turis sorbetur. farina qua chartae glutinantur calda in modum sorbitionis sumitur.

5   aqua in qua rosa et ruta et hyssopum decocta sunt vino miscetur et ita potui propinatur. marruvii scopae cum panico aqua decoquuntur eaque aqua bibitur.

6   uvae in vinaceis servatae aptae sunt excreantibus sanguinem. oleastri folia decoquuntur ex melle et dantur cochlearia tria.

7   palmae Thebaicae eduntur. cydonia matura devorantur cruda. nuclei amigdalorum cum amylo et mentastro devorantur. semen urticae aut myrti contritum in vino bibitur.

8   gummi optimum cum vino resolvitur et datur. si fieri potest, gummi ex amigdalis sit. ruborum in quibus mora nascuntur cauliculi teneri tunduntur, ex his sucus exprimitur, qui in sole ad crassitudinem mellis siccatur: hic haustus sanguinem efficacissime claudit.

9   eorundem ruborum caules ex vino austeri decocti eduntur idque vinum bibitur in potione. cornus cervini cinis in vino vetere potatur.

10 bubulinus sanguis cum aceto modice sumptus. haedini sanguinis recentis tres cyathi cum pari mensura aceti ferventes potui dantur. coagulum cervinum ex aceto datur; item coagulum leporinum eodem modo.

3   There are membranes which are thrown away in the bellies of chickens: the ash of these sprinkled in draughts dries catarrhs of the breast and wet coughs.

4   The ground shells of a raw snail are drunk in three *cyathi* of warm water. Snails ground with their shells with added saffron are eaten to soothe a cough.

5   Sheep's tallow decocted with dry wine assuages a cough. Cooked eggs ground with honey are given in food. Raw eggs beaten with an equal amount of raisin wine are drunk.

6   Red arsenic sulphide with turpentine resin put in a supping egg is eaten. Bear bile mixed through with honey. Draughts of horse's saliva heal when drunk three times in hot water for three days: they deliver the horse's death, but heal the person.

7   Deer lung with the gullet dried in smoke, and then pounded in honey so to be taken daily. You will give small draughts from *alica* well greased with goat tallow, or liquid pitch in an egg. A wolf's liver is given to eat.

25   *For bringing up blood*

1   If they were thrown from a height, *millefolium* is given to be drunk in vinegar. Five raw egg yolks are drunk in a *hemina* of wine for spitting blood.

2   And if there is purulent matter at the same time, a raw egg with an equal measure of chive's juice and the same of Greek honey is swallowed. Well-boiled snails are ground and drunk in water for spitting blood.

3   A draught of water in which quinces were decocted is beneficial. Unwashed snails are cooked in sea water and thus devoured. Snails ground with their shells and added saffron are eaten.

4   African sponge's ash is swallowed with chive's juice. Headed-leek's juice is swallowed with frankincense dust. The flour with which papers are glued is taken with hot water in the manner of a broth.

5   The water in which rose, rue, and hyssop were decocted is mixed with wine and thus given as a draught to be drunk. Horehound's twigs are decocted with Italian millet in water, and that water is drunk.

6   Grapes preserved in grape skins are suitable for spitting blood. Wild olive's leaves are decocted in honey and three *cochlearia* are given.

7   Theban dates are eaten. Raw, ripe quinces are devoured. Almond nuts are devoured with starch and catmint. Crushed nettle's or myrtle's seed is drunk in wine.

8   Top quality gum is dissolved with wine and is given. If it can, the gum should come from the almond. The tender stems of the bramble on which berries grow are crushed, the juice is squeezed from these, and is dried in the sun to the consistency of honey: this draught staunches blood effectively.

9   The same bramble's stems decocted in dry wine are eaten and that wine is drunk in a potion. Ash of deer horn is quaffed in old wine.

10   A moderate amount of ox blood taken with vinegar. Three *cyathi* of fresh kid's blood is given as a draught with an equal measure of boiling vinegar. Deer rennet is given in vinegar; likewise hare rennet in the same way.

26 *vomicae*

1   Vomicae plerumque in lateribus erumpunt in membranas supervacuas et ex languoribus natas umore concreto in tussimque converso, qui adeo fecunde subnascitur ut non tam excreetur quam evomatur.

2   eos itaque qui eam fortunam inciderint oportebit ambulare vectari ungui; lectus et requies. qui hunc morbum alunt, sustinendi erunt cibis firmis et glutinosis, avibus pinguibus, operibus pistoriis plus aequo mellitis, prout patientur facultates.

3   Vomicam sanat privatim id mel in quo sunt apes demortuae. ad hunc autem morbum facit optime potio haec: ovum crudum in vaso funditur, putamen eius repletur suco marrubii atque in eodem vase coicitur;

4   item repletur melle et similiter ibi adicitur, et ita permixta calefactaque ad teporem haec hausta vomicam rumpunt purgant ad sanitatem perducunt.

5   Multi medici se [medicos] adversum hoc malum non inveniunt. ego certe scio raro quemquam huic pesti ereptum qui se illis credidisset.

6   verum ita curatio eius expedita est ut etiam hieme asperrima explicari possit intra diem quadragesimum, vere autem vel aestate breviore tempore. aliquot a me curati sunt intra praefinitum tempus compositione ea quae infra scripta est:

7   mandragorae pondus denarii, hyoscyami pondus denarii, opii pondus denarii, turis pondus denarii, croci pondus denarii [singularum rerum omnium]. haec ex vino diligenter teruntur ad crassitudinem paulo spissiorem quam mellis.

8   ex hoc medicamento initio pondus victoriati in tribus cyathis aquae euntibus dormitum datur, mox deinde ex eodem modo aquae pondus denarii. prima potione profectus sentitur, deinde incredibili saltu explicatur curatio.

26 *For* vomica

1   *Vomicae* commonly erupt on the membranes surrounding the pleural cavity, and having been born from feebleness with congealed humour and transformed into a cough, that (the congealed humour) arises in such abundance that it is not so much coughed as it is vomited.

2   Therefore, those who have fallen to that fate will need to walk, be carried, and be rubbed; bed and rest (are needed). Those who develop this disease need to be sustained with strong and starchy foods, fatty birds, and pastries sweetened with more honey than usual, and as much as resources allow.

3   Honey in which bees died especially heals *vomica*. However, this potion is best made thus: raw egg is poured into a vessel, its shell is filled with horehound's juice and it is thrown into the same vessel;

4   it is again filled with honey and it is similarly added to it. And having been beaten and warmed to a mild temperature, these draughts rupture and cleanse *vomicae* and lead to health.

5   Not many doctors manage to treat this complaint. I certainly know that rarely was anyone set free from that plague by those he had trusted.

6   A treatment for it was developed so that even in the harshest winter it is possible to be freed by the fortieth day; however, in spring or summer within a shorter time. Some were cured by me within the determined time with that composition which was written below:

7   a *denarius* weight of mandrake, a *denarius* weight of henbane, a *denarius* weight of opium, a *denarius* weight of frankincense, a *denarius* weight of saffron. These are carefully ground in wine to a consistency a little thicker than honey.

8   A *victoriatus* weight from this medicament is first given in three *cyathi* of water when going to sleep, then afterwards a *denarius* weight in the same amount of water. Improvement is perceived with the first potion, and then the cure is unfurled with an incredible leap.

Liber II

capitula libri II

Book Two

Chapters of Book Two

1   *pthisicis*

1   Invenio iam desperatum pthisicum sanatum hoc modo. radicem decoquis in Punici mali cortice: mixtum ex aquae cyatho uno et lactis pari mensura cottidie sumptum profuit.

2   utilius est pthisicis et longis languoribus qui tenentur morari in saltibus ubi pix nascitur quam in mari navigare et marina loca visitare.

3   cancri fluviatiles ex iure in cibo sumpti ieiunis dantur. lacerta viridis decocta in vini sextariis tribus ad cyathum unum, singulis cochlearibus pthisico datis diebus singulis donec convalescat.

4   propinatur cochlearum cinis ex vino austero. suis feminae herba pastae laridum in cibo datur. carnes asini ex iure sumptae. suis fimi cinis ex passo propinatur.

5   adipis recentis pondo quadrans decoquitur in vini cyathis tribus; additur eo mel optimum, et pilulis gluttitur.

2   *syntexi*

1   Syntexis quoque nec periculo nec facie pthisi dissimilis morbus est. cui sic medetur. alicae cyathi III in passi sextarium et aquae congium commiscentur et sensim coquuntur donec aqua consumatur;

2   tunc suffunditur lactis ovilli sextarius aut caprini, quo subfervefacto fit genus sorbitionis. qua per se primis diebus curationis utuntur, procedentibus diebus et mel adiciunt. utillimum putant eos in aqua marina lavari.

3   *sciaticis*

1   Vermis terrenus effoditur et imponitur in catillum ligneum fissum ferro alligatum; aqua perfunditur rursusque in eo loco ex quo erutus est vivus suffoditur et ea aqua in eodem catillo bibitur.

2   cochleae crudae tritae ex vino Aminneo cum pipere bibuntur. lacerta viridis dempto capite et pedibus cum interaneis <ita> condita, ut fastidium abigat, in cibo datur.

3   rubiam qua pelles conficiuntur cottidie bibere utile est et lau<a>ri. genestae rami plurimis diebus in aceto macerantur, deinde tunduntur et coquuntur: ex eo suco cottidie cyathus potui datur.

4   fimus bubulus calefactus in cinere ferventi locis dolentibus in foliis cuiuscumque holeris imponitur.

1   For tuberculosis sufferers

1   I have already found this way to cure the desperate tuberculosis patient: you decoct pomegranate's root in its rind; taken daily, mixed with one *cyathus* of water and an equal measure of milk, it is beneficial.

2   There is greater benefit for tuberculosis patients and sufferers of extended feebleness who are kept in woodlands where pitch is produced to remain there than to sail on the sea or to visit seaside locales.

3   Riverine crabs in broth are given to fasting patients. A green lizard in three *sextarii* of wine is decocted to one *cyathus*, with a single *cochlear* given to the tuberculosis patient every day until he recovers.

4   Snails' ash is given to drink in dry wine. A grass-fed sow's bacon lard is given in food. Ass' flesh eaten in broth. Ash of pig's dung is given to drink in raisin wine.

5   A quarter of a pound of fresh grease is boiled down in three *cyathi* of wine; the best honey is added to this and it is swallowed in pills.

2   For syntexis

1   *Syntexis* is a disease dissimilar neither in danger nor appearance to tuberculosis. It is healed thus: 3 *cyathi* of *alica* are combined with a *sextarius* of raisin wine and a *congium* of water, and are slowly boiled until the water is reduced;

2   then a *sextarius* of sheep or goat milk is poured in which, having been simmered, makes a type of broth. This is used by itself in the first days of treatment, and in the following days they add honey. They believe it is most useful that patients be bathed in salt water.

3   For sufferers of hip-disease

1   An earthworm is dug out and placed into a wooden bowl that was split and bound with iron; it is doused with water, and alive it is reburied in that place from which it was uprooted, and that water is drunk from the same bowl.

2   Raw ground snails are drunk in Aminnean wine with pepper. A green lizard with its head, feet, and intestines removed, and seasoned in such a way that it prevents nausea, is given in food.

3   It is useful to drink madder with which hides are prepared daily and to be washed. Twigs of *genesta* are steeped in vinegar for many days, then they are beaten and cooked; a *cyathus* is given from this juice as a draught daily.

4   Ox dung warmed in hot embers is applied to the paining spot in the leaves of any vegetable.

4   *praecordiorum dolori*

1   In universo praecordia appellantur quae aliqui in plura vocabula dividunt, vocantes modo stomachum, interdum iecur, interdum praecordia. haec cum indurverint praeter gravissimum dolorem velocissimam mortem ingerunt.

2   His caninus catulus lactens subinde apponitur inque eum vitium transire constat: defunctum obrui moris est. bulbi triti inliniti ventri bene molliunt.

3   et ocimum tritum impositum praecordiis prodest. sextarius farinae lini seminis, sextarius feni Graeci cum pari mensura mellis ex aqua mulsa decocti calidi imponuntur saepius. aliqui malunt feniculi farinam cum pari mensura mellis decoquere et ita imponere.

4   cydonia cruda vel cocta ceroti modo in panno inlinuntur et calefacta praecordiis super imponuntur.

5   acori radix tusa cum vino efficacissime prodest. his quos linquit animus aut mens – et alienantur – quibusque vertigines fiunt cochleae singulae cum sua testa tritae ex passi cyathis ternis calefacta potione per dies VIIII dantur.

6   in eadem curatione aliqui dant per dies quinque in eodem modo passi primo die cochleam unam, sequenti duas, tertio tres, quarto duas, quinto unam: sic suspiria tollentur.

7   in his languoribus si febris non sit marina aqua lavari utile est. iocineri prodest in cibo viverra porcelli modo inassata. stomacho mede<n>tur cochleae si fieri potest Africanae in cibo sumptae:

8   coquuntur intactae ex aqua, deinde ex prunis torrentur, tunc ex vino et garo eduntur, impari numero stomachi dolori medentur. prosunt vivae cochleae ex aceto devoratae. [in hoc languore aqua marina lavari prodest].

9   Aestimo praecordiorum esse vitium cum cibus non continetur. certe quibus hoc accidit stomacho laborare dicuntur. horum potioni infricatur venter ossifragi arefactus. prodest etiam si teneatur in manu dum cibus sumitur.

10   Non est ab re compositionem operi convenientem ponere, quae stomachi fastidium et marcorem detergit celerrime.

11   in musti ex uvis albis congio coiciuntur cydonia quinque non purgata, totidem mala Punica, eo additur sorborum sextarius, roris Syriaci sextarius, croci Siculi semuncia, fici optimi semuncia.

12   sic coquitur usque ad crassitudinem mellis, inde in die lingula sumitur. servatur in vaso vitreo.

13   Fit efficacissima potio compositione ita scripta. apii seminis aridi drachmae sex, petroselini Macedonici drachmae IIII, spicae nardi drachmae IIII, myrrhae drachmae IIII, opii drachmae IIII, schoeni drachmae IIII, piperis longi drachmae V, piperis albi drachmae V.

14   haec una teruntur cum melle Graeco despumato quod satis est. servatur in vaso vitreo. a balneo dantur ieiuno in potione mulsi mixti ex aqua calida drachmae duae.

4   *For pain of the* praecordia

1   In general, *praecordia* are called by the many names into which one separates them: calling it at one time stomach, other times liver, and sometimes *praecordia*. When these have hardened they inflict the most grievous pain before a most swift death.

2   A suckling puppy is immediately applied to these and it is well known that the complaint transfers to it: dead, it is customary for it to be buried. Ground bulbs smeared onto the belly softens well.

3   And ground and applied basil is beneficial to the *praecordia*. A *sextarius* of linseed meal and a *sextarius* of fenugreek with an equal measure of honey decocted in mead are applied, hot, frequently. Some prefer to decoct fennel meal with an equal measure of honey and thus apply it.

4   Quinces, either raw or cooked in the manner of a cerate, are smeared on a cloth and applied hot over the *praecordia*.

5   *Acorus* root pounded with wine is most effectively beneficial. For those whose consciousness or mind leaves them – and they go insane – and for any who become dizzy, single snails ground with their shells are given in three *cyathi* of raisin wine as a hot draught for 9 days.

6   For the same cure, some give the same measure of raisin wine for five days and one snail on the first day, two on the following day, three on the third, two on the fourth, and one on the fifth day: thus shortness of breath will be removed.

7   For this faintness it is useful to be bathed with sea water if there is no fever. A ferret, baked in the manner of a suckling pig, is useful for the liver in food. Snails, if possible from Africa, eaten in food heal the stomach.

8   They are cooked intact in water, then roasted on coals, then eaten with wine and *garum* in an odd number, and they remedy a pain of the stomach. Swallowing live snails with vinegar is beneficial.

9   I consider it to be a complaint of the *praecordia* when food is not retained. It certainly is by those who are said to suffer this happening to the stomach. An *ossifragus'* dried stomach is rubbed into their drink. It is even helpful if it is held in the hand while food is eaten.

10   It is not disadvantageous to cite an appropriate composition in the text which quickly removes nausea and faintness from the stomach:

11   Five uncleaned quinces are laid in a *congius* of must made from white grapes, and as many pomegranates; to that is added a *sextarius* of sorb apples, a *sextarius* of Syrian sumach, half an *uncia* of Sicilian saffron, and an *uncia* of the best fig.

12   It is boiled continuously until it has the consistency of honey, and a *ligula* is taken from this daily. It is kept in a glass vessel.

13   A most effective potion is made from this recipe: six *drachmae* of dried *apium* seed, 4 *drachmae* of Macedonian parsley, 4 *drachmae* of spikenard, 4 *drachmae* of myrrh, 4 *drachmae* of opium, 4 *drachmae* of rush, 5 *drachmae* of long pepper, and 5 *drachmae* of white pepper.

14   These are ground together with a sufficient amount of skimmed Greek honey. It is stored in a glass vessel. Two *drachmae* are given to a fasting patient after a bath in a draught of honeyed wine mixed with hot water.

5   *ventri molliendo*

1   Menae salsae [id est pisces salsi] ventri molliendo cum felle tauri umbilico inlinuntur. lac caprinum potatum cum sale et melle. ventriculus suillus in quo sarda decocta sit.

2   porri capitati discocti per se in cibo sumuntur. urticae semen tostum pane colligitur. lens non percocta sorbetur. myrobalanus est genus cariotae nascens in Aegypto: haec os non habet; vino austeri trita et pota alvum citat.

3   fel lupi cum elaterio umbilico inlinitur. cydonia in melle servata cruda manducantur a ieiunis. pruna a ieiuno eduntur.

4   mororum maturorum sucus potui datur. ammoniacum potioni additur. ulmi corticis tunsi denarii pondus in hemina aquae frigidae etiam purgat. aqua bibitur in qua gallinacei decoxerint. hirundininus fimus adiecto melle suppositus.

5   salicis sucus ex vino mulso potatus. thalassomeli iucundissime purgat sine stomachi vexatione, et odore grato et sapore.

6   quod sic fieri debet [confectio thalassomelis]: aquae marinae et aquae caelestis eadem mensura et mel eiusdem portionis permiscetur, et servatur in vaso fictili picato.

6   *ventri sistendo*

1   Cancri fluviatiles triti ex aqua bibuntur. sativi siseris sucus in caprino lacte potatur. ocimum tritum ventri inlinitur. panicum in lacte caprino decoctum more sorbitionis <bis> in die sumitur.

2   vetus panis nauticus tunsus et iterum coctus ex aqua bibitur. in aqua cortices fabae ad tertias decoctae prosunt. lens ex aqua caelesti decocta sorbetur. acetum merum sumitur.

3   mala silvestria eduntur. aqua in qua pruna agrestia cocta sint bibitur. silvestrium prunorum bacae vel ex radice cortices in vino austeri decoquuntur ut tertia pars decidat, idque vinum bibitur merum, cyathus unus in die.

4   mororum sativorum inmaturorum sucus bibitur. sorbetur sucus seminis myrti. palumbus ferus ex pusca coctus in cibo datur. fimus columbinus cum melle ventri inlinitur.

5   bibitur anatum mascularum sanguis. flores vel cincinnos de avellana colligis et mittis in furno ut siccentur, et cum siccati fuerint teruntur et ex vino propinantur.

6   iuniperi bacae tritae ex vino nigro, id est ex uvis nigris expresso, potantur. flos hederae tribus digitis sumptus in vino austero bibitur bis in die. bacae acrifolii ex vino potantur.

7   ruborum in quibus mora nascuntur cauliculi ex vino austero decoquuntur et in cibo dantur. cochlearum quae vivae crematae sunt cinis potioni ex vino austeri inspargitur.

8   plantago editur ex aceto cocta. symphyti radix ex vino bibitur. gallinacei iecur assum in cibo sumitur.

5   *For opening the bowels*

1   Salted *menae* are smeared on the navel with bull's bile to open the bowel. Goat milk drunk with salt and honey. Pork belly in which a *sarda* was stewed.

2   Headed-leeks decocted by themselves are consumed in food. Toasted nettle's seed is combined with bread. Partially cooked lentils are swallowed. Behennut is a type of date native to Egypt; these have no stones: ground and drunk with dry wine, it moves the bowel.

3   Wolf's bile is smeared on the navel with *elaterium*. Raw quinces preserved in honey are nibbled by a fasting patient. Plums are eaten by a fasting patient.

4   The juice of ripe mulberries is given in a draught. *Ammoniacum* gum is added to drinks. Even a *denarius* weight of beaten elm bark in a *hemina* of cold water purges. The water in which hens were decocted is drunk. Swallow dung with honey suppository.

5   Willow's juice drunk in honeyed wine. *Thalassomeli* most pleasantly purges without disturbing the stomach, and has an agreeable smell and taste.

6   It ought to be made thus: an equal measure of sea water and rain water is mixed with the same proportion of honey, and stored in an earthenware vessel smeared with pitch.

6   *For stopping diarrhoea*

1   Ground riverine crabs are drunk in water. Cultivated skirret's juice is drunk in goat milk. Ground basil is smeared on the belly. Italian millet decocted in goat milk in the manner of a broth is consumed twice a day.

2   Old sailor's bread, crushed and cooked again, is drunk in water. Bean husks decocted in water to one-third are beneficial. Lentils decocted in rain water are drunk. Unmixed vinegar is consumed.

3   Wild apples are eaten. Water in which wild plums were cooked is drunk. The fruits of the wild plum tree or its root's bark is decocted in dry wine so that it reduces to one-third; that wine is drunk unmixed; one *cyathus* per day.

4   The juice of unripe cultivated mulberries is drunk. Myrtle seed's juice is swallowed. Wild wood-pigeon cooked in *posca* is given in food. Pigeon dung with honey is smeared on the belly.

5   Male ducks' blood is drunk. You collect the flowers or *cincinni* from the hazel and throw them into an oven so that they might be dried; when they were dried, they are ground and drunk in wine.

6   Ground juniper's berries are swallowed in dark wine, i.e. pressed from dark grapes. A three-finger-pinch of ivy's flower is drunk in dry wine twice a day. Holly's berries are swallowed in wine.

7   The shoots of the bramble on which berries grow are decocted in dry wine and given in food. Ash of snails which were burned alive is sprinkled into a potion of dry wine.

8   Plantain cooked in vinegar is eaten. Comfrey's root is drunk in wine. Roasted chicken's liver is consumed in food.

7   *cholerae*

1   Cholera ventris vitium est malum, praeceps, utpote quod et vomitu et per sedem exhauriat. adversus quam lactucae caules quanto maiores et amariores in patina coquuntur ex aqua et sic eduntur.

2   cydonia matura cruda in cibo sumuntur. optime facit et potio cuius compositionem cum de stomacho diceremus exposuimus.

3   bacae acrifolii tritae et ex vino datae. mororum de rubo sucus efficaciter bibitur. aqua marina calida clysterio infunditur. mirifice prodest compositio quae infra scripta est.

4   olivae quam veterrimae aqua calida eluuntur ita ut saporem salis amittant, et enucleatae cum pipere teruntur; quibus admiscentur coria mali in aceto decocta: oleum et acetum acerrimum cum triblas adicitur. oportebit autem qui curabitur potione quam diutissime abstinere.

8   *torminibus*

1   Lactuca discocta editur ex oleo cymino sale sinapi. ovum crudum diffunditur in vaso, putamen eius impletur oleo quod in vaso diffunditur; eadem ratione et vinum et mel: vinum sit austere.

2   haec permiscentur in unum cochleario, et bibitur. holera discocta ex sale eduntur. ruta cum hyssopo discoquitur eaque aqua ex vini potione miscetur.

3   panis cum lacte caprino decoctus bis in die sumitur more sorbitionis. in olei cyathis sex ruta decoquitur idque oleum bibitur. malum Punicum tusum ex tribus heminis vini coctum ad heminam emendat.

4   malum Punicum in olla addito operculo exustum in furno et tritum datumque in vini potione discutit. ruborum qui ferunt mora cauliculi teneri tunduntur et ex his exprimitur sucus, qui in sole ad crassitudinem mellis cogitur:

5   hic potus efficacissime prodest. lien pecudis tostus tritus ex vino bibitur. palumbus ferus in cibo datur decoctus in pusca.

6   anas viva apponitur ventri; in eandem morbus transit, itaque moritur. aqua marina calida clysterio infunditur. vinum tepidum addito coagulo leporis potui datur, creditur efficacissimum.

9   *tenesmo*

1   Tenesmo laborat si qui subinde concupiscit desurgere et nihil eicit. ad hoc vitium senectus anguium cum rosaceo in vaso stagneo decoquitur et ventri inlinitur.

2   et si exulceratio non sit, ostrea ex mulso decocta eduntur. lac bubulum potui prodest. ius piscium maritimorum in patina decoctorum cum lactucis sorbetur aut pane colligitur.

7   *For* cholera

1   *Cholera* is an injurious complaint of the belly; a critical danger since it exhausts by vomiting and diarrhoea. Against this stems of lettuce, the bigger and more bitter ones, are cooked in a pan with water and eaten thus.
2   Raw ripe quinces are eaten in food. The potion whose composition we recorded when we spoke about the stomach works very well.
3   Ground holly berries are given with wine. The juice of berries from the bramble is drunk to good effect. Hot sea water is injected as an enema. The composition which is written below is wonderfully beneficial.
4   The oldest possible olives are washed with hot water so that they lose the taste of salt, and having been pitted, they are ground with pepper; apple peels, decocted in vinegar, are mixed with these; oil and the sharpest vinegar are added by pressing. However, it will be necessary for the patient to abstain from drinking for as long as possible.

8   *For* colic

1   Lettuce decocted in oil with cumin, salt, and mustard is eaten. A raw egg is poured into a vessel, and its shell is filled with oil which is poured into the vessel; with the same measure, wine and honey. The wine should be dry.
2   These are mixed together into one with a spoon, and it is drunk. Cabbages decocted with salt are eaten. Rue is decocted with hyssop, and the water from this is mixed with a draught of wine.
3   Bread decocted with goat milk is taken in the manner of a broth twice a day. Rue is decocted in six *cyathi* of oil, and that oil is drunk. A pounded pomegranate boiled in three *heminae* until one *hemina* remains cures it.
4   A pomegranate in a jar with its lid on and burnt in a furnace, then ground and given in a draught of wine, disperses it. The soft stems of the brambles which bear berries are beaten and juice squeezed from them, which is congealed in the sun until it is as thick as honey.
5   This draught is most effectively useful. Toasted and ground spleen of livestock is drunk in wine. Wild wood-pigeon decocted in *posca* is given in food.
6   A living duck is applied to the belly; the disease moves into it, and it subsequently dies. Hot sea water is injected as an enema. Warm wine with added hare's rennet given as a draught is believed to be most effective.

9   *For* tenesmos

1   One suffers from *tenesmos* if one repeatedly desires to go to the stool and expels nothing. For this complaint snakes' slough is decocted with rose oil in a *stagnum* vessel and is smeared on the belly.
2   And if there is no ulceration, oysters decocted in honeyed wine are eaten. Ox milk is beneficial in a draught. A broth of marine fish decocted in a pan with lettuce is drunk or combined with bread.

3   holus [id est caules] discoctum editur cum sale. aqua marina ex alto hauritur; servatur in vetustatem, vires inde imponuntur: bibitur cum vino aut aceto, vomitu praecedente.

4   aquam marinam aliqui per se dant, sed raphanos supermandi iubent ex mulso aceto ut vomatur. pulticulam siliginis salsam bene sine oleo edendam dabis.

10 *dysenteriae*

1   Holera discocta cum sale eduntur. per se bulbi triti dantur in vino austero: potio miscetur caelesti aqua. coctum ocimum in cibo datur.

2   ruta cum caseo teritur in vino in modum moreti et ita editur. cera remissa in potione datur: puls fit ex alica tosta, priusquam detur in aqua; cum subigitur, cera remissa infunditur.

3   sarmenta in quibus acini uvarum haerent et acinorum lapilli comburuntur eorumque cinere aspergitur. sucus pampinorum vitium clysterio inmittitur.

4   cydonia matura cruda eduntur. myrti seminis pondus denarii in vino propinatur. vinum in quo folia myrti discocta sint potui datur.

5   galla Commagena comburitur, cinis eius extinguitur vino, inlinitur ventri: hoc et ad coeliacos facit. flos hederae tritus tribus digitis sumptus in vino austeri bis in die bibitur.

6   ruborum in quibus mora nascuntur cauliculi decoquuntur in vino austeri et per se eduntur.

7   lutea ovorum trium, lardi veteris unciae tres, mellis totidem, vini cyathi tres una conteruntur, et in nucis avellanae magnitudine ex aqua datur.

11 *coeliacis [id est torturae vel commissioni intestinorum]*

1   Bacae olivarum in vino propinantur. membranae gallinarum tostae in oleo et sale subfervefiunt, sic datae in cibo coeliacorum dolorem mulcent: abstinere a frugibus prius et gallinam et hominem oportet.

2   fimus columbinus tostus et tritus dysentericis in potione propinatur. palumbi in aceto discocti et dysentericis et coeliacis in cibo medentur.

3   dysentericos adiuvat turdus inassatus tritus in cibo sumptus cum myrti bacis. item in eundem modum merula sumitur.

4   gravissimum ventris vitium ileos appellatur: huic resistit discerpti vespertilionis sanguis inlitus ventri. dysentericis ova pridie in aceto macerantur, eorum lutea friguntur in oleo et devorantur.

5   ova ex aceto macerantur; ex his et farina et aqua panis coeliacis fit. quidam eadem ova resolvunt et in patinis tosta dant in cibo. caseus vetus ovillus in cibo prodest.

3   Decocted vegetable is eaten with salt. Sea water is drawn up from deep water; it is stored for a long time, and from that its potency is established: it is drunk with wine or vinegar, previously vomiting.

4   Some give sea water by itself, but they recommend eating radishes with honeyed vinegar beforehand, and it is vomited. You will give well-salted wheaten gruel without oil to be eaten.

10   For dysentery

1   Cabbage decocted with salt is eaten. Ground bulbs by themselves are given in dry wine: the potion is mixed with rain water. Cooked basil is eaten in food.

2   Rue is ground with cheese in wine in the manner of *moretum* and thus eaten. Melted wax is given in a potion: porridge is made from roasted *alica* before it is given in water; when it is prepared the melted wax is poured in.

3   Shoots on which the berries of grapes cling and the seeds of the grapes are burnt, and it is sprinkled with the ash of them. The juice of vines' shoots is inserted in a clyster.

4   Raw ripe quinces are eaten. A *denarius* weight of myrtle's seed is given to drink in wine. Wine in which myrtle's leaves were decocted is given in a draught.

5   Commagene oak-gall is burned; the ash of this is extinguished with wine, and is smeared on the belly: and this works for bowels. A three-finger-pinch of ground ivy's flower in dry wine is drunk twice a day.

6   Stems of the bramble on which berries grow are decocted in dry wine and eaten by themselves.

7   Three egg yolks, three *unciae* of bacon lard, the same amount of honey, and three *cyathi* of wine are pounded together, and it is given in the amount of a hazelnut in water.

11   For sufferers of bowel disease

1   Olives are given to drink in wine. The roasted skins of hens are heated from below in oil and salt; thus given in food, it soothes the pain of bowel disease patients. Beforehand it is necessary for the hen and the person to abstain from fruits.

2   Roasted and ground pigeon dung is drunk in a potion by dysentery patients. Wood-pigeons decocted in vinegar are good for dysentery and bowel disease patients in food.

3   Roasted, ground thrush with myrtle's berries taken in food helps dysentery patients. Likewise, blackbird is eaten in the same manner.

4   The most painful complaint of the belly is called *ileos*; blood of a torn apart bat smeared over the belly halts this. Eggs are steeped in vinegar the day before, and the yolks of these are fried in oil and gulped down by dysentery patients.

5   Eggs are steeped in vinegar; bread is made from these with flour and water for bowel disease patients. Some crack the same eggs, and roasted in pans, give them in food. Aged sheep cheese in food is beneficial.

6   sevum ovillum decoctum in vino austeri bibitur. hoc et coeliacis medetur.

7   cochleae duae teruntur cum suis testis et ova cruda ex passi cyathis duobus, aquae cyathis tribus, atque totum in novo vase calefactum ad temperamentum potionis bibitur.

8   cochlearum cum suo putamine combustarum cinis addito pusillo resinae ex vino bibitur. senectus serpentium decocta cum rosaceo in stagneo vaso ventri inlinitur.

9   dysentericis potiones ferro candenti calefieri debent. caseus vaccinus recens inmittitur. ad omnes epiphoras ventris caseum mollem [in cibo] imponi iubent, veterem autem tritum in modum farinae mensura cyathi addi in cyathos tres vini cibarii et ita devorari.

10   lac caprinum ad dimidias partes decoctum. infunditur gluten taurinum aqua calida resolutum. imponitur inflationi ventris vitulinus fimus in vino decoctus.

11   frequenter evenit ex causa aliqua latente ut ventri dolor subitus existat: qui numquam temptat habentem secum talum leporis.

12 *tineis*

1   Tineae quoque vitium ventris sunt. quae pelluntur poto cervini cornus combusti cinere. raphani decoquuntur ex aqua ad tertias et ea aqua vino miscetur.

2   radix inulae decoquitur, deinde sucus eius exprimitur et potui datur: cum eruta est inula terram non debet tangere. alium in oxymeli decoctum devoratur.

3   betae candidae decoctae devorantur cum alio crudo. aqua in qua lupini coxerint addita ruta et pipere bibitur.

4   bulbi genus est scilla, ex quo pusillum tritum cum oxymeli bibitur. malum Punicum tusum decoctum ex tribus heminis ad heminam tineas eicit potum.

5   acini hederae albae contriti tres ex oxymeli prosunt; in hac curatione convenit et ventri eos eadem ratione inlini.

13 *lieni sive spleni*

1   Solea piscis imponitur. idem praestat eodem modo torpedo. rombus cum est impositus vivus in mare remittitur.

2   aqua bibitur in qua holera decocta sint addito sale. eius qui cottidie ieiunus ervum ederit lienem consumi certum est.

3   sarmentorum cinis aceto conspersus binis cyathis ex aqua ei dabitur: is qui curabitur in lienem iacere debebit. acetum bibitur et in spongia apponitur. corymbi hederae poti vel inliti prosunt.

6 Sheep tallow decocted in dry wine is drunk. And this is good for bowel disease patients.

7 Two snails are ground with their shells and raw eggs with two *cyathi* of raisin wine and three *cyathi* of water; heated together in a new vessel to the temperature of a potion, it is drunk.

8 Ash of snails burnt with their own shells with a tiny amount of resin added is drunk in wine. Snakes' slough decocted with rose oil in a *stagnum* vessel is smeared over the belly.

9 Potions ought to be warmed with white-hot iron for dysentery patients. Fresh cow's cheese is injected. For all affluxes of the belly they prescribe placing soft cheese, while aged cheese, ground in the manner of meal, is to be added in the measure of a *cyathus* in three *cyathi* of table wine and is eaten thus.

10 Goat milk decocted to half the amount. Bull glue melted in hot water is administered. Calf dung decocted in wine is applied to the belly for flatulence.

11 It often happens for some unseen reason that a sudden pain in the belly arises: this never afflicts one who keeps a hare's anklebone with them.

12 For tapeworms

1 Tapeworms are also a complaint of the belly. These are expelled by drinking ash of burnt deer horn. Radishes are decocted in water to one-third, and that water is mixed with wine.

2 Elecampane's root is decocted, and then its juice is squeezed out and is given to drink: when the elecampane is dug up it must not touch the ground. Garlic decocted in *oxymel* is swallowed.

3 Decocted light beets are gulped down with raw garlic. Water in which lupines were boiled is drunk with added rue and pepper.

4 Squill is a type of bulb, and a tiny, ground piece from it is drunk with *oxymel*. Pomegranate, pounded and decocted from three *heminae* to one *hemina* and drunk, discharges tapeworms.

5 Three crushed berries of white ivy are beneficial with *oxymel*; with regards to this treatment it is appropriate that they be smeared on the belly in the same manner.

13 For a diseased spleen

1 A sole fish is applied. Likewise an electric ray in the same way is beneficial. When a living turbot is applied it is thrown back into the sea.

2 Water in which cabbages were decocted with added salt is drunk. It is said that the spleen of he who ate bitter vetch daily when fasting is reduced.

3 The ash of vine twigs sprinkled with vinegar will be given in two *cyathi* of water to him: he who is treated must lie on his spleen. Vinegar is drunk and applied in a sponge. Ivy's berries, drunk or smeared on, are beneficial.

4   hederaceis vasis in potione semper utendum est. pecudis lien recens super dolorem extenditur, dicente eo qui medebitur se lienem mederi, deinde in pariete dormitorii cubiculi tectorio includitur et ter novies subsignatur eademque dicentur.

5   caninus lien si viventi eximitur et laboranti in cibo datur, liberat de vitio lienis. catuli duum dierum datus ignoranti aegro in cibo ex aceto.

6   idem et lien erinacei praestat. cochlearum cinis cum lini semine et urticae addito melle imponitur donec persanetur.

7   lacerta viridis viva in olla ante cubiculum dormitorium suspenditur, ut egrediens et rediens manu tangat. sedat lienem fel apri vel suis potum, cervini cornus cinis potus ex aceto.

8   equi lingua inveterata ex vino bibitur. praesentaneo remedio lien bubulus assus recens vel elixus in cibo. alii capita XX tusa cum aceti sextario imponuntur.

9   haedi lien impositus idem praestat. radices violae lotae ex aceto inlinuntur. agarici oboli duo in aceto mulso poti per dies XXI consumunt lienem.

14 *lumborum dolori*

1   Acinorum nigrorum suci cyathus unus cum mulsi cyathis duobus potui datus lumbos dolentes sanat. itemque inulae foliorum sive radicis pulveris denarii duo ex vini cyatho uno bibiti emendant.

2   Pastinacae item radicis sive seminis denarii IIII in aqua mulsa decocti et potui dati lumborum et renum vitia emendant. item porri sectivi sucus ad cyathos duos in vini cyathis duobus bibitus sine mora sanat.

3   Itemque asparagi semen et cymini pari pondere tritum et ex vino vel aqua calida potui datum emendat. apii itidem radicis sucus ad cyathos duos ex vini cyathis tribus potui datus prodest.

4   Holusatri item radix in vino coquitur et ad cyathos duos potui datur. radix similiter asparagi trita et in vino potui data lumborum dolori medetur.

5   Item cataplasma ad idem. nasturcium cum polenta teritur calidumque imponitur. itemque ferulae viridis folia trita et in vino mixta et imposita mirifice sanant.

6   Lana sucida in oleo. pice liquida, sulphure vivo, nitro Attico fervefactis intincta quam fieri potest calidissima bis in die imponitur.

7   Item pil<ul>arum cupressi viridis sextarios tres in aquae sextariis tribus in olla nova decoques. ut sicut cera mollescat, et sublatis granis quae intus sunt atque proiectis ipsos teres diligenter et ut cataplasma panno induces lumbisque impones ac desuper fascias ligabis, et hoc per triduum facies ita ut cottidie mutetur. et de praedicto chalastico saepius lumbos confricabis et in balneo cum ipso sudet; sed et cum se collocat, fortius de ipso chalastico loca perungat quaecumque doluerint.

8   Item sulphur vivum imponitur cum adipe.

4   Vessels made of ivy ought to be used always for a potion. Fresh spleen of livestock is stretched over the pain, while he who will cure the patient states that he himself cures the spleen; it is then enclosed with plaster in the wall of the bedroom and is sealed thrice nine times, and they will say the same thing.

5   If a dog's spleen is removed when it is living and given to the patient in food, it frees the spleen from disease. A two-day-old puppy's spleen is given to an unwitting patient in food with vinegar.

6   Likewise, a hedgehog's spleen is beneficial. Snails' ash with added linseed, nettle's seed, and honey is applied until it is completely cured.

7   A living green lizard is hung in a pot in front of the bedroom so that he touches it with this hand when going back and forth. Wild boar's or pig's bile drunk or deer horn's ash drunk with vinegar allays the spleen.

8   A very old horse's tongue is drunk in wine. Fresh-baked or well-boiled ox spleen in food is a fast-acting remedy. Heads of garlic, 20, pounded with a *sextarius* of vinegar is applied.

9   Likewise, an applied kid's spleen is beneficial. Washed violet's roots are smeared on with vinegar. Two *oboli* of tree fungus with honeyed vinegar drunk for 21 days reduces the spleen.

14 For lower back pain

1   One *cyathus* of black berries' juice given as a draught with two *cyathi* of honeyed wine cures paining loins. Likewise, drinking two *denarii* of elecampane's leaves or powdered root in one *cyathus* of wine improves them.

2   Likewise, 4 *denarii* of parsnip's root or seed decocted in mead and given as a draught improve complaints of the loins and kidneys. Likewise, chive's juice, about two *cyathi*, drunk in two *cyathi* of wine heals without delay.

3   Likewise, ground asparagus' seed with an equal weight of cumin given as a draught in wine or hot water improves it. Likewise, the juice of *apium*'s root, about two *cyathi*, given as a draught in three *cyathi* of wine is beneficial.

4   Likewise, the root of alexanders is cooked in wine and about two *cyathi* are given as a draught. Similarly, ground asparagus' root given as a draught in wine cures pain in the lower back.

5   Likewise, a poultice of the same. Cress bruised with *polenta* is applied hot. Likewise, ground green giant fennel's leaves mixed with wine and applied cure marvellously.

6   Greasy wool dipped in boiled oil, liquid pitch, native sulphur, and Attic soda is applied as hot as possible twice a day.

7   Likewise, you will decoct in the same way that wax is made soft: three *sextarii* of green cones from a cypress in three *sextarii* of water in a new pot, and when the inner seeds which are removed and thrown away, you will carefully grind them and spread the poultice onto a cloth, and you will apply it to the lower back and bind bandages over it, and you do this for three days so it is changed daily. You will frequently massage the lower back with the aforementioned emollient and he should sweat himself in the bath; but indeed when he lays himself down, he should more vigorously rub whatever places hurt with that emollient.

8   Likewise, native sulphur is applied with grease.

15 *sedis vitiis*

1   Medicamentum ad anum, ad rhagadia, ad condylomata, ad tumores et ad inflationes: ammoniaci denarii VI, †lituematis† denarii VI, turis denarii VI, gallae Asianae denarii VI, croci denarii III, cerae denarii VI, terebintinae denarii III, olei ros<ac>ei denarii VI, quae terenda sunt.

2   sicca teris cum modico vino, ceram et terebintinam solvis cum rosaceo et misces pulveri, quem trivisti cum vino, et teris simul omnia, et cum opus fuerit, uteris.

3   Item ad condylomata quae in ano nascuntur: hyssopum tritum cum rosaceo commisces et teris atque uteris. item marrubii conbusti cinerem aspergito.

4   item folia rubi in quo mora nascuntur cum cera et cum oleo rosaceo sanant.

5   item adeps anserinus cum cerussa et rosaceo et cera Punica inponitur.

16 *coli dolori*

1   Ad coli dolorem pullorum ventriculos interiores purgabis et combures teresque cum pipere et ex aqua rutae dabis bibere. item tria grana alii infundis in aliquantulum aquae; dehinc levas et cum condito ea gluttis.

2   (Sunt occulti interaneorum morbi, de quibus mirum proditur. si catuli priusquam videant adplicentur triduo stomacho maxime ac pectori et ex ore aegri suctum lactis accipiant, transire vim morbi, postremo exanimari dissectisque palam fieri aegri causas;) defunctos obrui oportet.

3   Vespertilionis sanguine ventre contacto in totum annum caventur vitia interaneorum. cornus cervini teneri cinis cum cochleis Africanis cum testa sua tusis mixtus datur in potione vini.

4   facit optime ad colum potio cuius compositionem tradidimus in praecordiorum curatione subiectam operi. hederae et gladioli sucus pari mensura cum passo calefactus potui datur.

17 *condilomatis*

1   Oleum vetus, picem, pollinem decoquere oportet et quam calidissimum imponere. folia rubi in quo mora nascuntur cum cera et rosaceo sanant. radices eiusdem rubi decoquuntur ex vino ad tertias eoque vino foventur condylomata et omnia vitia sedis.

2   araneus dempto capite pedibusque et ita infricatus optime sanat condylomata. adeps anserinus cum cerussa et rosaceo et cera Pontica imponitur. adeps cygni et hoc et haemorroidas sedat.

15   *For complaints of the seat*

1   A medicament for the anus, cracks, *condylomata*, swellings, and flatulence: 6 *denarii* of *Ammoniacum* gum, 6 *denarii* of haematite, 6 *denarii* of frankincense, 6 *denarii* of Asian oak-gall, 3 *denarii* of saffron, 6 *denarii* of wax, 3 *denarii* of turpentine resin, and 6 *denarii* of rose oil which ought to be ground.

2   You grind the dry material with a little wine; you dissolve the wax and turpentine resin with the rose oil, and you mix in the powder which you ground with wine, and grind it all together, and you use it when it is needed.

3   Likewise, for *condylomata* which are formed on the anus: you mix and grind ground hyssop with rose oil and use it. Likewise, sprinkle burnt horehound's ash.

4   Likewise, the leaves of the bramble on which berries grow heal with wax and rose oil.

5   Likewise, goose grease is applied with white lead, rose oil, and Punic wax.

16   *For colon pain*

1   For colon pain you will cleanse pullets' gizzards, and you will burn and grind them with pepper, and give them to drink with water of rue. Likewise, you moisten three garlic seeds in a little water; then you smooth them and swallow them with spiced wine.

2   (There are hidden diseases of the intestines about which something strange is recorded. If puppies before they can see are applied for three days, especially to the stomach and chest, and they receive milk suckled from the mouth of the patient, the power of the disease transfers; finally they are killed, and having been dissected, the causes of the disease are made clear.) The dead ought to be buried.

3   They are protected for a whole year from complaints of the intestines by the belly having been touched with bat's blood. The ash of a young deer's horn mixed with African snails crushed with their shells is given in a draught of wine.

4   The potion whose composition we have recorded, placed under the treatment of *praecordia* in the work, acts best for the colon. Hot ivy and sword-lily juice is given in equal measure with raisin wine in a draught.

17   *For* condylomata

1   One ought to decoct old oil, pitch, and flour and apply it as hot as possible. Leaves of the bramble on which berries grow heal with wax and rose oil. The same bramble's roots are decocted in wine to one-third, and *condylomata* and all complaints of the seat are fomented with that wine.

2   A spider, with its head and feet removed, and thus rubbed in, best heals *condylomata*. Goose grease is applied with white lead, rose oil, and Pontic wax. Swan's grease soothes this and haemorrhoids.

18 *vesicae dolori et calculo*

1 Amyli semuncia conteritur et ovum; eiusdem ovi putamen ter impletur passo, idque <a> balneo subfervefactum datur adversum dolorem.

2 cicer arietinum in aqua discoquitur cum sale et ex aqua ea bibuntur bini cyathi per triduum in difficultate urinae: sic et calculi pelluntur. cariotae tritae dolori imponuntur.

3 adversus urinae difficultatem millefolium tritum ex aceto bibitur. murino fimo dolorem inlinire prodest. vermes terreni contriti bibuntur ex vino aut passo.

4 ad calculos comminuendos pellendosque cochleae inanes conteruntur combustae. earum cinis in potione calculos pellit. lapilli qui in gallinaceorum vesica aut in palumborum <ventriculo> inveniuntur contriti potioni insparguntur.

5 fimus palumborum in sorbitione ex faba fressa bibitur. turturum fimus in mulso decoctus imponitur.

6 cicadas tostatas in patella in vesicae dolore utile est bibere. contra omnes vesicae difficultates cinis plumarum palumborum ferorum ex aceto mulso bibitur. de nido hirundinis glebulae luti dilutae ex aqua calida bibuntur.

7 turdorum fimus ex mulso decoctus imponitur. convenit turdos esse cum bacis myrteis. aqua in qua decocti sunt pedes agnorum <potui datur>.

8 scorpio marinus in vino necatus vesicae vitia sanat et calculos pellit: ipse autem editur, vinum bibitur. lapillus qui invenitur in scorpionis marini cauda utiliter potatur.

9 inveniuntur in bacchi piscis capite quasi lapilli: hi poti ex aqua calculosis praeclare medentur. echini cum spinis suis tunduntur et singuli ex hemina vini bibuntur. difficultatibus urinae sucinum potum alligatumque prodest.

10 plantaginis vel folia vel radices potae ex passo prosunt. vesica apri in cibo elixa sumitur. leporis renes inveterati in vino poti calculos pellunt. ungulae equi cinis ex vino vel aqua bibitur.

19 *incontinentiae urinae*

1 Verrini genitalis cinerem potare ex vino dulci oportet, in canis cubile urinam facere et haec verba dicere, ne ipse urinam faciat ut canis in suo cubili.

2 ungulae apri vel suis cinis potioni inspargitur. leporis cerebrum in vino bibitur, et eiusdem testiculi tosti eduntur.

3 anserum trium linguae assae in cibo sumuntur. cochleae Africanae cum carne sua comburuntur cinisque earum ex vino bibitur.

18 *For bladder pain and stones*

1 Half an *uncia* of starch and an egg; the shell of the same egg is filled three times with raisin wine, and warmed from below, and is given after a bath for pain.

2 Ram's-head chickpeas are decocted with salt in water and two *cyathi* of that water is drunk at a time for three days for difficult urination, and thus stones are expelled. Ground dates are applied to the pain.

3 Ground *millefolium* is drunk in vinegar for difficult urination. It is useful to smear the pain with mouse dung. Ground earthworms are drunk with wine or raisin wine.

4 Burnt, emptied snails are crushed for the breaking and expelling of stones. Ash of those in a potion expels stones. Pebbles which are found in the bladder of chickens or the gizzard of wood-pigeons ground up are sprinkled into a potion.

5 Wood-pigeons' dung is drunk in a broth of crushed beans. Turtledoves' dung decocted in honeyed wine is applied.

6 It is useful to drink cicadas roasted in a dish for bladder pain. Ash of wood-pigeons' feathers is drunk with honeyed vinegar against all difficulties of the bladder. Little clods of mud from a swallow's nest diluted in hot water are drunk.

7 Decocted in honeyed wine, thrushes' dung is applied. It is appropriate to eat thrushes with myrtle berries. The water in which lamb's feet were decocted is given in a drink.

8 A sea-scorpion killed in wine cures all complaints of the bladder and expels stones. While it is eaten, the wine is drunk. The little stone which is found in the sea-scorpion's tail is usefully drunk.

9 Quasi-pebbles are found in the head of a *bacchus* fish: these, drunk in water, cure bladder stone sufferers splendidly. Sea-urchins are pounded, with their spines, and are each drunk with a *hemina* of wine. Amber, drunk or tied on, is useful for difficult urination.

10 Either plantain's leaves or roots are useful drunk in raisin wine. Boiled wild boar's bladder is taken in food. Dried hare's kidneys drunk in wine expel stones. Ash of a horse's hoof is drunk in wine or water.

19 *For urinary incontinence*

1 One ought to drink ash of boar genitalia in sweet wine, and urinate in a dog's bed and to speak these words: that he should not make urine like a dog in his own bed.

2 Ash of a wild boar's or pig's hoof is sprinkled into a draught. A hare's brain is drunk in wine, and the roasted testicles of the same are eaten.

3 Three baked goose tongues are taken in food. African snails are burnt with their flesh and the ash of these is drunk in wine.

20 *verendorum vitiis*

1   Si formicatio sit aut verrucae, arietini pulmonis sanies inlinitur. ceteris vitiis arietinorum vellerum cinis ex aqua, sevum ex omento pecudis praecipue ab renibus admixto pumicis cinere et sale imponitur, lana sucida ex aqua frigida.

2   caro pecudis combusta trita ex aqua frigida. mularum ungulae cinis, dentium caballinorum tunsorum farina inspargitur. ulceribus imponitur cum melle oesypum et plumbi scobis.

3   muricum vel purpurarum cum suis testis et carne combustarum cinis cum melle. carbunculos eorum salsamenta cum melle cocta restringunt singulariter.

4   cerebrum apri vel suis. sanat ea quae serpunt fel bubulum: cum alumine Aegyptio ac myrrha ad crassitudinem mellis subactum inlinitur. insuper beta cocta ex vino trita imponitur.

21 *testiculis et ramicibus*

1   Holus cum faba cocta aequis partibus dolori apponitur. bulbi triti ex vino mulso inliniti medentur.

2   rutam cum teneris lauri ramis contritam tumori imponunt, cyminum tostum contritum cum cera et melle <aut> rosaceo, farina<m> lini seminis cum resina et myrrha.

3   contra dolorem faba in vino cocta et contrita <adhibetur>. inflammationi beta ex aqua imponitur aut melle. ad idem faex vini [aut faba ex vino] inlinitur.

4   cupressi folia cum polenta trita ramici prosunt. pilulae de cupresso tenerae tritae cum axungia et lomento imponuntur. sucus de pilulis cupressi cum fico arida prius ademptis granis imponitur.

5   farina feniculi in hydromelle decocta addita axungia facit ad omnia. si decidit alter ex testibus, spuma cochlearum inlinitur.

6   taetris ulceribus ibi manantibus auxiliatur capitis canini recentis cinis, senectus anguium trita ex aceto. hydroceli<ci>s stelliones demptis pedibus et interaneis et capite inassati in cibo dantur.

7   tumores testium marina aqua utiliter foventur. si et dolor sit et tumor, pusca calida in spongia imponitur.

22 *inguinibus*

1   Negantur inguina intumescere eius qui habeat secum surculum ex myrto nec ferro nec terra tactum. cochleae minutae tritae ex melle inlinuntur.

2   inguina priusquam ex ulcere intumescant, in licio facere novem nodos oportet et ad singulos nominare singulas mulieres viduas, tum licium alligare ad talum vel cruri vel infra genu.

20 For complaints of the privates

1   If there are *formicatio* or warts, sanies of a ram's lung is smeared on. For other complaints the ash of ram fleeces with water, tallow of livestock from the caul, especially from the kidneys, mixed with pumice's ash and salt, or greasy wool in cold water, is applied.
2   Burnt and ground flesh of livestock with cold water. Ash of a hoof from molly-mules or the dust of crushed horses' teeth is sprinkled. For sores, wool grease and lead filings are applied with honey.
3   Ash of murex or purple-fish burnt with their shells and flesh with honey. Fish-pickles cooked with honey check *carbunculi* of these remarkably.
4   Wild boar's or pig's brain. Ox bile heals those sores which creep: it is applied, kneaded with Egyptian alum and myrrh to the consistency of honey. Moreover, beet cooked in wine and ground is applied.

21 For testicles and hernias

1   Cabbage with an equal amount of cooked beans is applied for pain. Ground bulbs smeared on with honeyed wine heal.
2   They apply to swelling ground rue with a laurel's tender twigs, roasted and ground cumin with wax and honey or rose oil, or linseed meal with resin and myrrh.
3   Beans cooked in wine and ground are used against pain. Beet with water or honey is applied to inflammation. Wine lees are smeared on for the same.
4   Cypress leaves with ground *polenta* are beneficial for a hernia. Ground tender cones from a cypress tree are applied with axle-grease and *lomentum*. The juice from the cones of the cypress is applied with a dried fig with seeds previously removed.
5   Fennel meal decocted in *hydromel* with added axle-grease is effective for everything. If one of the testicles drops, it is smeared with snails' mucus.
6   Fresh ash of a dog's head or the slough of snakes in vinegar helps foul weeping sores here. Roasted *stelliones* with feet, intestines, and head removed are given in food to sufferers of *hydrocele*.
7   Swellings of the testicles are usefully fomented with sea water. And if there is pain and swelling, hot *posca* is applied in a sponge.

22 For groins

1   Groins are said to not swell if one has with him a myrtle shoot touched by neither iron nor earth. Tiny, ground-up snails are smeared on with honey.
2   Before the groins swell because of a sore, one ought to make nine knots in a thread, and name an individual widowed woman at each knot; then tie the thread to the ankle or leg or below the knee.

3   si ab equitatu femina vexata sint, spuma equi ex ore feminibus inlinitur. inguinibus imponitur fimus suillus sub testa calefactus tritusque cum oleo.

4   myrtea virga quae ferro tacta non est in dolore inguinum circumligatur. absinthium habere in ventrali prodest. pollex eius pedis a quo inguen est proximo digito alligatus tumorem sedat.

23   *ulceribus in crure vel in tibiis*

1   Adeps ursinus admixta rubrica imponitur. quae serpunt curantur felle aprino cum resina et cerussa.

2   maxillarum apri vel suis cinere insparguntur.

3   fimus caprinus ex aceto subactus et subfervefactus imponitur. omnia in his locis ulcera purgantur, complentur, persanantur butyro ac medulla cervina, item felle taurino cum cyprino oleo aut irino.

[cruribus vel talis si tument vel dolent]

24   *talorum dolori et tumori*

1   Muscus ex oleo tritus imponitur. limus aquaticus ex oleo subactus mirifice prodest. fimus caprinus decoctus ex aceto et subactus cum melle.

25   *pernionibus et vitiis pedum*

1   Pulmo marinus imponitur. cancri marini cinis ex oleo imponitur. utiliter aqua foventur in qua ervum decoctum est.

2   ficus aridae decoctae cum cera liquida subactae ambustis, pernionibus impo-nuntur, ulceribus sevum pecudum cum alumine.

3   si pura sint ulcera, <cera> sanantur. fimi murini cinis ex oleo vetere imponitur. vermium terrenorum cinis ex oleo vetere imponitur.

4   cochlearum quae nudae inveniuntur vivarum combustarum cinere omnia vulnera pedum sanantur. fimi gallinaceorum aut columbarum cinis ex oleo exulcerationibus medetur.

5   attritus calciamentorum emendat veteris soli cinis ex oleo, aeque caprini cornus cinis ex oleo.

6   agninus pulmo vel arietinus imponitur. dentis caballini contusi farina sub-luviem emendat. lacertae viridis sanguis subtritos pedes inlinitus sanat. tegumenti testudinis cinis ex vino et oleo temperatus medetur. adeps ursinus addito alumine omnes rimas sarcit.

3   If thighs were tormented because of riding, the foam from a horse's mouth is smeared on the thighs. Swine dung warmed under a pot and ground with oil is applied to groins.

4   A myrtle twig which is untouched by iron is bound around on pain of the groins. It is beneficial to have wormwood in a belly-band. The big toe of the foot on the side the groin is swelling tied to the next digit allays swelling.

23   For ulcers on the shin or shanks

1   Bear grease mixed with red ochre is applied. Those which creep are cured by wild boar bile with resin and white lead.

2   They are sprinkled with the ash of wild boars or pig's jaw-bones.

3   Goat dung, kneaded with vinegar and warmed from below, is applied. All ulcers in these places are cleansed, filled, and fully healed by butter and also deer marrow, likewise by bull bile with Cyprian or iris oil.

24   For pain and swelling of the ankles

1   Ground moss is applied with oil. Watery muck worked with oil is wonderfully useful. Goat dung decocted in vinegar and kneaded with honey.

25   For chilblains and feet complaints

1   Sea-lung is applied. Marine crab's ash is applied with oil. They are usefully fomented with water in which bitter vetches were decocted.

2   Decocted dried figs kneaded with liquid wax are applied to burns and chilblains; livestock's tallow with alum to *ulcera*.

3   If *ulcera* are clean, they are healed by wax. Mouse dung's ash is applied with old oil. Earthworms' ash is applied with old oil.

4   All wounds of the feet are healed by ash of snails which are found naked and burnt alive. Ash of chickens' or pigeons' dung with oil heals ulcerations.

5   Ash of an old shoe sole in oil improves chafing from shoes; equally ash of goat horn in oil.

6   Lamb or ram lung is applied. A horse tooth crushed to powder improves foot-rot. Green lizard's blood smeared on heals chafing under the feet. The ash of a tortoise's shell combined with wine and oil heals. Bear grease with added alum restores all cracks.

26   *clavis et callis*

1   Plerumque pedibus innascuntur clavi aut calli, praecipue tamen in digitis et in manibus, quibusdam vero et in aliis corporis partibus. adversus quos monstrantur remedia talia.

2   Urina muli mulaeve cum suo luto inlinita tollit. fimus ovium imponitur.

3   iecur lacertae viridis vel sanguis impositus in flocco medetur. vermes terreni ex oleo. fimus columbinus decoctus ex aceto in modum malagmatis subactus imponitur.

4   fimus apri vel suis recens impositus et post diem tertium solutus prodest. faba in qua laser servatur in aceto missa et tumefacta et ita alligata.

5   si in facie nascantur, etiam lomenti assidua fricatione tolluntur [ex oleo]. pollinem ex oleo temperant et adiciunt: extrahit enim.

6   idem facit et hammoniacum. salicis ramorum primorum cortices exuruntur earumque cinis ex aqua impositus tollit.

7   utuntur et sevo bubulo cum turis polline. urina canis cum suo luto imponitur.

27   *podagrae dolori*

1   Muscus qui in aqua nascitur tritus impositus prodest. farina frumenti cocta ex aceto imponitur. utiliter dolor perungetur <oleo> in quo decocta sunt ranarum intestina.

2   ranae rubetae cinis cum adipe vetere. in palustribus lens nascitur quaedam in aqua non profluente, refrigeratoria sine comparatione: haec imponitur vel per se contrita vel cum polenta.

3   adipe viperino pedes perunguntur. sanguine milvi pedes perunguntur. hibisci radices coctas cum axungia misces et cataplasma pedibus ponis.

4   malvae erraticae coctae: pisas cum sale et pedibus ponis. lenticulam coquis, teris adiectis mellis cochlearibus tribus et pedibus imponis.

5   urtica trita cum columbarum sanguine apponitur. adipe vituli marini pedes perunguntur, cuius et pellibus calceari expedit. ranae aquaticae discerptae subinde recentes imponuntur.

6   lenit et plantago cum axungia. limus aquaticus cum oleo subactus mire prodest. ursino adipe, taurino sevo, cerae pari pondere decoctis utuntur.

7   bubulum fimum cum aceti faece magnificant. fimi caprini cinis cum axungia vetere prodest.

8   Cum autem pluribus malagmatibus utantur hi qui hoc malo laborant prout illa apud unumquemque commendat monstrantis auctoritas, ponam compositionem de qua nemo qui usus est questus est:

26   *For corns and calluses*

1   Generally, corns and calluses arise on the feet, but especially on digits and on hands, and indeed on certain other parts of the body. Against these the following remedies are advised.

2   A john- or molly-mule's urine smeared on with its own mud removes it. Sheep's dung is applied.

3   A green lizard's liver or blood applied on a tuft of wool is a remedy. Earthworms with oil. Pigeon dung, decocted in vinegar and kneaded in the manner of a poultice, is applied.

4   Fresh wild boar's or pig's dung applied and removed after the third day is useful. Beans in which *laser* is stored was thrown in vinegar and made to swell and thus bound on.

5   If they arise on the face, they are actually removed by an application of *lomentum* rubbed on. They mix flour with oil and apply it: it, in fact, removes it.

6   Likewise, *Ammoniacum* gum works. The bark of the tips of willow branches is burned and the ash of these applied with water removes it.

7   They use ox tallow with frankincense dust. Dog's urine is applied with its own mud.

27   *For* podagra

1   Moss which grows in water, ground and applied, is useful. Grain meal cooked in vinegar is applied. Pain will be usefully anointed with oil in which frogs' intestines were decocted.

2   Frog's or toad's ash with old grease. In marshes a certain lentil grows in stagnant water: cooling without comparison, this is applied crushed either by itself or with *polenta*.

3   Feet are anointed with viper grease. Feet are well anointed with kite's blood. You mix cooked marshmallow's roots with axle-grease and apply the plaster to the feet.

4   Cooked wild mallows: you may pound them with salt and apply them to the feet. You cook little lentils, grind them with three *cochlearia* of honey, and apply them to the feet.

5   Ground nettle is applied with pigeons' blood. Feet are anointed with seal's grease, and it is helpful to be shod with the hides of this. Aquatic frogs torn to pieces are applied fresh immediately.

6   Plantain with axle-grease alleviates it also. Watery muck worked with oil is marvellously beneficial. They use bear grease, bull tallow, and an equal weight of wax decocted.

7   They praise ox dung with vinegar lees. Ash of goat dung with old axle-grease is beneficial.

8   However, while those who are ill from this malady use many cataplasms in accordance with the authority of the advisor who recommends them to each, I will include a composition about which no-one who has used it has complained:

9   picis Bruttiae uncias V et scripulos VII, cerae Ponticae tantundem, resinae frictae tantundem, galbani Ǝ XI, hammoniaci semunciam:

10   omnia haec in cacabo novo componuntur, coquuntur ad unum fervore bono. in mortario autem teruntur haec:

11   euphorbii uncia I, s<t>ypteriae schistes tantundem, turis pollinis scripuli VIIII, opopanacis Ǝ VIIII, fellis taurini Ǝ VIII, salis Hammoniaci Ǝ VI.

12   his suffunduntur aceti acerrimi cyathi III, tum quod in cacabo coctum est mortario adicitur et pistillo permiscetur. cum eo utendum est, alutae inlinitur.

13   si induruit, modice ad ignem calefactum manibus perfricatur et ita mollescit. hoc medicamentum non inquinat, vires in usu non perdit, appositum reservari potest.

14   Sunt et qui potione podagra sint liberati, cuius compositionem subiciam et quemadmodum ea sit utendum. camedriae pondo libra, centauriae pondo unciae III, aristolochiae rotundae pondo unciae III, stoechados pondo unciae III, agarici pondo unciae IIII, cyperi seminis pondo quadrans, aloes pondo unciae III S.

15   haec pondera singularum expendi oportet et trita cribrata permisceri ex mellis Attici libris VI et in vitreum vas recondi.

16   usus huius potionis talis esse debet ut sumatur a ieiunis qui bene concoxerint et per numerum dierum anni, adiecto uno die.

17   si dies continuari non potuerint propter cruditatem aut languorem aliquamque causam, quotquot intermissi fuerint, totidem restituantur.

18   potionis vero mensura erit ut denarii argentei pondus bibatur ex tribus cyathis aquae semel in die.

19   Radix cucumeris erratici ex aceto coquitur et imponitur. mitigatur si secum habeat is qui vexabitur pedem leporis vivo abscisum.

20   Peractis singulorum membrorum malis et eorum remediis quae in proviso solent accidere percurremus eo ordine quo unaquaeque res succurrerit. incipiemus igitur a re podagrae proxima.

9   5 *unciae* and 7 *scripuli* of Bruttian pitch, as much of Pontic wax, and as much of roasted resin, 11 *scripuli* of *galbanum*, and half an *uncia* of *Ammoniacum* gum;

10 all these are put together in a new cooking pot, and they are decocted at a good heat. Now these are ground in a mortar;

11 1 *uncia* of *euphorbea*, as much of split alum, 9 *scripuli* of frankincense dust, 9 *scripuli* of *opopanax*, 8 *scripuli* of bull bile, and 6 *scripuli* of Ammoniac salt.

12 Poured on these are 3 *cyathi* of the sharpest vinegar, and then what was boiled in the cooking pot is added to the mortar and is mixed with the pestle. When this is to be used it is smeared on an adhesive patch.

13 If it hardens, it is warmed quickly near the fire, is rubbed with the hands, and thus becomes soft. This medicament does not stain or loses strength in use, and it can be stored.

14 There are some who are freed from *podagra* by a potion, the composition of which and in what way it ought to be used I will include below. A *libra* in weight of *camedria*, 3 *unciae* in weight of centaury, 3 *unciae* in weight of round *aristolochia*, 3 *unciae* in weight of French lavender, 4 *unciae* of tree fungus, a *quadrans* weight of galingal seed, and 3½ *unciae* weight of aloe.

15 These weights ought to be measured for each, and having been ground and sifted, ought to be mixed together with 6 *librae* of Attic honey and stored in a glass vessel.

16 The use of this potion must be as follows: it is taken by a fasting patient who digests well, and for the number of days in the year with an added day.

17 If the days were unable to be continuous because of indigestion or weakness or any reason, however many days were omitted, that many are made up.

18 However, the dose of the potion should be the weight of a silver *denarius* drunk with three *cyathi* of water once a day.

19 Wild cucumber's root is cooked in vinegar and applied. It is assuaged if he who will be tormented carries with him a hare's foot that was cut off while alive.

20 With the maladies of each part and their remedies completed, we will review those which are accustomed to occur unexpectedly in that order in which it comes to mind. Therefore, we will begin with the thing closest to *podagra*.

Liber III

capitula libri III

Book Three

Chapters of Book Three

– Preface on poisons –

1   *Ad nervos et articulos*

1   Amphisbaena mortua nervorum offensis alligatur. adeps vulturinus cum felle eiusdem perunguitur. iecur eiusdem arefactum et tritum cum axungia [eius] imponitur. senectus serpentium in corio taurino alligatur.

2   Beta ex melle et fico imposita morbis articularibus medetur. folia vitium trita et admixta hordeaceae farinae articularibus morbis imponuntur.

3   acrifolium tritum addito sale et oleo eidem rei prodest. incussos articulos aranei tela commodissime curat. articulis vexatis praesentaneum remedium est sevum pecudis cum cinere mulieris capillorum.

4   Nervorum nodis capitis viperini cinis cum oleo cyprino imponitur. ad idem faciunt terreni vermes triti cum melle, item galbanum per se. stirax inlinitur. fimum caprinum decoctum in aceto contritum cum melle.

5   tremulis utile est esse holera et panem ex aqua a balneo, perungui oleo in quo castoreum est additum. articulorum fracturis cinis ex femoribus pecudum cera admixta medetur.

2   *sanguini ex ulceribus sistendo*

1   Fimus caballinus cum ovorum putaminibus crematur isque cinis <ad>mixto melle spathomele imponitur plagae: <mire sistit>.

2   polypus tusus in pila in modum emplastri adhibetur. cortex vitium et folia arida tusa in farinam sanguinem sistunt et vulnus glutinant.

3   folia persici trita et imposita haemorrhogian sistunt. pilulae platani tusae ex aceto impositae.

4   ferulae cinis. hircini utris vinarii cinis cum pari pondere resinae ex aceto impositus sanguinem sistit et ulcera glutinat. haedinum coagulum ex aceto sanguinem sistit.

3   *recentibus vulneribus et nervis incisis*

1   Vermes terreni triti conglutinant, adeo ut etiam nervos incisos solident die septimo. idem arefacti in sole ex aceto triti vulneribus imponuntur et interposito biduo solvuntur.

2   cochleae exemptae de suis testis crudae tritae mirifice solidant. cochleae cum suis testis tusae cum myrrha et ture pari pondere etiam praecisos nervos sanant.

3   efficaces sunt et bulbi triti per se ad vulnera glutinanda: adiciebat tamen illis Damon medicus muscum qui in aqua gignitur et die quinto solvebat.

4   myrobalanum ut iam diximus genus est cariotae quod os non habet: haec ex vino austeri trita vulnera solidat.

5   et cupressi folia trita ad eundem effectum imponuntur. rubi sive platani vel flos vel mora sine collectionis periculo sanant.

1   *For tendons and joints*

1   A dead *amphisbaena* is tied on for injuries of tendons. Vulture grease is rubbed on with the bile of the same. Dried and ground liver of the same is applied with axle-grease. A snake's slough is tied on in bull hide.
2   Beet applied with honey and fig relieves joint diseases. Ground vines' leaves and added barley meal are applied for joint diseases.
3   Ground holly with added salt and oil is beneficial for the same thing. A spider's web heals struck joints most completely. The tallow of livestock with the ash of a woman's hair is an instantaneous remedy for injured joints.
4   For tendons' nodules, ash of a viper's head is applied with Cyprian oil. Ground earthworms with honey are useful for the same, likewise *galbanum* by itself. Storax is anointed. Goat dung decocted in vinegar and crushed with honey.
5   For those trembling, it is useful to eat vegetables and bread with water after a bath, and to be thoroughly rubbed with oil in which *castoreum* is added. Ash from the thighs of livestock is beneficial for fractures of joints mixed with wax.

2   *For staunching blood from wounds*

1   Horse dung is cremated with egg shells, and that ash is applied to the wound with added honey from a *spathomela*: it staunches marvellously.
2   A cephalopod beaten in a mortar is used like a plaster. Vines' bark and dried leaves beaten into a powder staunch blood and close a wound.
3   Peach's leaves ground and applied staunch a haemorrhage. Plane tree's catkins beaten with vinegar and applied.
4   Ash of giant fennel. Ash of a goat-leather wine-skin with an equal weight of resin applied with vinegar staunches blood and closes wounds. Kid rennet with vinegar staunches blood.

3   *For recent wounds and cut tendons*

1   Ground earthworms join (wounds); in the same manner they even unite cut tendons by the seventh day. The same dried in the sun and ground with vinegar are applied to wounds and are removed after two days.
2   Raw snails removed from their shells and ground, wonderfully reunite. Snails beaten with their shells and with myrrh and an equal amount of frankincense even heal tendons that are cut through.
3   Ground bulbs by themselves are effective for wounds that need to be closed, yet Damon the doctor added to these a moss which is produced in water, and it is removed on the fifth day.
4   We have already said that behen-nut is a type of date which has no stone: these ground in dry wine unite wounds.
5   Also ground cypress leaves are applied for the same effect. The flower or berries of the bramble or plane tree heal without the danger of an abscess.

6 et millefolium tritum vulneribus imponitur. centauriae radix tam efficax est ad plagas glutinandas ut etiam carnes cohaerescant quae cum ea coquuntur.

7 lana sucida infunditur in mel et acetum frigidum et oleum, deinde expressa imponitur. spongia ex aqua caelesti imposita recentia secta non patitur intumescere.

8 et caro vituli recentibus vulneribus arcet tumorem. idem fimum bubulum cum melle praestat.

9 recentes plagas ferro factas gluten taurinum liquefactum atque impositum neque ante diem tertium solutum efficacissime iuvat.

4 *ad ulcera et ad cancer quod noma vocatur*

1 Scio gratius futurum fuisse, si singulis generibus ulcerum nominatim dedissem titulos et remedia. sed cum aliquae res pluribus vitiis prosint, brevitatem secutus genus scripturae elegi quod subiectum est.

2 Vermes qui in ligno nascuntur vocantur cosses; hi triti in panno inlinuntur et ulceri apponuntur. idem combusti cum anethi pari pondere impositi noma<m> quod vocant cancer sistunt.

3 fimo ovium sub testa calefacto et subacto tumores sedantur, fistulae sanantur. noma<m> sistunt cochleae crudae de suo testo eiectae et in linteolo inlitae et appositae.

4 cacoethe emendat ulula avis cocta in oleo et contrita, cui miscetur butyrum ovillum et mel. eadem ratione curantur et cybio vetere, quod ut emplastrum panno inlini debet.

5 vermes ulceribus innati ranarum felle tolluntur. quae serpunt salsamento veteri tuso in modum emplastri curantur. radix peponis contrita ulcera sanat in modum favi concreta, quae ceria vocant.

6 semen raphani ex aqua tritum <et impositum> sistit ulcera quae phagedaenas appellant. porrus capitatus contritus ex melle ulcera purgat.

7 alium cum sulphure et resina fistularum vitia extrahit. vetera ulcera, etiam carcinomata, foveri debent aqua calida in qua cocta sint holera, deinde et ipsa holera trita imponuntur bis in die.

8 sic curantur fistulae et tumores, quos evo<ca>ri quosue tolli opus est. cruda holera trita veteribus ulceribus imponuntur. lini seminis farina in vino decocta prohibet serpere.

9 eadem farina cum melle eruptiones et pituitas emendat. pustulas ulcerum lenticula cocta rumpit. eadem collectiones sedat. eadem contra suppurantia cum polenta decocta imponitur.

10 lenticulae sucus ulceribus et oris et genitalium adhibetur, sed <is> cum rosaceo et cydonio trito. farina ervi serpere ulcera non patitur spathomele imposita.

6 Also, ground *millefolium* is applied to wounds. Centaury root is so effectual for closing wounds that even pieces of meat which are cooked with it cohere.

7 Greasy wool dipped into honey, cold vinegar, and oil, then squeezed, is applied. A sponge applied with rain water does not allow fresh cuts to become swollen.

8 Also calf's flesh prevents swelling in recent wounds. Likewise, ox dung with honey is excellent.

9 Bull glue, liquefied and applied to recent wounds made by iron and not removed before the third day, helps most effectively.

4   *For ulcers and for* cancer *which is called* noma

1 I know that it would have been more welcome if I had given the titles and remedies for all the types of ulcers by name. However, since some materials are beneficial for several conditions, I chose brevity and the following type of composition which is supplied below.

2 Worms which are born in wood are called *cossi*; these, ground, are spread on a cloth and applied to the ulcer. The same burnt with an equal weight of dill and applied, check *cancer* which they call *noma*.

3 Swellings are assuaged and fistulas cured by kneaded sheep's dung warmed under a pot. Raw snails removed from their shells, smeared on a small linen cloth and applied, check *noma*.

4 Screech owl cooked in oil and crushed, to which sheep butter and honey is mixed, improves *cacoëthes*. In the same way they are also healed by old tuna, which ought to be smeared on a cloth as a plaster.

5 Worms born in ulcers are destroyed by frogs' bile. Those which creep are cured by stale, beaten fish-pickle in the manner of a plaster. Crushed *pepon*'s root heals ulcers hardened like honeycomb, which they call *ceria*.

6 Radish's seed, ground and applied in water, checks ulcers which are called *phagedaena*. Headed-leek crushed with honey cleanses ulcers.

7 Garlic with sulphur and resin draws corruption out of fistulas. Old ulcers, even *carcinomata*, ought to be fomented with hot water in which vegetables were cooked, and then the ground vegetables themselves are applied twice in the day.

8 Fistulas and swellings which need to be drawn forth or removed are cured thus: ground raw vegetables are applied to long-standing ulcers. Linseed meal decocted in wine stops creeping.

9 The same meal with honey improves ruptures and mucus. Cooked lentils burst ulcers' pustules. The same assuage abscesses. Against suppurations, the same are applied with decocted *polenta*.

10 Little lentil's juice is applied to ulcers of the mouth and genitals, but that is with rose oil and ground quince. Bitter vetch meal applied with a *spathomela* does not allow ulcers to creep.

11   l<up>ini farina eodem modo imposita siccat. cinis vitium cum axungia vetere fistulas purgat et sanat. folia olivae commanducata et imposita ulceribus manantibus medentur.

12   cauliculi oleastri decocti cum melle impositi carnes quae ab ossibus recedunt comprimunt. contra collectiones folia oleastri ex vino trita imponuntur. his quae purganda sunt oleastri folia ex melle adhibentur.

13   ulcera manantia oleum amigdalinum cum vino expurgat. fici ramorum teneri cauliculi tusi imponuntur cum melle ulceribus quae ceria vocant.

14   carcinoma<ti>, si sine vulnere sit, quam pinguissimam ficum imponere singulare remedium est. nuces iuglandes perveteres commanducatae ulceribus medentur impositae.

15   glans roborea trita cum axungia duritias quas cacoethes vocant et evocat et emendat: melius si sit ilicina. ulceribus quae serpunt et quae in his excrescunt spondilium cum ruta inlinitur.

16   pix Bruttia cum melle ulcera purgat explet sanat. eadem pix cum uva passa et axungia ulceribus putrescentibus medetur. aqua in qua lentiscus decocta est ulcera quae serpunt utiliter foventur.

17   pilulae de platanis tusae emendant. vermes tollunt mala tusa ex melle. hedera ex vino decocta imponitur omnium generi ulcerum. idem praestat et lana sucida ex melle.

18   cinis fimi pecudum addito cinere ex ossibus femorum agnorum et nitrum tusum adhibetur ulceribus quae cicatricem non trahunt. pulmo arietinus carnes excrescentes in ulceribus exaequat.

19   ulcera quae serpunt et quae in his excrescunt cinis capitum menarum coercet. fistulae aperiuntur siccanturque salsamentis cum linteolo inmissis, intraque alterum diem omnem callum auferunt.

20   serpentium ulcerum coercet impetus calx non lota temperata ex rosaceo et aceto atque inlita, mox cera ac rosaceo permixta perducit ad cicatricem. symphitum omnia ulcera celerrime perducit ad cicatricem et sanat.

21   plantaginis sucus infunditur fistulis, et inmittitur isdem fel taurinum cum porri suco pari mensura. carcinomata curantur coagulo leporis cum pari mensura capparis, quod utrumque adsparsum vino teritur una.

22   gangraenis pinna inlinitur fel ursinum. his quae serpunt medetur <asini ungularum cinis>. caseus caprinus siccus ex aceto et melle purgat ulcera. quae serpunt cohibet sevum caprinum cum cera. idem additis [cum] sulphure et pice purgat.

5   *panis quas paniculas nos dicimus*

1   Nasturcium cum pice panas discutit. <maturis aut> maturescentibus imponitur lens ex aceto discocta. ervum cum melle tritum et impositum suppurare prohibet.

2   lupini ex aceto cocti aut minuunt aut maturant. ficum ex vino discoctam et tusam imponunt. viscum et resinam et ceram aequis ponderibus remissam imponunt. galbanum per se prodest.

11   Lupine meal applied in the same way dries. Vines' ash with old axle-grease cleanses and heals fistulas. Chewed and applied, olive's leaves cure weeping ulcers.

12   Wild olive's stems decocted with honey and applied close flesh which withdraws from bones. Against abscesses, ground wild olive's leaves are applied with wine. Wild olive's leaves are applied with honey to these which need to be cleansed.

13   Almond oil with wine cleanses weeping ulcers. Beaten tender stems of fig's boughs are applied with honey to ulcers which they call *ceria*.

14   For *carcinoma*, if it is without a sore, the only remedy is to apply the fattest fig possible. Chewed and applied, very old walnuts cure ulcers.

15   A ground acorn with axle-grease draws forth and improves indurations which they call *cacoëthes*: it is better if it is from a holm-oak. *Spondylium* is smeared with rue on ulcers which creep and the morbid growths that develop in these.

16   Bruttian pitch with honey cleanses, fills, and heals ulcers. The same pitch with a raisin and axle-grease cures putrid ulcers. Ulcers which creep are usefully fomented by water in which mastic was decocted.

17   Beaten catkins from plane trees improve them. Crushed apples with honey destroy worms. Ivy decocted in wine is applied to all types of ulcers. Likewise, greasy wool with honey is excellent.

18   The ash of livestock's dung with added ash from lambs' thighs and beaten soda is employed on ulcers which do not form a scar. Ram lung levels excrescences of the flesh in ulcers.

19   Ash of the heads of *menae* check ulcers which creep and the morbid growths which develop in these. Fistulas are opened and dried by fish-pickles inserted with little linen cloths, and during the second day it removes all hardened skin.

20   Unwashed lime, properly combined with rose oil and vinegar, and applied, checks the onset of creeping ulcers, then mixed with wax and rose oil it brings over a scar. Comfrey quickly brings a scar over and heals all ulcers.

21   Plantain's juice is poured into fistulas, and bull bile with an equal measure of leek's juice is likewise inserted. *Carcinomata* are cured by hare's rennet with an equal measure of caper, both of which are ground together sprinkled with wine.

22   Bear bile is smeared on gangrene with a feather. Ash of an ass' hooves heals those which creep. Dry goat cheese with vinegar and honey cleanses ulcers. Goat tallow with wax checks those which creep. Likewise, with added sulphur and pitch, it cleanses.

5   *For* pani *which we call* paniculae

1   Cress with pitch disperses *pani*. Lentils decocted in vinegar are applied to mature or maturing (*pani*). Ground and applied bitter vetch with honey prevents suppuration.

2   Lupines cooked with vinegar either lessen or mature. They apply a fig decocted in wine and beaten. They apply mistletoe, resin, and melted wax in equal weights. *Galbanum* by itself is beneficial.

3   feniculi farina ex hydromelle decocta addita axungia mitigat dolorem. aperit panas sevum pecudum cum sale tosto. discutit murinus fimus addito turis polline et sandaraca, lacerta divisa viridis imposita, cochleae tusae, cinis inanium cochlearum cera mixtus, fimus columbinus per se vel cum farina hordeacea impositus.

4   echinorum testae contusae ex aqua inlitae. cinis muricum vel purpurarum ex oleo vetere sive incipientes discutit sive concoctas aperit.

5   cancri fluviales triti medentur, salsamenta cocta et imposita. creta Cimolia trita ex aceto cohibet. ursinus sanguis discutit, item taurinus aridus tritus. ungulae equinae cinis cum oleo, bubulus <sanguis> inlinitur; fimum hircinum cum melle decoctum.

6   quidam ad panas utuntur hac compositione: cerae et turis drachmas vicenas, spumae argenti drachmas XL, muricum cineris drachmas X: permiscetur tusum et additur eo olei veteris hemina.

6   strumis [id est scrofae quae nascuntur in gutture]

1   Caprifici corticem intumescentem puer impubes si defracto ramo tollat dentibus et medulla ipsa alligetur ante solis ortum prohibere strumas constat. echinorum testae contusae cum alumine ex oleo vetere et pulte.

2   nasturcium cum lomento contritum superposito folio hederae. marrubium cum adipe. lens in aceto discocta. lupinum ex aceto coctum contritumque.

3   folia fici et ficus inmatura una tusa imponuntur. sucus pilulae cupressi ex fermento. galbanum per se exulceratis strumis imponitur. mustelae sanguis inlinitur. mustela ex vino discocta imponitur.

4   cochleae cum suis testis tusae; ad hoc faciunt optime quae salicibus adhaerent. cinis aspidis cum sevo taurino imponitur.

5   adeps anguis mixtus oleo. anguium cinis ex oleo. esse eos quoque praecipitur, abscisis a capite et a cauda digitis quaternis, aut cinerem crematorum bibere.

6   fimum columbinum imponunt alii mixta farina hordeacea ex aceto acri. talpae cinis ex melle imponitur. iecur talpae quidam inter manus contritum circumlinunt et triduo non abluunt.

7   talpae capita praeciduntur et cum terra a talpis egesta conteruntur et in pastillos rediguntur: qui si servantur in stagnea pyxide utiles ad omnia apostemata sunt.

8   vermes terreni totidem quot sunt strumae alligati cum his pariter arescunt. circumligantur lino quo vipera suspendio occisa est. milipedae imponuntur addita resinae parte quarta: non solum strumas sic curari praecipiunt sed et omnia apostemata.

9   calx viva cum resina liquida vel adipe suillo addito melle strumis utiliter auxiliatur. fel aprinum vel bubulum tepidum inlinitum discutit.

10 ungulae asini vel equi cinis ex aqua et oleo inlinitur. fimum caprinum ex aceto acri decoctum strumis inlinitur. bubulum sevum ex oleo imponitur. ebuli folia conteruntur et mixta cum faece cervisiae super additis foliis eiusdem ebuli in linteolo alliga<n>tur.

3   Fennel meal decocted in *hydromel* with added axle-grease mitigates pain. Livestock's tallow with roasted salt opens *pani*. Mouse dung with added frankincense powder and red arsenic sulphide, a green lizard split and applied, beaten snails, the ash of empty snails mixed with wax, or pigeon dung by itself or applied with barley meal disperse it.

4   Beaten sea-urchins' shells applied with water. Ash of murex or purple-fish with old oil either disperses the incipient or opens the matured (*pani*).

5   Ground riverine crabs or cooked and applied fish-pickles cure it. Cimolian chalk with vinegar checks it. Bear blood disperses it, likewise ground, dried bull blood. Ash of a horse's hoof with oil or ox blood is smeared on; goat dung decocted with honey.

6   Some use this composition: twenty *drachmae* of wax and frankincense, 40 *drachmae* of litharge, 10 *drachmae* of murex's ash; crushed, it is mixed and a *hemina* of old oil is added to this.

6   *For* strumae

1   If a prepubescent boy removes the swollen bark of the wild fig from a broken branch with his teeth and the inside itself is attached before the rising of the sun, it is known to prevent *strumae*. Beaten sea-urchins' shells with alum in old oil and porridge.

2   Pounded cress with *lomentum* and with an ivy leaf placed over. Horehound with grease. Lentils decocted in vinegar. Lupines cooked in vinegar and pounded.

3   Fig's leaves and unripe figs beaten together are applied. The juice of cypress' cones with leaven. *Galbanum* is applied to ulcerated *strumae* by itself. Weasel's blood is smeared on. Weasel decocted in wine is applied.

4   Pounded snails with their own shells; they best use those which adhere to willows for this. Asp's ash is applied with bull tallow.

5   Snake's grease mixed with oil. Snakes' ash with oil. It is also advised to eat these, with four fingers cut off from the head and tail, or to drink its burnt ash.

6   Others apply pigeon dung with barley meal mixed with sharp vinegar. Mole's ash applied with honey. Some spread around a mole's liver, having been crushed between the hands, and do not wash it for three days.

7   Heads of moles are cut off and pounded with earth expelled by moles, and are made into pastilles: if these are stored in a *stagneum* box, they are useful for all abscesses.

8   As many earthworms tied on as there are *strumae* dry up together with these. They tie around a thread with which a viper was killed by hanging. Millipedes are applied with an added fourth part of resin: not only do they advise that *strumae* are cured thus, but all abscesses are, too.

9   Quicklime with liquid resin or pork grease with added honey is effectively beneficial for *strumae*. Warm wild boar or ox bile smeared on disperses it.

10 Ash of a horse's or ass' hoof smeared on in water or oil. Decocted goat dung in sharp vinegar is smeared on *strumae*. Ox tallow is applied in oil. Dwarf elder's leaves are pounded and mixed with beer's dregs; they are tied on in a little linen cloth with additional leaves of the same dwarf elder over the top.

7   *furunculis*

1   Fimi gallinacei id quod rufum est recens inlinitur ex aceto. ventriculus ciconiae ex vino decoctus inlinitur. muscae impari numero infricantur digito minimo.

2   sordes ex auriculis pecudis inlinuntur. sevum arietis cum farina pumicis et salis aequis portionibus. nitrum cum resina mixtum extrahit.

3   nasturcium tusum cum fermento concoquit[ur]. novem granis hordei si quis furunculum circumducat singulis manu sinistra et omnia in ignem coiciat, confestim sanat.

4   ficus siccae decoctae ex vino et tritae imponuntur.

5   galbanum per se. sevum bubulum cum sale imponitur, aut si dolor sit sine sale liquatur cum oleo. simili modo facit caprinum sevum. limacis cinis aspersus purgat.

8   *carbunculis*

1   Fimus columbinus cum lini semine ex aceto mulso imponitur. mullorum salsorum cinis prodest.

2   ruta ex aceto trita. ervi farina ex vino imposita carbunculum rumpit. idem praestant et lupini triti. fimus pecudis incipientibus carbunculis imponitur.

3   ficus siccae in vino decoctae aut tritae et confricatae extrahunt. nuces iuglandes perveteres tritae impositae. pix Bruttia cum uva passa demptis nucleis addita axungia purgat.

4   herba sabina quae habet folia similia cupressi cum melle inlinitur. cerebrum suis feminae coctum et tostum imponitur.

9   *ambustis*

1   Fimus ovium cum cera ambustis imponitur. canini capitis cinis. cochlearum cinis ex oleo inlinitur. adeps verrinus. fimi columbini cinis ex oleo inlinitur.

2   garum infunditur nec nominatur. cancrorum marinorum vel fluvialium cinis ex oleo.

3   hordei cinis inspargitur. lens ex aqua semicocta imponitur: procedente curatione lens cruda teritur et cribratur eiectoque furfure coquitur et sic imponitur, novissime eo mel additur.

4   vitis cortex comburitur et cinis eius ex oleo inlinitur: et pilos reddit. prodest ambustis inlita faex vini sive sapae. olivarum carnes teruntur et imponuntur.

5   nigra oliva continuo si imponatur commanducata pustulas gigni prohibet. myrti foliorum cinis spargitur. flos hederae cum cera utiliter imponitur. hordeum tostum tritum ex albis ovorum addito adipe suillo mirifice prodest.

6   <ambusta> aqua ovis si statim occupentur ut elevantur, inde pustulae non sequuntur. ova in aqua decoquuntur, deinde in prunas coiciuntur donec putamina eorum comburantur, tunc lutea eorum ex rosaceo inlinuntur.

7   *For boils*

1   That which is red and fresh of chicken dung is smeared on with vinegar. Stork's gizzard decocted in vinegar is smeared on. An odd number of flies are rubbed in with the little finger.
2   Filth from the ears of livestock is smeared on. Ram's tallow with equal portions of pumice's dust and salt. Soda mixed with resin draws it out.
3   Beaten cress with leaven matures it. If one draws around the boil with nine grains of barley, one at a time with the left hand, and throws them all into a fire, it heals immediately.
4   Dried figs, decocted in wine and ground, are applied.
5   *Galbanum* by itself. Ox tallow is applied with salt, or if it is sore it is liquefied with oil without salt. One uses goat tallow in a similar way. Sprinkled slug's ash cleanses.

8   *For* carbunculi

1   Pigeon dung is applied with linseed in honeyed vinegar. Pickled mullet's ash is beneficial.
2   Ground rue with vinegar. Bitter vetch meal applied with wine bursts *carbunculi*. Likewise, ground lupines are also excellent. Livestock's dung is applied to incipient *carbunculi*.
3   Dried figs, decocted in wine or ground and rubbed, draw out. Applied very old ground walnuts. Bruttian pitch with deseeded raisin and axle-grease cleanses.
4   The herb savin which has leaves similar to the cypress is smeared on with honey. A sow's brain, boiled and roasted, is applied.

9   *For burns*

1   Sheep's dung with wax is applied to burns. Ash of a dog's head. Snails' ash is smeared on in oil. Boar grease. Pigeon dung's ash is smeared on with oil.
2   *Garum* is poured on and not mentioned. Marine or riverine crabs' ash in oil.
3   Barley's ash is sprinkled on. Lentils par-boiled in water are applied; as the healing progresses, raw lentils are ground and sifted, with the bran cast out, and are boiled and applied, and lastly honey is added to this.
4   Vine's bark is cremated and the ash of that is smeared on with oil; it restores hair. Smeared on wine lees or must are beneficial for burns. The flesh of olives is ground and applied.
5   If chewed, black olives are immediately applied and prevent blisters from forming. Ash of myrtle's leaves is sprinkled on. Ivy's flower is usefully applied with wax. Toasted and ground barley with added egg whites and pork grease is wonderfully beneficial.
6   If scalds are immediately spread over with eggs when raised, then blisters do not follow. Eggs are boiled in water, then are thrust among coals until their shells are burnt, and then their yolks are smeared on with rose oil.

7   oleum addito sale pustulas reprimit. eis quae ferventi aqua exusta sunt ranarum cinis aspersus adeo prodest ut etiam pilos reddat.

8   efficax est fibrinarum [ferarum] cinis pellium. magnes lapis crematus tritusque inspargitur. fimus leporis et caprae inlinitur aequis ponderibus.

9   gluten taurinum remissum sicuti solet a fabris remitti sine cicatrice sanat: optimum est ex auribus taurorum et genitalibus sordes applicare.

10   *canis rabiosi morsui*

1   Salsamentum imponitur. rutae suci pondus denariorum XV ex vino bibitur. plagae imponuntur rutae folia trita cum sale et melle vel cum pice et aceto.

2   folia nigrae ficus trita ex aceto medentur. rosae silvestris radix pota efficacissime abigit aquae pavorem. plantago pota et imposita facit et adversus canis rabiosi morsum et adversus omnium bestiarum.

3   lana sucida indita morsum sanat post diem septimum soluta. cinis capitis canini inlitus abigit aquae pavorem, aut caput canis devoratum.

4   vermis de cadavere canis adalligatus pavorem tollit. est limus sub lingua canis rabiosi; qui datus in potione hydrophoviam prohibet.

5   omnia praecedit ut iecur eiusdem canis qui momorderit devoretur, si fieri potest crudum, si minus quoquo modo coctum. crista gallinacei contrita imponitur plagae.

6   anseris adeps cum melle. salliuntur a quibusdam canes qui rabiosi fuerint ut in remedium carnes eorum edantur.

7   lactens catulus eiusdem sexus qui momorderit in aqua necatur eiusdemque iecur crudum devoratur.

8   fimus gallinacei rufus ex aceto morsui imponitur. glebulae ex hirundinis nido solutae ex aceto inlinuntur. catulus lactens priusquam videat aperitur eiusdemque coagulum bibitur, ita ut is qui bibit in defluenti aqua stet usque ad umbilicum.

9   pavescentibus aquam totam faciem perungunt adipe vituli marini. aquam expavescentes usta plaga ferro continuo sanantur.

11   *morsui canis non rabiosi*

1   Nitrum et axungia et resina aequis portionibus ex aceto imponuntur. allex cruda in linteolis concerptis. alium cum melle tritum. menta cum melle contrita.

2   marrubium tritum cum axungia vetere. urtica trita addito sale.

3   cinis vitium cum oleo. acetum calidum in spongia. ramorum fici cauliculi teneri triti. nuclei amigdalini cum melle triti. nucum iuglandium carnes cum cepa et sale et melle contritae.

4   easdem carnes nucum ab ieiuno homine commanducatas imponi iubent.

5   spongiae minutae conciduntur et imponuntur infusae vel ex aceto vel ex aqua vel ex melle. faex aceti cum melanthio plagae imponitur.

7   Oil with added salt prevents blisters. For those who were burned by boiling water, sprinkled frog's ash is so beneficial that it even restores hair.

8   Ash of beaver pelts is effective. Burnt and ground magnet is sprinkled. Hare's and nanny-goat's dung is smeared on in equal amounts.

9   Melted bull glue, as is usually dissolved by carpenters, heals without a scar: it is best to apply the filth from bulls' ears and genitals.

10 For a rabid dog's bite

1   Fish-pickle is applied. A weight of 15 *denarii* of rue's juice is drunk in wine. Ground rue leaves are applied to the bite with salt and honey or with pitch and vinegar.

2   Black fig's ground leaves cure with vinegar. Drunk wild rose's root drives away the fear of water most effectively. Plantain used in drink and applied helps against a rabid dog's bite and against the bite of all beasts.

3   Greasy wool put on the bite heals when removed after the seventh day. Ash of a canine head smeared on drives away the fear of water, or a dog's head devoured.

4   A worm from a dog's corpse tied on destroys the fear. There is slime under a rabid dog's tongue which, given in a potion, prevents hydrophobia.

5   It surpasses everything when the liver of the same dog which bit is eaten, raw if it is possible to do so, or cooked in whatever way if not. A pounded rooster's comb is placed on the bite.

6   Goose's grease with honey. Dogs which are rabid are salted by some in order that their flesh can be eaten as a remedy.

7   A suckling puppy of the same sex as the victim of the bite is killed in water and its raw liver is devoured.

8   Chicken's red dung is applied in vinegar to the bite. Dissolved lumps from a swallow's nest are smeared on with vinegar. A suckling puppy before it can see is opened and its rennet is drunk, while he who drinks it stands in flowing water up to the navel.

9   For fearing water, the whole face is thoroughly anointed with seal's grease. Those afraid of water are healed immediately by burning the wound with iron.

11 For a non-rabid dog's bite

1   Soda, axle-grease, and resin in equal portions are applied with vinegar. Raw *allex* on small, torn linen pieces. Ground garlic with honey. Pounded mint with honey.

2   Ground horehound with old axle-grease. Ground nettle with added salt.

3   Vines' ash with oil. Hot vinegar in a sponge. Ground soft shoots of fig's boughs. Ground almonds with honey. The flesh of walnuts pounded with onion, salt, and honey.

4   They recommend that the flesh of the same nuts, chewed by a fasting person, be applied.

5   Tiny sponges, wet with vinegar or water or honey, are cut up and applied. Vinegar lees are applied to the wound with *melanthium*.

12 *cicatricibus quibus color reddi debet*

1   Arietinus pulmo recens quam frequentissime imponitur. sevum eiusdem cum nitro efficax est. adeps leoninus ex rosaceo. utuntur senectute anguium ex vino decocta.

2   fimus columbinus cum melle. fel scorpionis marini. erucae semen cum felle bubulo. lupini ex aceto cocti. sevum asini impositum. fel vituli adiecta myrrha et oleo et croco extenvat: servatur in pyxide aerea, calefactum imponitur.

13 *frigore exustis*

1   Ituri per nivem farinam opopanacis bibere debent eaque perungui: vim enim habet mirifice excalefactoriam. si facta sint vulnera, frumentum tostum in ferro et tritum ex vino praesentaneo remedio est.

2   rutae folia in oleo cocta imponuntur. leporini pili cinis. pulmo leporis adalligatur. aristolochia[m] ex oleo excalefactoriam vim habet. axungia porcina.

14 *extrahendis his quae corpori fixa sunt*

1   Mus vivus discerptus imponitur. lacertae caput concussum et cum sale tusum. lacerta viva discerpta. cochleae exemptae de testis suis et contritae cum leporis coagulo.

2   testarum sepiae cinis. alium elixum cum pice harundines extrahit. nasturcium cum pice impositum. farina lini seminis cum radice silvestris cucumeris una trita. urticae radix <cum sale> trita et imposita.

3   <harundinis radix trita et imposita> filicem extrahit, item filicis radix eodem modo harundinem extrahit.

4   radix acrifolii coquitur et teritur et sic imponitur. blattae sine pedibus et capite et pennis tritae inlinuntur.

5   cancri fluviatiles triti. testarum purpurarum cinis ex aceto. fimus caprae ex vino. coagulum quodcumque [est], sed maxime leporis, cum pari pondere turis aut visci.

15 *quartanis*

1   Caput clavi quo aliquis in crucem fixus est alligatur panno, vel spartum de cruce.

2   fimi bubuli cinis spargitur. urina pueri inlinuntur primi digiti in manibus et pedibus. leporis cor adalligatur coagulumque eius bibitur ante accessionem, leonis in cibo datur.

3   viperae caput abscisum in linteolo adalligatur. muri vivo rostellum primum et auriculae summae deciduntur et in russeo panno adalligantur, et ipse mus vivus dimittitur.

12   *For scars which need to have their colour restored*

1   Fresh ram lung is applied as frequently as possible. Tallow of the same with soda is effective. Lion grease with rose oil. They use snakes' slough decocted in wine.

2   Pigeon dung with honey. Sea-scorpion's bile. Rocket's seed with ox bile. Lupines cooked in vinegar. Applied ass' tallow. Calf's bile with added myrrh, oil, and saffron reduces it: it is stored in a bronze box and is applied heated.

13   *For frostbite*

1   Those about to walk through snow ought to drink *opopanax* powder and be thoroughly anointed with the same, for it has a wonderfully warming power. If wounds were formed, grain toasted on iron and ground with wine is an instantaneous remedy.

2   Rue's leaves cooked in oil are applied. Ash of hare fur. A hare's lung is tied on. *Aristolochia* in oil has a warming power. Pork axle-grease.

14   *For extracting matter which is stuck in the body*

1   A live mouse torn to pieces is applied. A struck lizard's head ground with salt. A live lizard torn to pieces. Snails removed from their shells and pounded with hare's rennet.

2   Ash of cuttlefish's shells. Well-boiled garlic with pitch extracts reeds. Cress applied with pitch. Linseed meal ground with wild cucumber's root. Nettle's root ground with salt and applied.

3   Ground and applied reed's root extracts fern, likewise fern's root extracts reed in the same way.

4   Holly's root is cooked and ground, and thus applied. Ground cockroach with feet, head, and wings removed are smeared on.

5   Ground riverine crabs. The ash of purple-fish's shells with vinegar. Nanny-goat's dung with wine. Whatever rennet, but the best is hare's, with an equal weight of frankincense and mistletoe.

15   *For quartan fevers*

1   The head of a nail with which someone was fixed onto a cross is tied on in a cloth or a rope from a cross.

2   Ash of ox dung is sprinkled. The first digits on the hands and feet are smeared with a child's urine. A hare's heart is tied on and its rennet drunk before the onset; a lion's (heart) is given in food.

3   A viper's cut off head is tied on in a little linen cloth. The end of the muzzle and the tips of the ears are cut from a living mouse and tied on in a reddish cloth, and the living mouse itself is released.

4   ranae in trivio decoquuntur cum oleo; carnibus earum proiectis eo oleo utun-
     tur ad unctionem. alii elixi caput unum cum laserpicii obolo in vino austeri
     bibitur.

5   hirundinis fimi drachma una trita ex lactis caprini aut ovilli aut passi cyathis
     tribus ante accessionem propinatur. rubetae ranae cor vel iecur adalligatum in
     panno leucopeo.

6   semen anethi tribus digitis comprehensum et feniculi tantundem ex aceti
     mulsi cyatho uno potui datur.

7   in charta virgine scribis quod in dextro brachio ligatum portet ille qui patitur:
     "recede ab illo Gaio Seio, tertiana, Solomon te sequitur".

8   item panem et salem in linteo de licio alliget et circa arborem licio alliget et
     adiuret per ter panem et salem: "crastino hospites mihi venturi sunt, suscipite
     illos". hoc ter dicat.

16 *tertianis*

1   Spongiae Africanae cinis ex oleo vel aceto in fronte inlinitur. ante solis ortum
     cancri fluviatilis oculi eruti adalligantur, ipse cancer in aqua remittitur.

2   pulei ramus in lana involutus ante accessionem olfaciendus datur aut stratis
     subditur.

3   urticae autumnalis radix adalligatur: is qui eam effodiet debet nominare eum
     cui medetur et quibus parentibus natus sit.

4   herba quae in fluminibus aut rivis nascitur adalligatur in laevo brachio quid
     sit nescienti, tertianas discutit: legi debebit ante solis ortum sic ut eum qui
     colligit nemo videat.

5   lacerta viridis viva adalligatur in vaso quod eam capiat.

6   aranei tela cuilibet emplastro infrica[n]tur idemque emplastrum ut libet in
     aluta tamquam anaco<l>lema imponitur ante accessionem et aquae frigidae
     decem unciae bibuntur.

17 *febribus periodicis [id est febres quae de accessione nascuntur]*

1   Iecur delphini ante accessionem gustandum datur. in aselli piscis capite lapilli
     qui plena luna inventi sunt adalligantur in linteolo. utile est urgui oleo et sale.

2   cancris fluviatilibus tritis in oleo et aqua ante accessionem perungui oportet.

3   oculus lupi dexter salsus adalligatur. ante meridiem dantur aquae heminae
     tres potui, in quibus additae sint tres guttae sanguinis ex vena asini quam in
     auricula habet. recidivas prohibet lacerta viridis viva adalligata in vascello
     quod eam capiat.

4   Frogs are decocted with oil at the crossroads; when the flesh of these is expelled from the oil they use it as an ointment. One head of well-boiled garlic with an *obolus* of *silphium* juice is drunk in dry wine.

5   One ground *drachma* of swallow's dung in three *cyathi* of goat or sheep milk or raisin wine is given to drink before the onset. A toad's or frog's heart or liver is tied on in an ash-coloured cloth.

6   A three-finger pinch of dill's seed and just as much of fennel's seed is given in a one *cyathus* draught of honeyed vinegar.

7   You write on a clean piece of paper which he who suffers should carry, tied on the right arm: "Withdraw from him, Gaius Seius, tertian. Solomon follows you!"

8   Likewise, he should bind bread and salt in a cloth with thread and with the thread he should tie it around a tree and he should swear three times by bread and salt: "Tomorrow guests are going to come to me; receive these!" He should say this three times.

16 *For tertian fevers*

1   An African sponge's ash is smeared on the forehead in oil or vinegar. A riverine crab's plucked eyes are tied on before the rising of the sun; the crab itself is returned to the water.

2   A twig of pennyroyal rolled up in wool is given to be smelled or placed under beds before the onset.

3   Autumnal nettle's root is tied on: when whoever digs it up he ought to name him for whom the remedy is for, and from which parents he was born.

4   A plant which grows in rivers or streams is tied on the (patient's) left arm without their knowledge it disperses tertian fevers; it ought to be gathered before the rising of the sun in such a way that no one sees him who collects it.

5   A living green lizard is tied on in a vessel which holds it.

6   A spider's web is rubbed into any plaster, and the same plaster you choose is applied in an adhesive patch, just like an adhesive plaster, before the onset, and ten *unciae* of cold water is drunk.

17 *For periodic fevers*

1   A dolphin's liver is given to eat before the onset. The little stones which were found in a hake's head during the full moon are tied on in a little linen. It is beneficial to be anointed with oil and salt.

2   It is necessary to be thoroughly anointed with ground riverine crabs in oil and water before the onset.

3   A wolf's salted right eye is tied on. Before midday, three *heminae* of water are given in a draught, in which there were added three drops of ass' blood from a vein which it has in the ear. A living green lizard tied on in a little vessel which holds it prevents recurring (fevers).

18 *lethargicis*

1   Cimices septem triti in aquae cyatho uno dantur si vir sit, si puer sit in eodem modo aquae cimices quattuor.

2   castoreum fronti inlinitur. ruta ex aceto datur olfacienda. sisymbrium capiti infunditur ex aceto. urtica pedes caeduntur et frons.

3   spondilium capiti instillatur. mustelae iecur exuritur ad olfactum faciendum. pulmo pecudis calidus circa caput adalligatur.

4   palumbi tres putrefacti lethargum excitant odore. euphorbio ex aceto nares tanguntur. capri cornus usti nidor dormire eum non patitur.

5   vulturis nervos tollis et eos nervos circa manus laborantis ligabis. aristolochium rotundum cum adipe vulturino teris et ex eo manus fricabis.

19 *phreneticis [qui sensum perdunt] et qui somnum non capiunt*

1   Rosaceo et castoreo et peucedano peruncto capite somnus accedit. alium elixum in cibo datur.

2   sucus rutae tritae ex aceto instillatur in tempora. spondilium infunditur capiti. suffitus lanae sucidae prodest. pulmo pecudis calidus circa caput alligatur.

3   adipe gliris frontem lini et dormit. pellem de lepore albo nescienti sub capite pone.

4   lauri folia tria nescienti sub capite ponis et dormit. semen papaveris, semen lactucae, dactylos tres in aqua coquis ad tertias, das bibere et dormit.

5   seminis lactucae cochlear dimidium teris cum vino et per imbricem supino pone et dormit.

20 *cardiacis*

1   Aqua potui datur in qua holera discocta sunt addito sale. ruta ex aceto et melle cum farina hordeacea pectori imponitur.

2   rutae fasciculus cum rosaceo ex aceto decoquitur adiecta aloes uncia una: id oleum perunctione[m] <sudorem sistit>.

3   radix ferulae ex aceto et oleo perunctorum sudorem inhibet. vinum merum in spongia mammae sinistrae imponitur.

4   myrti semen cum polenta ex vino imponitur mammae sinistrae. folia rubi in quo mora nascuntur per se trita imponuntur eidem mammae.

5   sucus mororum quae in rubo nascuntur potui datur. cornus cervini et caprini cinere ex oleo myrteo adversus sudorem perunguntur. pulvis ex myrti foliis tostis inspersus sudorem statuit. [lapillus qui in ventriculo hirundinis invenitur gestatur.]

18 *For lethargic patients*

1   Seven ground bedbugs are given in one *cyathus* of water if he is a man; if he is a child, it is four bedbugs in the same measure of water.

2   *Castoreum* is smeared on the forehead. Rue in vinegar is given to smell. Water mint is poured on the head with vinegar. The feet and forehead are struck with nettles.

3   *Spondylium* is poured onto the head. A weasel's liver is burned to produce a smell. The hot lung of livestock is tied around the head.

4   Three putrefied wood-pigeons wake a lethargy patient by the smell. Nostrils are touched with *euphorbea* in vinegar. The fume of a goat's burnt horn does not permit him to sleep.

5   You remove the tendons of a vulture, and you will tie these tendons around the hands of the sufferer. You grind round *aristolochia* with vulture grease and you will rub down the hands with this.

19 *For phrenetic patients and who do not capture sleep*

1   Sleep approaches when the head is thoroughly anointed with rose oil, *castoreum*, and sulphurwort. Well-boiled garlic is given in food.

2   Ground rue's juice is poured on the temples with vinegar. *Spondylium* is poured on the head. A fumigation of greasy wool is beneficial. The hot lung of livestock is tied around the head.

3   Smear the forehead with a dormouse's grease and he sleeps. Place the hide from a white hare under the head, without the patient's knowledge.

4   You place three laurel leaves under the patient's head without his knowledge, and he sleeps. You boil in water poppy's seed, lettuce's seed, and three *dactyli* to a third; you give this to drink and he sleeps.

5   You grind one-and-a-half *cochlearia* of lettuce's seeds with wine and place it along the nasal septum while on his back, and he sleeps.

20 *For* cardiacus disease

1   Water in which vegetables were decocted with added salt is given in a draught. Rue in vinegar and honey with barley meal is placed on the breast.

2   A bundle of rue is decocted with rose oil in vinegar with one added *uncia* of aloe: that oil checks perspiration by thorough anointing.

3   Giant fennel's root in vinegar and oil inhibits perspiration of those thoroughly anointed. Unmixed wine is applied to the left breast in a sponge.

4   Myrtle's seed with *polenta* is applied in wine to the left breast. Ground leaves of the bramble on which berries grow are applied by themselves to the same breast.

5   Juice of berries which grow on the bramble is given in a draught. Against perspiration they are thoroughly anointed with deer or goat horn ash in myrtle oil. The sprinkled powder from the parched leaves of myrtle stops perspiration.

21   *comitialibus*

1   Testiculi ursini in cibo prosunt. testes aprini crudi triti ex aqua bibuntur. cum primum quis cecidit, in eo loco quo caput eius fuit clavus ferreus figatur: non repetit.

2   dantur carnes edendae bestiae occisae eo ferramento quo homo ante occisus est. <lapillus qui in ventriculo hirundinis invenitur gestatur.>

3   hirundinis sanguis cum ture vel eiusdem cor recens devoratur. lapillus de nido hirundinis adalligatus ad collum iacentem recreat et ab hoc periculo tutum praestat.

4   <alium> elixum subinde in cibo et in potione sumitur. tenentes in manu anethum comitiali morbo non appetuntur. testiculi arietini inveterantur et ex his dimidii denarii pondus datur in hemina aquae tritum.

5   abstinentia vini utendum est diebus quinque ante et totidem postea. sanguis pecudis utiliter bibitur. sed et humanus sanguis hoc vitio liberat.

6   fel agninum cum melle vel cochleari vel ligula sumitur. catulus lactens absciso capite et pedibus, exsectis interaneis, ex vino et myrrha coctus editur.

7   viverra sumpta in cibo prodest. lacerta viridis ablato capite et pedibus et interaneis in cibo datur ita condita ut fastidium abigat.

8   cochlearum cinis addito lini semine et urticae ex melle inlinitur cum sale. iecur vulturis tritum cum suo sanguine propinatur ter septenis diebus.

9   melius prodest si ea avis cum occiditur satura erit humano cadavere. fel testudinis naribus inlitum iacentem erigit.

10   coagulum vituli marini bibitur cum lacte equino aut mali Punici suco aut mulso aceto. castoreum in aceti mulsi cyathis tribus ieiunis datur.

11   his qui saepius cadunt clystere infunditur hoc: castorei drachmae duae, mellis hemina, olei hemina, aquae sextarius I.

12   mustelae marinae iecur in cibo bene sumitur. carnes caprinae in rogo hominis tostae hunc morbum depellunt. caprini vel cervini cornus usti nidor adhibetur.

22   *hydropicis*

1   Lapidem achatem hydropicus si secum portaverit, liberabitur. vomitus canini ventri inlinuntur.

2   sablone calido marino obruuntur. spongiae Afrae siccae apponuntur. adeps delphini liquatus ex vino bibitur, propter graveolentiam naribus obturatis aut unguento optimo tactis.

3   cancri marini vel fluviatiles in cibo ex iure. alium viride cum fico duplici alvum evacuat.

21 *For epileptics*

1 Bear testicles in food are beneficial. Raw, ground wild boar testes are drunk in water. After anyone first fell, an iron nail, if it is fixed in that place where the head was: it (the disease) does not return.

2 They are given to eat the flesh of a beast killed with an iron weapon with which a man was killed previously. A little stone which is found in a swallow's gizzard is carried.

3 A swallow's blood with frankincense or the fresh heart of the same is eaten. A little stone from a swallow's nest, tied to the neck, revives the fallen and keeps them safe from this danger.

4 Well-boiled garlic is repeatedly consumed in food and drink. Holding dill in the hand, they are not seized by the comitial disease. Ram testicles are aged, and half a *denarius* weight, ground, is given in a *hemina* of water.

5 Abstinence from wine should be employed for five days before and as many after. The blood of livestock is usefully drunk. Yet human blood frees them from this disease.

6 Lamb bile with honey is consumed either in a *cochlear* or a *ligula*. A suckling puppy with its head and feet cut off, and intestines removed, cooked in wine and myrrh is eaten.

7 Ferret consumed in food is beneficial. A green lizard with the head, feet, and intestines removed is given in food, seasoned in such a way that it removes nausea.

8 Snails' ash with added linseed and nettles in honey are applied with salt. Ground vulture's liver with its own blood is drunk three times for seven days.

9 It is more beneficial if, when that bird is killed, it has eaten from a human cadaver. Tortoise's bile smeared on the nostrils will rouse the fallen.

10 Seal's rennet is drunk with horse milk or pomegranate's juice or honeyed vinegar. *Castoreum* in three *cyathi* of honeyed vinegar is given while fasting.

11 To those who fall often, this is administered in an enema: two *drachmae* of *castoreum*, a *hemina* of honey, a *hemina* of oil, and 1 *sextarius* of water.

12 A sea-weasel's liver is well consumed in food. Goat flesh roasted on a human pyre banishes this disease. The fume of burnt goat and deer horn is used.

22 *For the dropsical*

1 A dropsical person will be freed if he carried an agate stone with him. Dog's vomit is smeared on the belly.

2 They are buried in hot marine sand. Dried African sponges are applied. Liquefied dolphin's grease is drunk with wine, with the nostrils stopped up or touched with unguent because of the foul smell.

3 Marine or riverine crabs in food with broth. Fresh garlic with a split fig evacuates the bowel.

4   scilla subiecta linguae sitim compescit. scillae bulbus torretur, deinde purgatur
    et medium eius in aqua coquitur. cum madidum est eximitur, ex eo tres oboli
    dantur potui ex melle et aceto: evacuatur per urinam.

5   sinape[m] et ficus et cyminum aequis partibus tusa ventri imponuntur. ficus
    siccae coquuntur et ex vino et absinthio suffunduntur; farina hordeacea addito
    nitro: omnia in unum conteruntur et ita imponuntur.

6   folia myrti in vino decocta conteruntur et ex eo vino duo cyathi potui dantur.
    radices sambuci in vino decoquuntur et ex eodem vino duo cyathi poti
    exinaniunt.

7   est hedera quae chrysocarpos appellatur propterea quod fert grana aurei
    coloris: haec grana XX in vini sextario conteruntur et ex eo vino terni cyathi
    bibuntur qui per urinam exinaniunt.

8   testudo decisis pedibus et capite et cauda, intestinis abiectis, in cibo datur ita
    condita ut citra fastidium sumi possit.

9   fimus vituli masculi ventri inlinitur. vincae pervincae aridae tusae farinae
    cochlearis mensura ex aqua data celerrime reddit sanitatem.

10 elleborum contusum ut sit pulvis: deinde commiscebimus illud radicibus et
    super ventrem in linteolo imponimus, ita ut pulveris pusillum supra spargas.
    adalligatum habeas licet biduum vel triduum unum adalligamentum.

23 *morbo regio*

1   Sordis de auriculis aut de mamma pecudis pondus denarii cum myrrhae
    pusillo ex duobus cyathis vini hauriuntur.

2   vermes terreni cum myrrha in aceto mulso propinantur. cerebrum perdicis in
    tribus cyathis vini bibitur.

3   cineres interaneorum palumborum <ad> cochlearia bina bibuntur ex mulso.
    salsamentum in cibo ex pipere sumitur servata carnis abstinentia.

4   alium tritum in potione vini propinatur. erucae silvestris tria folia sinistra
    manu decerpta ex aqua mulsa bibuntur.

5   cicer arietinum decoquitur in aqua et duo cyathi potui dantur vel ex melle in
    cibo. nuces Graecae cum absinthii semine teruntur, deinde pilulae ex aceto
    eduntur.

6   rubia qua pelles inficiuntur in aqua mulsa bibitur. herba sabina, quae habet
    folia cupressi similia, trita ex vino potui datur.

7   canini capitis cinis in mulso propinatur. gallina si sit luteis pedibus, aqua
    pedes ei purificantur, deinde vino colluuntur idque vinum potui datur. folia
    oleastri in vino trita imponuntur.

8   spondilium ex vino bibitur. fimus pulli asinini quem primum edidit a partu
    datur ex vino ad magnitudinem fabae: triduo medetur.

9   idem praestat equini pulli fimus eadem ratione. cyminum ex vino albo a
    balneo datur.

4   Squill placed under the tongue suppresses thirst. A squill's bulb is roasted, then it is cleansed, and the middle of it is boiled in water. When it is soft boiled it is removed, and from this three *oboli* are given in a draught with honey and vinegar: it is purged through urine.

5   Mustard, fig, and cumin pounded in equal amounts are applied to the belly. Dried figs are cooked and suffused with wine and wormwood; barley meal with added soda: everything is pounded together into one and thus applied.

6   Myrtle's leaves decocted in wine are pounded, and from that wine two *cyathi* are given in a draught. Elder's roots are decocted in wine and a drink from that wine of two *cyathi* drains.

7   There is ivy which is called *chrysocarpi* because it bears berries of a golden colour: 20 of these are pounded in a *sextarius* of wine, and from that wine three *cyathi* are drunk, which drains through urine.

8   Tortoise, with its feet, head, and tail cut off and intestines removed, is given in food, having been spiced in such a way that it is possible to eat without nausea.

9   A male calf's dung is smeared on the belly. The measure of a *cochlear* of dried and crushed periwinkle flour in water most quickly restores health.

10 Hellebore is pounded so that it is dust; then we will mix that with roots and apply it in a little linen over the belly in such a way that you sprinkle a tiny amount of dust above. Having been tied on, you can wear one dressing for two or three days.

23   For jaundice

1   A weight of a *denarius* of filth from the ears and udder of livestock with a tiny amount of myrrh is swallowed in two *cyathi* of wine.

2   Earthworms are drunk with myrrh in honeyed vinegar. A partridge's brain is drunk in three *cyathi* of wine.

3   Ashes of wood-pigeons' intestines, about two *cochlearia*, are drunk in honeyed wine. Fish-pickle is eaten in food with pepper, while continuing to abstain from meat.

4   Ground garlic is drunk in a potion of wine. Three leaves of wild rocket, plucked with the left hand, are drunk with mead.

5   Ram's-head chickpeas are decocted in water and two *cyathi* are given in a draught or in food with honey. Almonds are ground with wormwood's seed, and then pills are eaten with vinegar.

6   Madder, with which hides are dyed, is drunk in mead. Ground savin herb, which has leaves similar to cypress, is given in a draught with wine.

7   Ash of a dog's head is drunk in honeyed wine. A hen, if it has yellow feet, its feet are cleansed with water, then they are thoroughly washed with wine, and that wine is given to drink. Ground wild olive's leaves are applied in wine.

8   *Spondylium* is drunk in wine. Dung of an ass' foal, which is the first put forth after its birth, is given in an amount the size of a bean in wine; it cures in three days.

9   Likewise, the dung of a horse's foal is beneficial in the same way. Cumin is given in white wine after a bath.

24 *igni sacro*

1   Vermes terreni ex aceto inlinuntur. serpentium senectus cum bitumine et felle sive fimo agnino ex aqua inlinitur a balneo.

2   alii cinis ex oleo et garo inlinitur. ruta ex aceto et oleo inlinitur. lens ex aqua marina decocta imponitur.

3   amurca olivae nigrae infunditur. herba sabina tusa quae habet folia quasi cupressus cum melle inlinitur.

4   ova cocta trita cum oleo imponuntur et operiuntur foliis betae, ovorum trium candidum cum amyli pari mensura contritum imponitur. hyssopum cum pompholica et rosaceo inlinitur.

5   grillus contritus manu ab eo qui non sit eo vitio apprehensus eum qui hoc fecerit in totum annum ab hoc malo liberat: oportet autem eum erui ferro cum cavernae suae terra.

6   anseris adipe perunguitur vitium. viperae caput aridum combustum ex aceto superlinitur.

7   spongia ex aceto imponitur tam grandis ut sanas quoque partes tegat. ursinus aut suillus adeps. adicitur fimus vitulinus vel bubulus. ramenta pellis cervinae delecta pumice ex aceto trita imponuntur.

8   Est genus sacri ignis quod zoster vocatur, quoniam occidit eum quem appetit si praecingat. huic occurrit imposita plantago cum creta Cimolia.

9   Aqua cisternina aut certe dulcis solvitur ex oleo, locus deinde penna perunguitur: eadem die liberat. ovi medium quod est rufum teritur, sublato albo, in vaso cupreo, perinde pistillo de cupro, et sic dolor penna inlinitur.

25 *ossibus fractis*

1   Caninum cerebrum linteolo inlitum imponitur, superpositis lanis quae subinde oleo suffundantur: quarto decimo die solidat. cinis silvestrium murium imponitur cum melle.

2   cinis terrenorum vermium cum melle etiam minuta ossa extrahit. laridum elixum circumligatum mira celeritate solidat.

3   articulorum fracturis cinis de femoribus pecudum cum cera, costis fractis imponitur caprinus fimus ex vetere vino: aperit extrahit sanat.

26 *scabiei*

1   Plurimum prosunt asini medullae inlitae. urina asini cum suo luto imposita sedat.

2   fimus bubulus impositus. sanguis bubulus recens impositus: cum aruit, alter super inlinitur, postero die abluitur cinere lixivo.

3   sanguis caninus inlinitur. alumen liquidum imponitur admixto nitro et melanthio. ocustarum pratensium pedes cum sevo hircino triti medentur.

24 *For erysipelas*

1   Earthworms are smeared on with vinegar. Snakes' slough with bitumen and bile or with lamb dung with water is smeared on after a bath.

2   Garlic's ash is smeared on with oil or *garum*. Rue is smeared on with vinegar and oil. Lentils decocted in sea water are applied.

3   Black olive's *amurca* is poured on. Pounded savin herb which has leaves like cypress is smeared on with honey.

4   Ground, boiled eggs are applied with oil and are covered over with beet leaves. Three egg whites, beaten with an equal amount of starch, are applied. Hyssop is smeared on with *pompholyx* and rose oil.

5   A cricket crushed by hand by one who was not taken by that disease; one who did this is set free from this complaint for a whole year. However, it is necessary that it be dug up with iron and with earth of its own hole.

6   The disease site is thoroughly anointed with goose's grease. A burnt, dried viper's head is smeared over with vinegar.

7   A sponge so large that it will also cover the healthy parts is applied with vinegar. Bear or pork grease. Calf or ox dung is applied. Ground scrapings of deer hide removed by a pumice stone are applied with vinegar.

8   There is a type of erysipelas which is called "the belt" because it kills him whom it assails if it encircles. Plantain applied with Cimolian chalk relieves this.

9   Stored rain water, or at least fresh water, is dispersed in oil, then the site is thoroughly anointed with a feather; it frees on the same day. The middle of an egg which is red, with the white removed, is ground in a copper vessel with a pestle also of copper, and thus the painful site is smeared with a feather.

25 *For broken bones*

1   Dog brain smeared on a little linen is applied, with wool placed over which is repeatedly wet underneath with oil; it knits by the fourteenth day. Ash of field-mice is applied with honey.

2   Earthworms' ash with honey even extracts tiny bones. Thoroughly boiled bacon lard fastened around knits with remarkable speed.

3   Ash from livestock's thighs for fractures of the joints with wax. Goat dung with old wine is applied to broken ribs; it opens, extracts, and heals.

26 *For* scabies

1   Applications of ass' marrow are the most beneficial. Ass' urine applied with its own mud assuages it.

2   Applied ox dung. Fresh ox blood is applied; when it dries, it is smeared over again, and on the following day it is washed off with ash lye.

3   Dog blood is smeared on. Liquid alum is applied with soda and *melanthium* mixed in. Meadow locusts' ground feet heal with goat tallow.

27 *papulis <et pruritui>*

1   Lupinorum farina ex aceto subacta in balneo papulis inlinitur. pruritus sedant cochleae minutae tritae impositae.

2   nitrum candens vino austeri extinguitur, deinde conteritur et sine oleo in balneo aspergitur. pruritum et scabiem sedat oleum in quo pastinacae marinae decoctae sint.

3   aluminis liquidi pars tertia, duae partes mellis in balneo papulis inlinuntur. aeque papulis inlinitur creta Cimolia in balneo.

4   pustulis suilli fimi cinis vel cornus cervini cinis ex aqua inlinitur. sulphur tritum mixtum liquamine in balneo utiliter inlinitur.

28 *varis*

1   Folia porri sectivi trita imposita tollunt varos. farina ervi ex aqua imposita sanat et toto corpore maculas emendat. oleum amigdalinum ex melle inlinitur.

2   adeps gallinaceus cum cepa contritus imponitur. naevos tollit farina avenae ex aceto cocta et imposita.

29 *verrucis*

1   Verrucae abolentur urina recenti canis cum suo luto inlita, fimi canini cinere cum cera [et cepa] imposito, fimo ovium inlito, sanguine murium recenti, erinacei felle, sanguine lacertae, fimo gallinacei cum oleo et nitro.

2   efficaciter tolluntur [cymino] ocimo cum atramento sutoricio, inmaturarum ficorum lacte cum axungia mixto, capitum menarum cinere cum alio trito, cinere fimi vitulini ex aceto, asini urina cum suo luto.

30 *livoribus et tumoribus*

1   Recenti livori cortex raphani ex melle tritus imponitur. alium ustum tritum ex melle. holus crudum tritum per se. apium viride tritum cum albo ovi.

2   sinapis Alexandrini heminam triti, adipis anserini uncias IIII, mellis selibram in mortario commisceri oportet et in panno induci et parti quae ex contusione in dolore est imponi, et mirifice remediat.

3   percussa in facie aut discorticata pane ex melle sanantur. acrifolii radix decoquitur, teritur et imponitur livori et tumori.

4   pulmones pecudum in tenvissima frusta conciduntur, deinde coniecta in aquam ferventem calida subinde tumoribus imponuntur.

5   columbino fimo contrito utuntur. aqua marina calida utiliter tumores foventur, deinde postea aceto aequo calido. plantagine cruda et contrita si tumor sive duritia cataplasmetur, efficaciter sedatur: quod remedium et alia huius modi curat et canceromata.

27 *For* **papulae** *and itching complaints*

1   The meal of lupines kneaded with vinegar is smeared on *papulae* in the bath. Ground, small snails applied assuage itch.

2   Boiling-hot soda is extinguished with dry wine; it is then pounded and sprinkled on in the bath without oil. Oil in which stingrays were decocted assuages itch and *scabies*.

3   A third part of liquid alum and two parts of honey are smeared on *papulae* in the bath. Cimolian chalk is also smeared on *papulae* in the bath.

4   Swine dung's ash or the ash of deer horn is smeared on *pusulae* with water. Ground sulphur mixed with *liquamen* is usefully smeared on in the bath.

28 *For pimples*

1   Ground and applied chive's leaves remove pimples. Bitter vetch meal applied with water heals and improves moles on the whole body. Almond oil is smeared on with honey.

2   Chicken grease pounded with onion is applied. Oatmeal cooked with vinegar and applied removes *naevi*.

29 *For warts*

1   Warts are killed by fresh dog's urine smeared on with its own mud, ash of dog dung applied with wax, smeared on sheep's dung, the fresh blood of mice, hedgehog's bile, lizard's blood, or chicken's dung with oil and soda.

2   They are effectually destroyed by basil with cobbler's black, latex of unripe figs mixed with axle-grease, the ash of *menae*'s heads with ground garlic, calf dung ash with vinegar, or ass' urine with its own mud.

30 *For bruises and swellings*

1   Ground radish's skin is applied to a recent bruise with honey. Burnt, ground garlic with honey. Raw ground vegetable by itself. Ground fresh *apium* with egg white.

2   It is necessary for a *hemina* of ground Alexandrian mustard, 4 *unciae* of goose grease, and half a *libra* of honey to be mixed together in a mortar, spread on a cloth, and placed onto the part where there is pain because of a contusion, and it heals wonderfully.

3   Strikes to the face or removed skin are healed by bread with honey. Holly's root is decocted, ground, and applied to a bruise and swelling.

4   Lungs of livestock are cut into the thinnest slices, then thrown, hot, into boiling water, and they are immediately placed on swellings.

5   They use ground pigeon dung. Swellings are usefully fomented by hot sea water, then afterwards also with hot vinegar. If there is swelling or hardness, a plaster from raw ground plantain; it is effectually assuaged. That remedy also cures *cancer* and other problems of this type.

6   sal in saccum linteum coicitur, deinde intinctus in aquam ferventem et ita
    calefactus crebro imponitur. livorem ab ictu recentem spongia ex aqua salsa
    calida saepius imposita tollit.

7   mirifice facit adversus tumores fimum suillum sub testo calefactum tritumque
    cum oleo. vitiatis ex percussu fimum aprinum decoctum ex aceto imponitur.

8   eiusdem fimi arida farina inspersa potioni eversis utilissima est. aliqui
    putant melius esse eiusdem fimi farinam ex aqua bibere. itaque sic curantur
    agitatores tracti a quadrigis et rotis pressi.

9   proximam huic putant suillo fimo vim inesse. luxatis recens fimum vel apri-
    num vel suillum vel vitulinum imponitur.

10 verris spuma recens cum aceto inlinitur. fimum caprinum cum melle. bubula
    caro trita. ruptis convulsisque inlinitur fel ovillum cum lacte mulieris. cancri
    fluviatiles triti cum lacte asinino.

11 Ponimus hoc loco compositionem emplastri quo Sagares uti solebat, pancra-
    tiastes de nobilissimis, adversus omnia quae in eiusmodi certamine solent
    inferri. quod praeterea furunculis strumis vulneribus collectionibus podagris
    quoque medetur.

12 in cacabum novum fictilem coicitur spumae argenti tusae cribratae libra, olei
    veteris sesquilibra. haec coquuntur et subinde tudicula permiscentur: modus
    est ut fiat crassitudo glutinis fabrilis.

13 tunc additur picis siccae pondo quadrans, sevi taurini diligenter contriti
    pondo uncia, et interposita horae dimidia parte cum desederit tudicula, in
    aqua frigida +missa et amota digitis inquinata retollitur+ et cum opus fuerit
    in linteolo spisso imponitur ita ut oleo non tangatur.

14 Nero initio imperii sui quotiens in nocturnis grassaturis in faciem verberatus
    esset, tapsia cum ture et cera caesa inliniebat et postero die sine ullis argu-
    mentis rixae populo Romano vultum suum spectandum praebebat.

15 si sanguis suffuderit, farina frumenti pollinis ex aqua temperatur, eaque
    tantam habet potentiam ut sanguinem perducat usque fascias.

31 *paralyticis*

1   Nullus tam idoneus est paralyticis cibus quam holera. rubia salubriter ab his
    bibitur, sed ut usus sequatur balnei.

2   aliqui solent solia temperare addito euphorbio. pingue glirium et soricum
    decoctorum ex aqua dant edendum.

6 Salt is poured into a linen bag, then, having been dipped into boiling water and thus warmed, it is repeatedly applied. A sponge frequently applied with hot salted water removes a recent bruise caused by a blow.

7 Swine dung warmed under a pot and ground with oil works wonderfully against swelling. Wild boar dung decocted in vinegar is applied to damage caused by a beating.

8 Dried powder of the same dung sprinkled into a potion is most helpful for those knocked down. Some think that it is better to drink the powder of the same dung with water. Thus charioteers, dragged by a four-horse chariot and run over by wheels, are cured.

9 They believe that the next in potency is swine dung. Fresh wild boar, swine, or calf dung is applied to a dislocation.

10 Fresh boar's foam is smeared on with vinegar. Goat dung with honey. Ground beef. Sheep bile with breast milk is smeared on ruptures and wrenches. Ground riverine crabs with ass milk.

11 We place in this position the composition of a plaster which Sagares, one of the most respected pancrationists, was accustomed to use for everything which is likely to be inflicted in a contest of this type. Besides which, it also cures boils, *strumae*, wounds, abscesses, and *podagra*.

12 A *libra* of crushed and sifted litharge is poured into a new earthen cooking pot, with one-and-a-half *librae* of old oil. These are boiled, and immediately afterwards they are mixed in a *tudicula*; this is until the consistency becomes that of carpenter's glue.

13 Then a quarter *libra* by weight of dry pitch is added with an *uncia* of carefully pounded bull tallow, and after half an hour elapsed while it settled in the *tudicula*, having been thrust into cold water and contaminants removed with fingers, it is withdrawn; and when it is needed it is placed on a thick linen cloth so it is not touched by oil.

14 At the beginning of his reign, because Nero had often been struck in the face during nocturnal prowlings, he smeared the blows with *thapsia* together with frankincense and wax, and on the following day he presented his face to be seen by the Roman people without any evidence of the brawl.

15 If blood suffused, the dust of finely ground grain is combined with water and it has so much power that it even draws blood into bandages.

31 For paralytics

1 Nothing is as suitable for paralytic patients as eating vegetables. Madder is advantageously drunk by these, but in the bath so that benefit might result.

2 Some are wont to combine baths with added *euphorbea*. They give the fat of dormice and shrew-mice decocted in water to be eaten.

32 *psilotrum*

1   Sunt qui vel suis pilis vel servorum suorum in balneo offendantur, sine ulla quidem ratione; sed illorum quoque persuasioni occurrendum est et monstrandum quemadmodum effici possit ut evulsi pili non renascantur.

2   nam omni psilotro sic utendum est ut, priusquam adiciatur, resina auferantur.

3   Sanguisugae vivae tostae in vaso fictili ex aceto inlinuntur per horas tres, deinde in balneo abluuntur. lacte canis primi partus inlinitur.

4   amerinae nigrae semen cum spumae argenti pari pondere inlinitur a balneo. sanguis vespertilionis. vipera exemptis ossibus in tribus heminis olei discoquitur et teritur: hoc peruncti psilotrantur.

5   fel erinacei inlinitur. et tithymalli sucus <cum> oleo inlinitur in sole frequenter et hyaenae sanguis inlinitur quoque.

33 *praef. venenis et venenatis morsibus*

1   Cum adversus omnes morborum incursus fuerimus diligentissimi, non ideo tamen habebimus spem certam salutis, cum ex inproviso serpentes saeviant, mures aranei, phalangii, et his omnibus nocentiores sint venefici hominis morsus.

2   adversus haec itaque convertendus est animus in instrvendis remediis, ut appareat benignitatem naturae etiam ea mortifera esse noluisse.

33 *antidotum contra venena*

1   Antidotum Mithridaticum laudant medici eiusdemque compositiones diversas afferunt et ad commendanda migmata pretiosa propter raritatem ingentes pecunias poscunt.

2   appendunt namque singulas libras vicenis sestertiis et infelicium credulitatem hoc quoque ingenio circumveniunt ut illis persuadeant emere quae noceant.

3   alia namque stomachum laedunt, alia caput adgravant, alia pallorem afferunt et corporis maciem. itaque frequenter accidit ut hi qui illorum antidotis usi sunt miserius morerentur quam si bibissent venenum.

4   Pompeius autem Magnus Mithridate devicto invenit in scrinio eius ipsius manu scriptam compositionem, qua ille praesumpta adversus omnia veneficia in totum diem tutum se incolumemque praestabat: nuces iuglandes duae, ficus siccae duae, rutae folia XX, salis granum I in unum contunduntur et devorantur a ieiuno.

5   Electrum est aurum in quo quinta pars argenti invenitur. ex quo si quis vaso potatorio utatur, insidias veneni vitabit. discurrunt enim in eo arcus caelestibus similes cum igneo stridore, eoque modo duplici ratione deprehenditur scelus.

32 *Depilatory*

1   There are those who are offended by either their own hair or that of their slaves at the bath, indeed without any reason; but their belief also ought to be addressed and shown how it can be brought about that plucked hairs do not regrow.

2   Every depilatory should be used in such a way that they (the hairs) are removed with resin before it is applied.

3   Living leeches roasted in an earthen vessel are smeared on with vinegar for three hours, then washed off in the bath. It is smeared with milk of a bitch which has had her first litter.

4   Black Amerian willow's seed is smeared on with an equal weight of litharge after a bath. Bat's blood. A viper with its bones removed is decocted in three *heminae* of oil and is ground; having been thoroughly anointed with this they are treated with a depilatory.

5   Hedgehog's bile is smeared on. Spurge's juice is repeatedly smeared on with oil in the sun, and hyena's blood is also smeared on.

33 *Preface: For poisons and venomous bites*

1   Since we were most diligent against every attack of disease, we will not have a reliable expectation of health because snakes, shrew-mice, and *phalangia* unexpectedly strike, and more harmful than all these, are the poisonous bites of a man.

2   Therefore attention ought to be directed towards the preparation of remedies against these, so that it appears that even the benevolence of nature did not want these to be deadly.

33 *Antidotes against poisons*

1   Doctors praise the Mithridatic antidote and they publish their different compositions, and they demand vast amounts of money for recommending expensive mixtures because of their rarity.

2   For they weigh each *libra* for twenty-thousand *sesterces*, and they defraud the credulity of unfortunate people also with this trick so that they persuade them to buy that which harms them.

3   Some injure the stomach, others make the head heavy, and others still cause pallor and thinness of the body. Accordingly, it frequently happens that those who lamentably use their antidotes die as if they had drunk poison.

4   However, Pompey the Great found, when Mithridates was defeated, a composition written in his own hand in a case, by the consumption of which he made himself safe and sound from all poisons for the whole day: two walnuts, two dried figs, 20 rue leaves, and 1 grain of salt are pounded together and consumed by a fasting individual.

5   *Electrum* is gold in which one-fifth of silver is found. If someone makes use of a drinking vessel made from this, he will avoid the trap of poison. For bows run to and fro in it, like those in the sky, with a fiery crackle, and in that manner crime is detected in a double fashion.

6 est et electrum fictum in auro addita argenti parte quinta, sed hoc tantum praestat quantum illud naturale.

7 Ergo monstravimus quo antidoto venenum non admittatur et quo vasculo arguatur. nunc et remedia suggeram.

8 Centaurion potum omnia mala medicamenta exigit per alvum. aristolochiae radicis pondus denarii ex hemina vini bibitur. sanguis caninus hauritur adversus toxica.

9 coagulum agninum in potione, ventriculus ciconiae cum lacte ovium in cibo datur. mustela vulgaris inveterata drachmis binis potatur.

10 sanguis anatum Ponticarum servatur spissus et diluitur ex vino. asinini sanguinis potus venena rest[r]ing<u>it. haedi sanguis utiliter bibitur.

34   *contra leporem marinum et pastinacam*

1 Saeviunt quidam et marino lepore. qui cum sit genus piscis, mortem infert in cibo inpactus, non subitam sed quae trahatur quantum plerique existimant totidem diebus quot dictus lepus vixit.

2 atque qui has insidias inciderit ipse suo corpore ostendit veneficium: habet namque odorem piscis. hoc periculo liberabitur cancris marinis coctis et in cibo sumptis. ostrea fricta in cibo sumpta.

3 malva cum sua radice coquitur et sucus eius potui datur. sanguis anserinus aequa cum olei portione bibitur. ad omnium marinorum ictus coagulum leporis et haedi vel agni bibitur ex vino cyathis tribus.

35   *contra murem araneum*

1 Mus araneus exiguus est ultra modum, longo rostello, oculorum acie obtusa, et ideo quantum existimo iners e<s>t huius natura ut non possit transire orbitam. morsum venenatum habet, cui sic occurritur.

2 coagulum agninum ex vino bibitur. ungulae arietinae cinis cum melle imponitur. ipse mus araneus divulsus imponitur. terra quam in orbitam rota depressit plagae imponitur. talpa discerpta imponitur.

36   *contra phalangium*

1 Phalangium praecipue in leguminibus et in hort<ensi>is observatur, sed et araneus et alia genera bestiolarum mortifera, quorum morsus non sentiuntur sed pruritu intelleguntur.

2 adversus haec omnia vinum merum bibitur. acetum calidum <in> spongia quam amplissima imponitur, ita ut tres sextarios aceti habeat, sextantem sulphuris. radicis hederae sucus bibitur.

3 sucus bibitur mororum de rubo. gallinacei cerebrum cum piperis exiguo additur in puscae potione. fimi pecudum cineres ex aceto <inponuntur>.

6   And *electrum* is fashioned by adding a fifth part of silver to gold, and in truth this is as excellent as that which is natural.

7   Now we have shown by which antidote poison is not admitted and by which vessel it is betrayed. Now I will provide remedies.

8   A centaury draught expels every bad drug through the bowel. The weight of a *denarius* of *aristolochia*'s root is drunk in a *hemina* of wine. Dog blood is drunk against *toxica*.

9   Lamb rennet is given in a potion, and stork's gizzard is given in food with sheep's milk. Preserved common weasel is drunk in a two *drachmae* dose.

10 Pontic ducks' thickened blood is preserved and diluted in wine. A drink of ass' blood mitigates poisons. Kid's blood is usefully drunk.

34   *Against sea-hares and stingrays*

1   Some are maddened by sea-hare. While it is a type of fish, inserted in food it brings death, not suddenly, but it is assumed, as the majority thinks, after as many days as the said hare had lived.

2   And whoever has fallen to these snares himself shows the poisoning on his own body: insomuch as it has the odour of fish. He will be freed from this danger by cooked marine crabs consumed in food. Roasted oysters consumed in food.

3   Mallow is cooked with its root and its juice is given in a draught. Goose blood is drunk with an equal amount of oil. Hare's, kid's, or lamb's rennet is drunk in three *cyathi* of wine for the strikes of every marine creature.

35   *Against the shrew-mouse*

1   The shrew-mouse is tiny beyond measure with a long muzzle, dull eye-sight, and, as I think, its nature is so weak that it is unable to cross a wheel-rut. It has a venomous bite, which is cured as follows.

2   Lamb rennet is drunk with wine. Ram hoof's ash is applied with honey. The same shrew-mouse, torn apart, is applied. The earth which the wheel has depressed in a rut is applied to the bite. A mole, torn to pieces, is applied.

36   *Against a* phalangium

1   A *phalangium* is chiefly seen among legumes and in gardens, but so is the spider and other deadly types of small animals, the bites of which are not felt but are perceived through itching.

2   Unmixed wine is drunk against all these things. Hot vinegar is applied in as large a sponge as possible, so that it holds three *sextarii* of vinegar and one-sixth of sulphur. Juice of ivy's root is drunk.

3   The juice from the bramble's berries is drunk. Chicken's brain with a tiny amount of pepper is added into a potion of *posca*. Ashes of livestock's dung are applied with vinegar.

37 *contra serpentis et hominis morsum*

1 Serpentes praecipitem morsum inferunt. quos sanare in promptu est, quin etiam ipsas fugare [sit] facillimum vulturinarum pinnarum suffitu, ebuli fumo, nidore usti cornus cervini.

2 viperae qui iecur coctum hauserit negatur umquam a serpentibus feriri. erucis ex aceto tritis perunctos non mordent. habentem secum cor vulturis nec serpentes nec ferae appetunt.

3 Nunc remedia morsibus subiciemus. raphanus sativa ex aqua coquitur et trita plagae imponitur. alium tostum cum restibus suis et tritum ex oleo adicitur.

4 radix ferulae ex vino medetur imposita. farina milii cum pice liquida optime facit. ervum tritum ex aceto et ad serpentium morsus et ad omnium ferarum et hominis mirifice medetur.

5 vinum merum in spongia imponitur. mori folia trita recentia – si arida sint, decocta et aeque trita – imponuntur. hyssopi semen bibitur.

6 eius qui percussus est vertex inciditur eoque additur euphorbium: medetur quacumque parte corporis periculum est.

7 centauriae radicis pondus denarii in tribus cyathis vini bibitur. vettonica herba trita morsui imponitur. agarici oboli quattuor in duobus cyathis aceti mulsi propinantur.

8 aristolochiae radicis pondus denarii in vini hemina saepius bibitur. et ipsa ex aceto contrita imponitur plagae. fimus pecudis recens <in> vino decoctus imponitur.

9 mus discerptus adicitur. viperae morsui viperae cuiuslibet tritum et appositum caput efficacissime prodest. carnibus gallinaceorum discerptorum ita ut tepeant extrahitur venenum.

10 item columbarum cerebrum vel gallinaceorum plagae imponitur. sal cum origano et hyssopo ex melle. fraxini tenerorum foliorum sucus bibitur et ipsa super plagam adiciuntur.

11 Non omittenda theriaca qua Antiochus rex adversus omnes serpentes utebatur praeter aspidem. quae adeo probata est experimentis ut Coi in templo Aesculapii incisa sit in lapide.

12 quam sic componi oportet. opopanacis serpulli mei singulorum binae drachmae, trifolii seminis pondus denarii unius, anethi et feniculi seminis et amuli et apii singulorum pondus denariorum senum, ervi farinae pondus denariorum duodecim.

13 haec singula trita cribrata, deinde mixta ex vino teruntur et digeruntur in pastillos ponderis victoriati, deinde in vaso vitreo ponuntur. cum utendi necessitas venit, singuli pastilli dantur ex vino mixti cyathis tribus.

14 Hominis morsui carnes bubulae, efficacius vituli imponuntur neque ante diem quintum solvuntur. sordes ex humanis auribus inlinuntur plagae.

37 *Against snake- and human-bite*

1 Snakes inflict a dangerous bite. It is easy to heal these, but it is easiest to drive these away with the fumigation of vulture feathers, the smoke of dwarf elder, or the fume of burnt deer horn.

2 It is said that whoever consumed a cooked viper's liver is never struck by snakes. They do not bite those thoroughly anointed with ground rocket with vinegar. Neither snakes nor wild animals approach one while carrying a vulture's heart with himself.

3 Now I will supply remedies for bites. Cultivated radish is boiled in water, and ground, it is applied to the wound. Garlic, roasted with its own leaves and ground, is applied with oil.

4 Applied giant fennel's root is a cure. Millet meal with liquid pitch works best. Ground bitter vetch with vinegar is extraordinarily good for the bites of snakes, of all wild animals, and of man.

5 Unmixed wine is applied in a sponge. Fresh ground mulberry's leaves, if they are dried, decocted, and similarly ground, are applied. Hyssop's seed is drunk.

6 The crown of he who was struck is cut open and *euphorbea* is inserted in it; it heals whichever part of the body where there is danger.

7 The weight of a *denarius* of centaury's root is drunk in three *cyathi* of wine. Ground betony herb is applied to the bite. Four *oboli* of tree fungus are given to drink in two *cyathi* of honeyed vinegar.

8 The weight of a *denarius* of *aristolochia*'s root is frequently drunk in a *hemina* of wine. And itself pounded is applied to the wound with vinegar. Fresh livestock's dung, decocted in wine, is applied.

9 A torn apart mouse is applied. Any viper's head, ground and applied, is most effectively beneficial for a viper's bite. Venom is removed by the flesh of torn apart chickens (applied) while they are warm.

10 Likewise, pigeons' or chickens' brain is applied to the wound. Salt with oregano and hyssop with honey. Juice of an ash tree's tender leaves is drunk and they themselves are applied over the wound.

11 Not omitting the theriac which king Antiochus used against all snakes except asps. Indeed it was so proven by experiments that it was inscribed in stone on the temple of Asclepius on Cos.

12 It ought to be made thus: two *drachmae* each of *opopanax*, tufted thyme, and spignel; the weight of one *denarius* of trefoil's seeds; the weight of six *denarii* each of dill's and fennel's seeds, starch, and *apium*; and the weight of twelve *denarii* of bitter vetch meal.

13 These are ground and sifted alone, then mixed and ground with wine, and divided into pastilles of a weight of a *victoriatus*, then placed in a glass vessel. When it becomes necessary to use these, pastilles are each given, mixed with three *cyathi* wine.

14 Beef flesh, a calf's is more effective, is applied to human-bites and not removed before the fifth day. The filth from a man's ears is smeared on the wound.

38 *contra aspidem*

1   Adversus aspidis morsum unum refugium habebant priores ut percussus urinam suam biberet.

2   intra paucos annos casu inventum est et alterum remedium. namque is qui utrem plenum aceti ferebat percussus ab aspide dolorem non sensit, donec fatigatus requiescendi gratia utrem deposuit.

3   quo facto perniciem sentire coepit, rursusque imposito sibi utre desiit. intellectum est quod, si acetum bibisset, posset sanari. ex eo experimento palam factum est hanc potionem esse efficacissimam.

4   si autem morsum aspidis secutus est sanguis, nulla de eo qui percussus est spes superest.

38 *Against the asp*

1   Forebears had one refuge against an asp's bite: that the struck individual drank his own urine.

2   A few years ago a second remedy was discovered by chance. In fact, one who was struck by an asp while carrying a skin full of vinegar did not feel pain until he put the skin down to take a rest.

3   With this act, he began to feel the bane; again it stopped when he carried the skin. It was thought that if he had drunk the vinegar, he might be cured. From that experiment it is well known that this potion is most effective.

4   However, if blood accompanied the asp's bite, there is no hope left for him who was bitten.

Commentary

Abbreviations used

Editions of the most popular ancient works cited are available in the Loeb Classical Library (Cambridge MA, Harvard University Press), publishing the Greek or Latin text with an English translation. References that read "LCL: *Volume Title*, Page Number" (e.g. LCL: *Celsus II*, 200 or LCL: *Galen Method of Medicine I*, lxxxviii–ix) refer to notes, translations, or introductions in one of these editions. Additional publications of these texts and other sources can be found in the editions referred to below.

Ael. – Aelian
Ael. *NA* – Aelian, *On Animals*.
Brodersen, K. (ed. & tr.) (2018). *Tierleben*. Berlin, De Gruyter.
Ael. *VH* – Aelian, *Historical Miscellany*.
Brodersen, K. (ed. & tr.) (2018). *Vermischte Forschung*. Berlin, De Gruyter.

Aët. – Aëtius
Daremberg, C. & Ruelle, C. E. (eds.) (1897). "Iatricorum Liber XI." *Oeuvres de Rufus d'Ephèse: texte collationné sur les manuscrits, traduit pour le première fois en français, avec une introduction*. Paris, Imprimerie national: 85–126, 568–81.
Kostomiris, G. A. (ed.) (1892). Ἀετίου λόγος δωδέκατος. Paris, Klincksieck.
Olivieri, A. (ed.) (1935). *Aëtii Amideni libri medicinales i-iv*. Leipzig, Teubner.
Olivieri, A. (ed.) (1950). *Aëtii Amideni libri medicinales v-viii*. Berlin, Akademie.
Zervos, S. (ed.) (1901). *Gynaekoloie des Aëtios (Iatricorum Liber XVI)*. Leipzig, Fock.
Zervos, S. (ed.) (1906). "Ἀετίου Ἀμιδηνοῦ περὶ δακνόντων ζῴων καὶ ἰοβόλων." *Athena* 18: 264–92.
Zervos, S. (ed.) (1909). "Ἀετίου Ἀμιδηνοῦ λόγος δέκατος πέμπτος." *Athena* 21: 7–138.
Zervos, S. (ed.) (1911). "Ἀετίου Ἀμιδηνοῦ λόγος δέκατος ἔνατος." *Athena* 23: 273–390.

Alex. – Alexander of Tralles
Alex. *Therap.* – Alexander, *Therapeutica*
Alex. *Lumbric.* – Alexander, *De Lumbricos*
Puschmann, T. (ed.) (1963). *Alexander von Tralles*, Vols. 1–2. Amsterdam, Hakkert.

Antidot. Brux. – *Antidotaria duo codicis Bruxellensis*
Rose, V. (ed.) (1894). "Antidotaria duo codicis Bruxellensis." *Theodori Prisciani Euporiston Libri III cum Physicorum Fragmento et Additamentis Pseudo-Theodoreis*. Leipzig, Teubner: 363–96.

Ps-Apul. – Pseudo-Apuleius
Brodersen, K. (ed. and tr.) (2015). *Apuleius' Heilkräuterbuch/Apulei Herbarius*. Wiesbaden, Marix.
Howald, E. & Sigerist, H. (eds.) (1927). *Antonii Musae De herba Vettonica liber, Pseudo-Apulei Herbarius, Anonymi De taxone liber, Sexti Placiti Liber medicinae ex animalibus*. Leipzig, Teubner: 15–217, 287–98.

Archig. – Archigenes
Brescia, C. (ed.) (1955). *Frammenti medicinali di Archigene*. Naples, Libereria Scientfica Editrice.

Aret. – Aretaeus
Aret. *CA* – *Aretaeus De curatione acutorum morborum* (Books 5–6).
Aret. *CD* – *Aretaeus De curatione diuturnorum morborum* (Books 7–8).
Aret. *SA* – *Aretaeus De causis et signis acutorum morborum* (Books 1–2).
Aret. *SD* – *Aretaeus De causis et signis diuturnorum morborum* (Books 3–4).
Hude, K. (ed.) (1958). *Aretaeus*, 2nd edn. Berlin, Akademie.

Aristophanes of Byzantium, *Epit.* – Aristophanes of Byzantium, *Epitome of On Animals*.
Lampros, S. (ed.) (1885). *Excerptorum Constantini De Natura Animalium libri duo; Aristophanis Historiae Animalium epitome abiunctis Aeliani Timothei aliorumque eclogis*. Berlin, Reimer.

Arist. – Aristotle
Arist. *Hist. an.* – Aristotle, *History of Animals*.
Arist. *Part. an.* – Aristotle, *Parts of Animals*.
Arist. *Gen. an.* – Aristotle, *Generation of Animals*.
Arist. *[Pr.]* – Aristotle, *Problems*.

Cassius – Cassius Felix
Rose, V. (ed.) (1879). *Cassii Felicis De Medicina Ex Graecis Logicae Sectae Auctoribus Liber Translatus*. Leipzig, Teubner.

Cels. – Celsus

Cod. Sang. – Codex Sangallensis
Cod. Sang. 751: A compendium of 39 medical texts (9th Century). St. Gallen, Stiftsbibliothek. Viewed 20 April 2017, <www.e-codices.unifr.ch/en/list/one/csg/0751>.
Cod. Sand. 752: Manuscript compilation: Pliny the Younger's chapter on medicine; Gargilius Martialis, the Medicinae ex oleribus et pomis by Gargilius Martialis; treatise Oxea et chronia passions Yppocratis, Gallieni et Urani; etc. (c. 900 CE). St. Gallen Stiftsbibliothek. <www.e-codices.unifr.ch/en/list/one/csg/0752>.

Crateuas
Wellmann, M. (ed.) (1914). "Fragmenta." *Pedanii Dioscuridis Anazarbei De materia medica libri quinque*. Berlin, Weidmann: 144–6.

Cyran. – Cyranides
Kaimakes, D. (ed.) (1976). *Die Kyraniden*. Meisenheim am Glan, Hain.

Damig. – Damigeron
Abel, E. (ed.) (1881). *Orphei Lithica: Accedit Damigeron De Lapidibus*. Berlin, Apud S. Calvary et Socios: 161–95.
Brodersen, K. (ed. & tr.) (2016). *Heilende Steine/De Lapidibus*. Wiesbaden, Marix.

Diocl. – Diocles of Carystus
van der Eijk, P. (ed.) (2000). *Diocles of Carystus: A Collection of the Fragments With Translation and Commentary, Vol. I*. Leiden, Brill.

Diosc. – Dioscorides
Diosc. *Eup.* – Dioscorides, *Euporista*
Diosc. *MM* – Dioscorides, *De Materia Medica*
Beck, L. (tr.) (2017). *De Materia Medica*. Hildesheim, Olms.
Wellmann, M. (ed.) (1906–14). *Pedanii Dioscuridis Anazarbei De materia medica libri quinque*. Berlin, Weidmann.

Ps-Diosc. – Pseudo-Dioscorides
Ps-Diosc. *Alex.* – Pseudo-Dioscorides, *Alexipharmaca*
Ps-Diosc. *Lapid.* – Pseudo-Dioscorides, *De Lapidus*
Ps-Diosc. *Ther.* – Pseudo-Dioscorides, *Theriaca*
Ruelle, C. (ed.) (1898). "De lapidibus." *Les lapidaries de l'antiquité et du Moyen Age, Vol. 2.1*. Paris, Leroux: 179–83.
Sprengel, K. (ed.) (1830). *Pedanii Dioscorides Anazarbei, Vol. 2*. Leipzig, Knobloch.

DMAC – *De morbis acutis et chroniis.*

Garofalo, I. (ed.) (1997). *Anonymi medici De morbis acutis et chroniis.* Leiden, Brill.

Gal. – Galen

Ad Glauconem de medendi methodo libri ii, K11.1–146.

De alimentorum facultatibus libri iii, K6.453–748.

De antidotis libri ii, K14.1–209.

De compositione medicamentorum per genera libri vii, K13.362–1058.

De compositione medicamentorum secundum locos libri x, K12.378–1007; K13.1–361.

De locis affectis libri vi, K8.1–452.

De methodo medendi libri xiv, K10.

De naturalibus facultibus, K2.101–257.

De sanitate tuenda libri vi, K6.1–452.

De simplicium medicamentorum temperamentis ac facultatibus libri xi, K11.379–892; K12.1–377.

De theriaca ad Pisonem, K14.210–294.

Ps-Gal. – Pseudo-Galen

De fasciis liber, K18a.768–827.

De remediis parabilibus libri iii, K14.311–581.

De theriaca ad Pamphilianum, K14.295–310.

Definitiones medicae, K19.346–462.

Introductio seu medicus, K14.674–797.

Everett, N. (2012). *The Alphabet of Galen: Pharmacy from Antiquity to the Middle Ages: A Critical Edition of the Latin Text With English Translation and Commentary*. Toronto, University of Toronto Press.

Kühn, K. (ed.) (1821–33). *Galeni Opera Omnia*. Leipzig, Knobloch. (the volume number of Kühn's edition is abbreviated as K; this includes works of Galen & Pseudo-Galen).

Leigh, R. (2013). *On Theriac to Piso, Attributed to Galen, a Critical Edition With Translation and Commentary*. Ph.D. Thesis, University of Exeter.

Garg. – Gargilius Martialis

Maire, B. (2002). *Gargilius Martialis: Les Remèdes tirés des légumes et des fruits*. Paris, Les Belle Lettres.

Rose, V. (ed.) (1875). "Medicinae ex Oleribus et Pomis." *Plinii Secundi quae fertur una cum Gargilii Martialis Medicina*. Leipzig, Teubner: 132–208 (the *recensio altera* is printed below the main text).

Ps-Garg. – Pseudo-Gargilius

Lommatzsch, E. (ed.) (1903). "Curae Boum ex Corpore." *P. Vegeti Renati Digesta artis mulomedicinae Accedit Gargili Martialis De Curis Boum Frangmentum*. Leipzig, Teubner: 307–10.

Geopon. – Geoponica
Beckh, H. (ed.) (1895). *Geoponica.* Leipzig, Teubner.

Harpocrat. – Harpocration
Boudreaux, P. (1912). *Catalogus codicum astrologorum graecorum, Vol. 8.3: Codices Parisini.* Brussels, Lamerton: 134–51.

Herod. – Aelius Herodianus
Lentz, A. (ed.) (1965). "De prosodia catholica." *Grammatici Graeci, Vol. 3.1.* Repr. Hildesheim, Olms: 3–547.

Hesych. – Hesychius
Hansen, P. (ed.) (2005). *Hesychii Alexandrini lexicon, Vol. III.* Berlin, De Gruyter.

Hippiatr. – Hippiatrica
Hippiatr. Berol. – Hippiatrica Berolinensia
Hippiatr. Cant. – Hippiatrica Cantabrigiensia
Hippiatr. Paris. – Hippiatrica Parisina
Hoppe, K. & Oder, E. (eds.) (1924–7). *Corpus hippiatricorum Graecorum,* Vols. 1–2. Leipzig, Teubner.

Hippoc. – Hippocrates
Hippoc. *Acut. (Sp.)* – Hippocrates, *Regimen in Acute Diseases (Appendix)*
Hippoc. *Aff.* – Hippocrates, *Affections*
Hippoc. *Aphor.* – Hippocrates, *Aphorisms*
Hippoc. *Art.* – Hippocrates, *On Joints*
Hippoc. *Epid.* – Hippocrates, *Epidemics*
Hippoc. *Fist.* – Hippocrates, *Fistulas*
Hippoc. *Haem.* – Hippocrates, *Haemorrhoids*
Hippoc. *Int.* – Hippocrates, *Internal Affections*
Hippoc. *Liq.* – Hippocrates, *Use of Liquids*
Hippoc. *Morb.* – Hippocrates, *Diseases*
Hippoc. *Morb. mul.* – Hippocrates, *Diseases of Women*
Hippoc. *Morb. Sacr.* – Hippocrates, *On the Sacred Disease*
Hippoc. *Prorrh.* – Hippocrates, *Prorrhetic*
Hippoc. *Reg.* – Hippocrates, *Regimen*
Hippoc. *Reg. Health* – Hippocrates, *Regimen in Health*
Hippoc. *Ulc.* – Hippocrates, *Ulcers*

Isid. – Isidorus Hispalensis
Isid. *Etym.* – Isidorus, *Etymologiae*
Lindsay, W. (ed.) (1911). *Isidori Hispalensis Episcopi Etymologiarum siue Originum libri XX.* Oxford, Clarendon Press.
Migne, J. (ed.) (1850). *De differentiis verborum.* Paris, Garnier.

Iul. Afr. – Iulius Africanus
Wallraff, M. *et al.* (ed.) (2012). *Cesti the Extant Fragments/Iulius Africanus*. Berlin, De Gruyter.

Leo – Leo, *Conspectus medicinae*
Ermerins, F. (ed.) (1963). "Conspectus medicinae." *Anecdota medica Graeca*. Amsterdam, Hakkert: 80–86, 89–217.

Marc. – Marcellus Empiricus
Epist. – Epistula Plinii Secundi ad amicos de medicina (Helmreich 13–14, Liechtenhahn 34–36).
Helmreich, G. (ed.) (1899). *De Medicamentis Liber*. Leipzig, Teubner.
Liechtenhan, E. (ed.) (1968). *De medicamentis liber, post Maximilianum Niedermann Iteratis curis*, 2 vols. Corpus Medicorum Latinorum 5. Kollesch, J. & Nickel, D. (trs.). Berlin, Akademie.

Med. Plin. – Medicina Plinii
Brodersen, K. (ed. & tr.) (2015). *Plinius' Kleine Reiseapotheke*. Stuttgart, Steiner.
Önnerfors, A. (1964). *Plinii Secundi Iunioris qui feruntur De medicina libri tres*. Corpus Medicorum Latinorum III. Berlin, Akademie.
Rose V. (1875). *Plinii Secundi quae fertur una cum Gargilii Martialis medicina*. Leipzig, Teubner.

Metrod. – Metrodora
Del Guerra, G. (ed.) (1953). *Il Libro di Metrodora: sulla malattie delle donne e il recettario di cosmetica e terapia*. Milan, Cheschina.

Mulomed. Chiron. – Mulomedicina Chironis.
Oder, E. (ed.) (1901). *Mulomedicina Chironis*. Leipzig, Teubner.

Ps-Musa – Pseudo-Antonius Musa
Howald, E. & Sigerist, H. (eds.) (1927). *Antonii Musae De herba Vettonica liber, Pseudo-Apulei Herbarius, Anonymi De taxone liber, Sexti Placiti Liber medicinae ex animalibus*. Leipzig, Teubner: 3–11.

Nic. – Nicander
Nic. *Ther.* – Nicander, *Theriaca*
Nic. *Alex.* – Nicander, *Alexipharmaca*
Nicander (1953). *Poems and Poetical Fragments*. Gow, A. & Scholfield, A. (trs.) Cambridge, Cambridge University Press.

Orib. – Oribasius
Orib. *CM* – Oribasius, *Collectionum medicarum*
Orib. *EM* – Oribasius, *Eclogae medicamentorum*

Orib. *Eun.* – Oribasius, *Libri ad Eunapium*

Orib. *Syn.* – Oribasius, *Synopsis ad Eustathium*

Raeder, J. (ed.) (1928–33). *Collectionum medicarum reliquiae, Vols. I-IV (incl. eclogae medicamentorum)*. Leipzig, Teubner.

Raeder, J. (ed.) (1926) *Synopsis ad Eustathium: Libri ad Eunapium*. Leipzig, Teubner.

Orphic *Lithica*

Halleux, R. & Schamp, J. (eds.) (1985). "Lithica kerygmata." *Les lapidaries grecs*. Paris, Les Belles Lettres: 146–77.

Pall. *Agric.* – Palladius, *Opus Agriculturae*

Brodersen, K. (ed. & tr.) (2016). *Das Bauernjahr*. Berlin, De Gruyter.

Rodgers, R. (ed.) (1975). *Palladii Rutilii Tauri Aemiliani viri inlustris Opus agriculturae de veterinaria medicina de insitione*. Leipzig, Teubner.

Pap. Oxy. – Papyrus Oxyrhynchus

Hunt, A. (1911). *The Oxyrhynchus Papyri, Pt. VIII*. London, Egypt Exploration Society.

Paul. Aeg. – Paulus Aegineta

Heiberg, J. (ed.) (1921–4). *Paulus Aegineta, 2 vols*. Leipzig, Teubner.

Paul. Nic. – Paulus Nicaeensis

Ieraci Bio, A. (ed.) (1996). *Paulo di Nicea: Manuele Medico*. Naples, Bibliopolis.

PGM – Papyri Graecae Magicae

Preisendanz *et al.* (1973–4). *Papyri Graecae Magicae: Die griechischen Zauberpapyri*. Stuttgart, Teubner.

Philum. – Philumenus.

Wellmann, M. (ed.) (1908). *Philumeni De venenatis animalibus eorumque remediis*. Leipzig, Teubner.

Physiologus – Physiologus Graecus

Sbordone, F. (ed.) (1976). *Physiologus*. Hildesheim, Olms.

Plac. – Sextus Placitus

Howald, E. & Sigerist, H. (eds.) (1927). *Antonii Musae De herba Vettonica liber, Pseudo-Apulei Herbarius, Anonymi De taxone liber, Sexti Placiti Liber medicinae ex animalibus*. Leipzig, Teubner: 235–86.

Plin. – Pliny the Elder

Mayhoff, K. (ed.) (1892–7). *C. Plini Secundi Naturalis Historiae*, Vols. III-IV. Leipzig, Teubner.

Prom. – Aelius Promotus
Prom. *Coll.* – Aelius Promotus, *Medicinalium Formularum Collectio*
(Δυναμερόν)
Prom. *Ther.* – Aelius Promotus, Περὶ τῶν ἰοβόλων θηρίων καὶ δηλητηρίων
φαρμάκων
Crismani, D. (ed.) (2002). *Elio Promoto Alessandrino, Manuale della salute*
(Δυναμερόν). Alessandria, Edizioni dell'Orso.
Ihm, S. (ed.) (1995). *Der Traktat* περὶ τῶν ἰοβλων θηρίων καὶ δηλητερίων
φαρμάκων *es sog: Aelius Promotus*. Wiesbaden, Reichert.

Ruf. – Rufus Ephesius
Daremberg, C. & Ruelle, C. (eds.) (1879). "De renum et vesicae morbis."
*Oeuvres de Rufus d'Ephèse: texte collationné sur les manuscrits, traduit
pour le première fois en français, avec une introduction.* Paris, Imprimerie
national: 1–63.

Schol. in Opp. – Scholia in Oppianum
Bussemaker, U. (ed.) (1849). "Scholia et paraphrases in Nicandrum et
Oppianum." Dübner, F., *Scholia in Theocritum.* Paris, Didot: 171–449.

Scribon. – Scribonius Largus
Brodersen, K. (ed. & tr.) (2016). *Compositiones*/Der gute Arzt. Wiesbaden, Marix.
Helmreich, G. (ed.) (1887). *Scribonii Largi Compositiones.* Leipzig, Teubner.

Seren. – Quintus Serenus
Brodersen, K. (ed. & tr.) (2017). *Liber medicinalis/Medizinischer Rat.* Berlin,
De Gruyter.
Pépin, R. (ed. & tr.) (1950). *Liber medicinalis.* Paris, Presses Universitaires de
France.
Vollmer, F. (ed.) (1916). *Quinti Sereni Liber medicinalis.* Leipzig, Teubner.

Serv. – Servius Grammaticus
Thilo, G. & Hagen, H. (ed.) (1884). *Servii Grammatici qui Fervuntur in Vergilii
Carmina Commentarii, Vol. II.* Leipzig, Teubner.

Solin. – Solinus
Brodersen, K. (ed. & tr.) (2014). *Collectanea rerum mirabilium/Wunder der
Welt.* Darmstadt, Wissenschaftliche Buchgesellschaft.
Mommsen, T. (ed.) (1895). *C. Iulii Solini Collectanea Rerum Memorabilium.*
Berlin, Weidmann.

Soran. – Soranus
Ilberg, J. (ed.) (1927). *Sorani Gynaeciorum libri IV, De signis fracturarum, De
fasciis, Vita Hippocratis secundum Soranum.* Leipzig, Teubner.
Rose, V. (ed.) (1882). *Sorani Gynaeciorum Vetus Translatio Latina.* Leipzig,
Teubner.

Suda
Adler, A. (ed.) (1931). *Suidae lexicon, Vol. 2*. Leipzig, Teubner.

Suppl. Mag. – Supplementum Magicum
Daniel, R. & Maltomini, F. (1990). *Supplementum Magicum, Vol. 1*. Opladen, Westdeutscher Verlag.

Tatian. – Tatianus
Goodspeed, E. J. (1915). *Die ältesten Apologeten*. Göttingen, Vandenhoeck & Ruprecht: 268–305.

Theod. – Theodorus Priscianus, *Euporista*
Rose, V. (ed.) (1894). *Theodori Prisciani Euporiston Libri III cum Physicorum Fragmento et Additamentis Pseudo-Theodoreis*. Leipzig, Teubner: 1–257.

Ps-Theod. *Ad.* – Pseudo-Theodorus, *Additamenta*
Ps-Theod. *Simp.* – Pseudo-Theodorus, *De Simplici Medicina*
Rose, V. (ed.) (1894). *Theodori Prisciani Euporiston Libri III cum Physicorum Fragmento et Additamentis Pseudo-Theodoreis*. Leipzig, Teubner: 261–359, 403–23.

Theophr. – Theophrastus
Theophr. – Theophrastus, *Enquiry into Plants*

Thessal. – Thessalus
Friedrich, H.-V. (ed.) (1968). *Thessalos von Tralles*. Meisenheim am Glan, Hain.

Veget. *Mulomed.* – Vegetius, *Mulomedicinae*
Lommatzsch, E. (ed.) (1903). *P. Vegeti Renati Digesta artis mulomedicinae Accedit Gargili Martialis De Curis Boum Frangmentum*. Leipzig, Teubner.

Commentary on Book One

Prologus

This prologue is essential to understanding this text; it introduces readers to the author, his biases, and the principles which guided his writing. The prologue also provides a description of what he thought a good "first aid kit" ought to have looked like.

§§1–2. *frequenter – occasionem.*
Comparandum: Marc. *Epist.* 1.
Grassor: used to describe the approach of doctors, this has a negative connotation (including potential overtones relating to attack, ambush, and cunning) which cannot be encapsulated in an English translation.

For how this rhetoric is similar to Pliny's see Doody (2009, 97–100).

Önnerfors (1963, 21) estimated that only one-sixth of the material contained within was sourced from elsewhere than Pliny.

§3. *ante – praestat.*

Comparanda: Plin. 23.40.82; Diosc. *MM* 1.30.2; Marc. *Epist.* 2.

§4. *et – potest.*

Comparanda: Plin. 31.34.67; Marc. *Epist.* 2.

§5. *oxymeli – resolutis.*

Comparandum: Marc. *Epist.* 2.

This recipe significantly differed from Pliny's (23.29.60), using a different honey to vinegar ratio (1:6 instead of Pliny's 1:3) and omitting salt and water. The omission of water might have occurred because it was assumed that people diluted the preparation; compare Galen's comparison between *oxymel* dosages and mixing wine (K6.272).

The omission of salt might suggest the use of a Greek source other than Dioscorides. Galen (K6.272–4) described *oxymel* as made in accordance to the individual patient's taste, and therefore not pre-prepared, but he provided a provisional ratio from which to start: 2:1:4 of honey, vinegar, and water, with the option to use equal parts of honey and vinegar resulting in a 1:1:2 ratio. Paulus Aegineta's recipe (7.11.9) for a simple *oxymel* was one *sextarius* of honey, one *sextarius* of vinegar, and two *sextarii* of water; a 1:1:2 ratio. More complicated and specialised *oxymels* were developed over time in Greek medical literature (e.g. Aët. 3.77–80), but none included salt, so it is possible that the *Medicina Plinii* draws from a Greek tradition.

§5. *thalassomeli – venerimus.*

Comparandum: *Med. Plin.* 2.5.5–6.

§6. *opus – frangitur.*

Comparanda: Plin. 18.14.72–3; Marc. *Epist.* 2.

Polenta: not the modern grain dish, but pearl or peeled barley, possibly prepared as porridge (LCL: *Pliny Natural History V*, 237).

The *Medicina Plinii* simplifies Pliny's directions. Wetting barley and drying it for one night was a process used by Greeks prior to parching and milling. Pliny made no reference to the amount of barley, and no other extant source described this preparation.

§7. *in – sunt.*

Comparanda: Plin. 29.38.128, 29.39.143; Marc. *Epist.* 3.

Pliny did not specify this as a general medical norm, but instead recommended it to treat eyes and ears.

§7. *quo – collo*.
Comparanda: Plin. 29.9.33; Diosc. *MM* 2.73.1; Marc. *Epist.* 3.

§8. *iubemur – ferventi*.
Comparanda: Plin. 29.32.98; Marc. *Epist.* 3.
Argilla: a specialist, white, potters clay.

§9. *omnibus – utemur*.
Comparandum: Marc. *Epist.* 3.

§9. *oportet – X*.
Comparanda: Plin. 21.109.185; Marc. *"Item de ponderibus et mensuris medi-camentorum ex libro XXI Plinii Historiarum Naturalium", "De mensuris et ponderibus medicinalibus ex Graeco translatus iuxta Hippocratem"*.
The weights and measures given in the *Medicina Plinii* all derived from Pliny with the exceptions of *cochlear, scripulus*, and the description of a *sextarius* having ten *unciae*. Marcellus described *drachmae* as containing two *cochlearia* and *denarii* containing three *scripuli*. Pliny's exclusion of the smaller measures might have been deliberate given his rhetoric against tiny medicament measures (22.56.118).
Pliny described the post-Neronian silver *denarius* as close enough to the Attic *drachma*, and provided weights based on its weight. The use of the "silver *denarius*" as a base measure in the *Medicina Plinii* might have led to its readers giving incorrect doses because the weight of silver *denarii* changed over time. Nero's *denarius* normally weighed approximately 3.45 grams, whereas the median weight of *denarii* under Commodus (187–92 CE) was 3.06 grams (Butcher & Ponting 2012, 68), its average weight under Gallienus (253–65 CE) was 1.94 grams (Oman 1916, 53), and silver *denarii* had ceased to be produced in the late third century. If readers were relying on circulation coinage, this measuring system was problematic.
Sextarius: 546 millilitres. It contained 12 *cyathi*, eight *acetabuli*, two *heminae*, and 48 *cochlearia*. A *congius* contained six *sextarii*.
Other weights which the author used but did not describe are the Roman pound, *libra* (327.45 grams), which contained 12 *unciae*, and four *quadrans*.

§10. *nunc – capite*.
This general approach was also used by other Latin medical writers including Marcellus and Serenus.

1. *capitis dolori*

The author followed the typical *euporista* "head-to-toe" format, commencing with a chapter devoted to pains of the head. See the Introduction for further details on this approach. Many medical texts differentiated between varieties of head pain (e.g. Cels. 4.23, Marc. 1–3), but the *Medicina Plinii* only provides occasional references to particular types in a single chapter.

§1. *capitis – auriculas.*

Comparanda: Plin. 20.21.45; Marc. 1.59; Ps-Theod. *Ad.* II,14(44).

Porrum sectivum: literally "cut-leek", but identified as chive. Chives were not referred to in Greek literature except once (Diosc. *MM* 2.149.2), leek was instead. Dioscorides (*Eup.* 1.3.1) recommended pouring leek and honey into the nose as a nasal drench.

Nasal drenches were fairly commonly recommended (e.g. Scribon. 7; Aret. *CD* 1.2.6; Gal. K12.582–7).

§1. *veteres – emendantur.*

Comparanda: Plin. 20.27.69; Marc. 1.94, 3.3.

Dizziness was associated with some headaches (e.g. Orib. *CM* 12.π.14; Ps-Theod. *Ad.* II,14(44)), and they shared some treatments (see Aret. *CD* 1.2.4). Beets were more commonly used as a nasal drench (e.g. Scribon. 7; Diosc. *Eup.* 1.3; Gal. K12.582, 585–6).

§1. *in – aceto.*

Comparanda: Plin. 20.20.73; Garg. 12; Marc. 1.92, 3.3; Ps-Theod. *Ad.* II,14(44).

Endive was recommended topically with other medicaments (e.g. Diosc. *Eup.* 1.2.1; Ps-Gal. K14.321; Aët. 6.41; Alex. *Therap.* 1.469).

Vinegar and rose oil used topically were extremely common: alone (e.g. Cels. 2.10.1, 4.2.6; Ps-Gal. K14.315; Cassius 1; Alex. *Therap.* 1.481; Paul. Aeg. 2.43.1; Paul. Nic. 14); and with other medicaments (e.g. Diosc. *Eup.* 1.2.1; *Med. Plin.* 1.1,4,5,7; Orib. *EM* 1.2).

§1. *ocimum – imponitur.*

Comparanda: Plin. 20.48.121; Ps-Apul. 118.1; Marc. 1.74.

Celsus (2.10.1, 2.33.2) described basil as suitable because of its cooling properties.

It was also recommended with rose oil and vinegar (e.g. Diosc. *Eup.* 1.2.1; Orib. *EM* 1.2; Paul. Aeg. 3.4.2).

§2. *ruta – bibitur . . .*

Comparandum: Plin. 20.51.135.

§2. . . . *et – rosaceo.*

Comparandum: Diosc. *Eup.* 1.2.3.

Almost all other authors mixed rue with both rose oil and vinegar for topical applications (e.g. Diosc. *MM* 3.45.3, *Eup.* 1.2.1; Plin. 20.51.135; *Cyran.* 5.16; Gal. K12.514, 550–1; Ps-Gal. K14.516; Garg. 3; Ps-Apul. 9.14; Marc. 1.73, 1.95).

The use of rue was known well enough in society to be punch-line in an epigram (*Anthologia Palatina*, 11.74).

§2. *corona – imponita.*

Comparanda: Plin. 20.54.152; Marc. 1.76; Ps-Theod. *Ad.* II,14(44).

Aëtius (5.118) recommended smelling pennyroyal. Celsus (2.33.2) described
it as cooling, and it was used in numerous ways (e.g. Prom. *Coll.* 5.4; Gal.
K12.520, 564; Ps-Gal. K14.398; Orib. *EM* 1.2; Aët. 6.48; Paul. Aeg. 2.43.1).

§2. *pollinem – alligetur.*

Comparandum: Marc. 1.60.

Fascia pedalis: a bandage measuring a foot (a little under 30 cm), likely in
width rather than length because most head circumferences are greater than
a Roman foot.

Binding the head might reflect a different tradition. Pliny stated that a woman's
"band", *fascia*, relieved headaches (28.22.76); Hippocrates (*Liq.* 1) referenced the use of linen bandages; and Athenaeus (15.675d) referred to wrap-
ping the head as a cure.

§2. *anethum – inguitur.*

Comparanda: Ps-Apul. 122.3; Marc. 1.61.

This might have been a misreading of Pliny (20.73.190) who described boiling *anesum* with oil and pouring drops of this on the head. *Anethum* refers
almost always to dill (*Anethum graveolens*), although it can sometimes be
anise, whereas *anesum/anisum* is anise (*Pimpinella anisum*). Both plants
are members of the *Apiaceae/Umbelliferae* family, but their appearance is
markedly different, so this confusion is the result of the similarity of their
names.

Both anise and dill appear in Greek headache remedies, but dill and its oil was
more common (e.g. Ps-Gal. K14.316; Orib. *EM* 1.1; Aët. 6.42; Paul. Nic. 14).

§3. *serpyllum – temporibus.*

Comparanda: Plin. 20.90.246; Ps-Apul.100.1; Marc. 1.93.

Tufted thyme was used like this with rose oil added to vinegar (e.g. Diosc. *MM*
3.38.2, *Eup.* 1.2.1). It was also recommended with oil (Gal. K12.365; Orib.
Eun. 4.2.7; Aët. 6.48). Its use might be owing to cooling properties (Cels.
2.33.2).

§3. *et – oportet.*

Comparanda: Plin. 23.42.54; Marc. 1.62, 1.77, 1.93.

Almond oil was described as soothing, but not associated with sleep (Diosc.
MM 1.33.2, *Eup.* 1.1; Orib. *EM* 1.1; Cassius 1).

§3. *tempora – inlinuntur.*

Comparanda: Plin. 20.23.54; Garg. 18.

Garlic was also used with rocket seeds for headaches (Gal. K12.587), and
included in two compounds for migraines (Orib. *EM* 1.9; Paul. Aeg. 3.5.6).

§3. *nucleorum – inlinitur.*

Comparanda: Plin. 23.67.132; Garg. 44; Marc. 1.77; Ps-Theod. *Ad.* II,14(44).

Promotus similarly used peach kernels for migraines (*Coll.* 4.2), and they were
  included in compounds (*Coll.* 4.8; Cassius 1).

§3. *nuclei – febre.*

Comparanda: Plin. 23.75.144; Cels. 2.10.2; Ps-Gal. K14.500; Marc. 1.62,
  1.77; Aët. 5.118.

Almond applications and plasters were very popular, but with additional
  materials (e.g. rose oil and vinegar: Diosc. *MM* 1.23.1, *Eup.* 1.2.1–2;
  Gal. K12.553; Orib. *CM* 11.α.44; or other medicaments: Scribon. 3; Gal.
  K12.579, 581; Orib. *EM* 1.2; Aët. 6.50; Paul. Aeg. 3.4.2, 3.4.9).

§3. *bacae – instillantur.*

Comparanda: Plin. 23.80.156; Marc. 1.50, 1.78; Ps-Theod. *Ad.* II,14(44).

Laurel oil and leaves were also used (e.g. Gal. K12.503–4, 588; Orib. *Syn.*
  8.17.1; Alex. *Therap.* 1.475; Paul. Aeg. 3.4.4).

§4. *si – imponitur.*

Comparanda: Plin. 24.10.15; Gal. K12.502–3; Marc. 1.62.

Celsus described cypress as cooling (2.33.4), and he recommended cooling
  plasters for heat-provoked headaches and recognised the sun's role in causing headaches (4.2.3).

§4. *hederae – inlinitur.*

Comparanda: Plin. 24.47.75; Ps-Apul. 99.8; Marc. 1.79.

Celsus (2.33.4) described ivy leaves as cooling; Galen (K12.588) recommended their use in a nasal drench with oil.

More commonly used were ivy berries (e.g. Scribon. 2; Gal. K12.561; Orib.
  EM 1.2; Cassius 1; Alex. *Therap.* 1.491), and ivy juice (e.g. Scribon. 7;
  Diosc. *MM* 2.179.1; Gal. K12.586; Aët. 6.50).

§4. *herba – sedat.*

Comparanda: Plin. 24.106.170; Marc. 1.43; Ps-Theod. *Ad.* II,14(44). Cf. Marc.
  2.20.

This was a magical treatment employing *similia similibus* (like-to-like) to
  choose the plant, then using it as an amulet. The use of red threads to tie on
  amulets was not uncommon (Anon. 2018).

§4. *panacis – perunguitur.*

Comparanda: Plin. 25.84.134; Marc. 1.80.

Panax: any kind of all-heal or woundwort. There were multiple varieties.
  While some texts specified the variety (Theophr. 9.11.2; Diosc. *MM* 3.48.4),
  often it was not (e.g. Gal. K12.555; Orib. *EM* 2.3; Aët. 6.26).

§5. *veratrum – instillatur.*

Comparandum: Plin. 25.89.139.

There are only four other references to the use of hellebore which are in no way similar (Scribon. 10; Diosc. *Eup.* 1.3.1; Gal. K12.584; Aët. 3.27).

§5. *peucedano – unguntur.*

Comparanda: Plin. 25.89.139; Marc. 2.19.

"Pains on one side of the head": migraines.

Sulphurwort was recommended for migraines by Promotus (*Coll.* 4.3), Aëtius (6.50), and (Paul. Aeg. 3.5.4). It was also used for headaches (e.g. Diosc. *MM* 2.78.2; Plin. 32.23.68; Gal. K12.579–81; Orib. *CM* 12.π.14; Cassius 1; Aët. 6.46; Alex. *Therap.* 1.495; Paul. Aeg. 2.4.3).

§5. *ossa – prodest.*

Comparanda: Plin. 29.36.112; Plac. 23.2; Marc. 1.81; Ps-Theod. *Ad* II,14(44).

Magical texts provide variations on this: *Cyranides* (3.9) described hanging them on purple thread from the elbow; *Vulture Epistles* recommended they be worn in deer skin (Mackinney 1943, 495; Cumont 1926, 25).

§5. *gallinaceus – dolentis.*

Comparanda: Plin. 29.36.112; Marc. 1.82.

§6. *surculus – aegro.*

Comparanda: Plin. 29.36.113; Marc. 1.83; Ps-Theod. *Ad.* II,14(44).

The insistence of the author that the patient be ignorant added another magical element to Pliny's advice. Cf. *Medicina Plinii* 3.19.3–4.

§6. *murinarum – inlinitur.*

Comparanda: Plin. 29.36.113; Marc. 1.84.

§6. *cochleae – suspenditur.*

Comparanda: Plin. 29.36.114; Seren. I l. 21; Marc. 1.85.

The author simplified Pliny's directions for this amulet.

§6. *fracto – dolorem.*

Comparanda: Plin. 29.36.114; Marc. 1.86.

§7. *aqua – potetur.*

Comparanda: Plin. 28.46.166; Marc. 1.58.

The non-magical drinking of water was recognised as assisting headaches (e.g. Cels. 4.2.8; Gal. K12.517). It was not often cited, perhaps because it was considered obvious advice. Drinking this three times was likely an attempt to improve the treatment's power by using the magical number three.

§7. *cervini – prodest.*
Comparanda: Plin. 29.46.166 (either vinegar or rose oil); Marc. 1.58.
Galen advised applying burnt deer horn with wine (K12.503–4); Placitus
(1α.3) recommended drinking it with wine and water.

2. *pthiriasi et prurigini [id est pediculos in capite]*

The author shifted from internal pain to the head's external surface conditions,
addressing parasites first, then moving onto other surface conditions of the head.
While the scalp is higher on the body than a headache, standard *euporista* texts
start with headaches before moving on to address parasites and scalp conditions,
just as the author does here and in the following chapter.

While some of the terminology is similar to that used at *Medicina Plinii* 3.27,
the conditions treated are different. In addition to louse-associated conditions,
this chapter addressed dandruff without naming it, incorporating it within "itch".

Pthiriasis/phthiriasis, φθειρίασις: the "the disease of the lice". The term was
used to describe two very different conditions: the fatal disease famously suffered
by the Roman dictator Sulla which corrupted his whole body internally with lice
(Plin. 26.86.128; Plutarch *Sulla*, 36.2–3); or a disorder where lice were "born"
between the eye-lashes (Cels. 6.6.15A). It was believed that lice were generated
within the host's body (Arist. *Hist. an.* 5.31). The placement of the chapter suggests the eye-lash complaint was meant, but treatments included treated both
forms. The Sullan form of the disease was still diagnosed into the 1870s, and
the hypothesis has been advanced that it was a form of burrowing mite which
advances in human hygiene has prevented (Bondeson 1998, 333–4).

Pediculus in capite: head lice.

§1. *pthiriasis – vino.*
Comparanda: Plin. 20.40.102 for dandruff; Marc. 4.1.
Bulbus: often translated as "bulb". Jones (LCL: *Pliny Natural History VI*, 60)
  suggests that Pliny's description of "other bulbs" *ceteri bulbi* at the start
  of his discussion of bulbs was probably a reference to varieties of onions,
  chives, garlic, or similar plants, influenced by the immediately preceding
  discussion of squills. Dalby (2003, 64) points out that this word is erroneously translated as onion.
Sulphur was commonly included in Greek dandruff treatments (e.g. Gal.
  K12.478; Orib. *Syn.* 8.26.2, *Eun.* 4.10.2; Aët. 6.66; Paul. Aeg. 3.3.3), and
  included in a treatment for both *phthiriasis* and dandruff (Orib. *CM* 10.21.2).

§1. *item – inlinuntur.*
Comparanda: Plin. 24.11.18 for *phthiriasis* and dandruff; Diosc. *Eup.* 1.101.1;
  Seren. 3 l. 40, 5 l. 67; Marc. 4.2; *Geopon.* 18.16.2.
Cedar resin was used to remove lice and nits (Diosc. *MM* 1.77.2; Gal. K12.17;
  Orib. *EM* 6.1, *Eun.* 4.11.2; Aët. 1.189; Paul. Aeg. 3.3.8, 7.3.10).

§1. *alium – infricatur.*

Comparanda: Plin. 20.23.53 for *phthiriasis* and dandruff; Marc. 4.2; Ps-Theod. *Ad.* I,6(15).

Soda was a common treatment. It was often included with many of the other medicaments recommended in the *Medicina Plinii* for dandruff and lice (e.g. Cimolian chalk: Aët. 6.73: vinegar: Cels. 6.2.2; sulphur: Plin. 35.50.177; stavesacre: Gal. K12.463; Orib. *Syn.* 4.11.3; Cassius 3; Aët. 6.67).

§1. *farina – purgat . . .*

Comparanda: Plin. 24.120.187; Marc. 4.3.

The author often confused fenugreek for fennel when he read Pliny 24.120.187–8 (cf. *Med. Plin.* 2.21.5, 3.5.3). It recommended *farina feniculi* "meal of fennel" instead of *farina feni*, the term used by Pliny throughout his discussion regarding the use of fenugreek. Rose (1875, 12) went so far as to replace *farina feniculi* with *farina feni graeci* as a result.

Serenus (3 ll. 35–6) recommended fennel, soda, and sulphur.

§1. . . . *et – aceto.*

Comparanda: Seren. 3 ll. 37–8, 5 l. 68.

Furfur can be "bran" or a dermatological condition named after bran; Greek uses a similar naming convention with πίτυρον. This might account for Marcellus' (4.3) corrupted version of this treatment. Bran was occasionally used to treat itch (e.g. Orib. *EM* 77.1; Paul. Aeg. 4.4.1) and dandruff (e.g. Gal. K12.477).

Pliny (23.27.55) recommended the use of vinegar to treat scurf.

§2. *idem – suffusque.*

Comparandum: Plin. 25.84.133 for dandruff.

Pliny also recommended hellebore juice with oil applied to the whole body to treat Sullan *phthiriasis* (26.86.138) and white hellebore juice with milk (25.25.61).

Hellebore (usually white) was recommended elsewhere to treat *phthiriasis* (e.g. Gal. K12.463; Orib. *CM* 10.21.3; Marc. 4.66; Cassius 6; Aët. 6.67) and itch (Orib. *EM* 78.11; Paul. Aeg. 4.4.1).

§2. *hyssopum – pruritibus.*

Comparanda: Plin. 25.87.136; Marc. 4.4.

Hyssop was rarely used. Galen (K12.493) used it in a compound to treat dandruff.

§2. *ova – tollunt.*

Comparanda: Plin. 20.11.47; Marc. 4.5.

For more on *scabies*, see *Medicina Plinii* 3.2.

One Greek dandruff compound treatment included egg, wine, and soda (Gal. K12.496).

§3. *prurigines – inarescat.*

Comparanda: Plin. 29.35.111 for dandruff; Diosc. *MM* 2.78.3–4; Marc. 4.6.

Cimolian chalk (or earth) has been identified as either hydrated magnesium silicate, i.e. talc, of calcium montmorillonite type (Pittinger 1975, 194) or hydrous silicate of aluminium i.e. kaolin (Sparkes 1982, 233).

Cimolian chalk was known for its cleansing properties (Plin. 35.57.198).

Cimolian chalk and bull's bile were also recommended with soda to treat itch (Diosc. *Eup.* 1.124.1), with beet juice for dandruff (Aët. 6.66), and with vinegar for dandruff (Gal. K12.461; Ps-Gal. K14.323).

§3. *lendes – necantur.*

Comparanda: Plin. 31.33.65; Diosc. *MM.* 5.11.1, *Eup.* 1.101.1; Orib. *Eun.* 4.11.3 for *phthiriasis*; Seren. 5 l. 69; Aët. 6.67; Ps-Theod. *Ad.* I,5(12).

Cassius (3) and Oribasius (*Syn.* 5.57.1) described first washing the head with sea water before treatment, and sea water was used with other medicaments by Galen (K12.463). Other recommendations for bathing in sea water relate to the *phthiriasis* occurring on the eyelids (e.g. Ps-Gal. K14.415; Aët. 7.67; Paul. Aeg. 3.22.15).

§3. *item – oleo.*

Comparanda: Plin. 31.46.117; Diosc. *Eup.* 1.101.1; Theod. 1.5.12; Alex. *Therap.* 1.459.

Named after its island of origin, Samos, Samian earth was exported for use medicinally. It might have contained higher amounts of borates which would have been medicinally useful (Photos-Jones *et al.* 2015, 261), but these are not pediculicides.

Samian earth was also used to treat dandruff (e.g. Gal. K12.490; Ps-Gal. K14.325; Aët. 6.68; Paul. Aeg. 3.3.3).

§3. *nitrum – tollit.*

Comparanda: Plin 31.46.122; Marc. 4.7.

While alum was described by Dioscorides (*MM* 5.106.6) as treating both dandruff and lice, it was rarely referred to elsewhere (only Diosc. *Eup.* 1.101.1; Gal. K12.493; Aët. 6.67).

3. *ulceribus in capite manantibus*

The author's shift from itches and *phthiriasis* to weeping head sores here was logical as extreme scratching creates sores on the scalp. This transition might reflect the author's understanding that sores were a complication of itching, but this is not supported by the text.

Ulcus has been translated as "sore", but it can also refer to ulcer (see introductory commentary on *Med. Plin.* 3.2).

Greek medical literature rarely referred to "sores on the head", using instead ἄχωρ, a term commonly translated as scurf or dandruff. A number of treatments for it were referred to in the previous chapter's commentary owing to similarities between conditions. This identification relies upon the correlations between treatments recommended by Pliny and Dioscorides, and Galen's inclusion of ἄχωρ among his discussion of types of sores or ulcers (K12.481).

§1. *ulcera – infestant.*
Comparandum: Marc. 4.8.

§1. *quae – inlinuntur.*
Comparanda: Plin. 28.46.164; Marc. 4.8.
The author misread Pliny's advice that calf bile healed weeping sores, and that calf bile and vinegar removed nits.
Galen (K12.476) also recommended wiping these with bull's urine.

§2. *sevum – est.*
Comparanda: Plin. 29.46.165; Diosc. *Eup.* 1.99.2.
Marcellus (4.9) recorded this as a treatment for *phthiriasis*.

§2. *testarum – inlinuntur.*
Comparanda: Plin. 32.23.68; Marc. 4.10.

§2. *alium – imponitur.*
Comparanda: Plin. 20.23.51; Garg. 18; Marc. 4.11.
Aëtius (6.68) recorded a similar treatment using burnt garlic germander (σκόρδιον) instead of burnt garlic (σκόρδον); it could be a copyist's error.

§2. *menta – siccat.*
Comparanda: Plin. 20.53.148 healing sores on children's heads; Ps-Apul. 121.2.

§3. *oleum – expurgat.*
Comparanda: Plin. 23.42.85; Diosc. *MM* 1.33.2; Marc. 4.12. Cf. *Med. Plin.* 3.4.13.

§3. *galbanum – melle.*
Comparandum: Plin. 24.13.21.
Galbanum: the resinous juice of all-heal, *Ferula galbaniflua*.

§3. *folia – impomuntur.*
Comparanda: Plin. 24.73.118; Diosc. *MM* 4.37.1; Marc. 4.37.1.
Aëtius (6.68) recommended the use of bramble leaves with pine resin.

§3. *misy – superponitur.*
Comparandum: Plin. 34.31.121.
Misy: a form of copper ore found in Cyprus' copper works according to Pliny.
    Spencer (LCL: *Celsus II*, 1938a, lv) identifies it as antimony sulphide, whereas

Beck (2017, 377) describes it as a copper ore. Celsus described it as cleansing (5.5.2), and recommended its use in a compound to treat ulcers (6.6.22). It was included in a compound recommended by Galen (K12.486) for ἄχωρ.

§3. *malva – dessicat.*
Comparanda: Plin. 20.84.224; Diosc. *MM* 2.118.1, *Eup.* 1.99.1; Marc. 4.14.
Human urine was used in the treatment of ἄχωρ (e.g. Aët. 2.108), and mallow was used without urine (e.g. Gal. K12.496; Aët. 6.68).

§§4–5. *omnia – mixtum.*
Comparanda: Marc. 4.15; Ps-Theod. *Ad.* I,6(15).
Spuma agenti: literally "foam of silver" and commonly translated as litharge. This is lead oxide created as a "waste" product during the final stage of silver smelting. For details regarding its production and use see Dioscorides (*MM* 5.87.3–12) and Rehren *et al.* (1999, 299–308).
Cerussa: white lead; lead carbonate or lead acetate. Pliny (34.54.175–6) described its production and toxic nature when consumed.
The combination of litharge and white lead was included in various compounds (e.g. Gal. K12.485–9; Aët. 6.68).

4. *alopeciis*

Like the preceding chapter, this addresses the external surface of the head. This discussion of *alopecia* included a cosmetic focus, beginning a shift from medical concerns to issues of beauty which continued into the subsequent chapter on hair dye.

Alopecia, ἀλωπεκία: named after the skin disease which affected foxes. Celsus (6.4.2) described it as spreading without a defined configuration on the hairy scalp and beard. When fox mange, an infection of *Sarcoptes scabei* mites, transfers to humans it does not affect the hairy parts of the head, so *alopecia* was not fox mange, but looked somewhat like it (Gal. K10.82). The term alopecia today refers to baldness, especially "spot baldness".

§1. *alopeciae – diminuuntur.*
Comparandum: Marc. 6.15.
The author's reference to the price of slaves suggests that he might have been a slave trader. Such a profession would explain his interest in travel; at the time of composition there was a significant slowing in this trade because of the shrinking of the Roman empire which resulted in fewer prisoners of war entering the slave market (Scheidel 2011, 287–310). This change in conditions might have led to more slavers travelling to reduce the use of middlemen and increase their margins.

§1. *itaque – sparso.*
Comparanda: Plin. 20.34.109; Seren. 8 l. 108; Marc. 6.15; Ps-Theod. *Ad.* I,7(18).
Viper was used in other ways (Aët. 6.55; Paul. Aeg. 7.3.4).

§1. *nasturcium – emdendat.*

Comparanda: Plin. 20.50.129; Marc. 6.11; Cassius 5.

When mustard and cress were used together it was normally with other medic-
    aments, especially *thapsia* (e.g. Gal. K12.391; Orib. *Eun.* 4.5.8; Aët. 6.55).

§2. *cydonia – restituunt.*

Comparanda: Plin. 23.54.101; Marc. 6.12.

§2. *roboris – emendant.*

Comparanda: Plin. 24.7.18; Seren. 8 l. 109; Marc. 6.17.

Roboris pilulae: catkins or globules of hard oak. These are similar to oak-gall
    (Plin. 16.10.28–16.11.30; Marc. 6.17) which were used in Greek medicine
    instead (e.g. Gal. K12.402; Orib. *EM* 4.1; Aët. 6.55).

The use of bear fat was extensive (e.g. Diosc. *MM* 2.76.18; *Cyran.* 2.1; Prom.
    Coll. 3.4; Gal. K12.331, K12.399, K12.417; Orib. *EM* 4.1; Aët. 2.152, 6.56;
    Alex. *Therap.* 1.443; Paul. Aeg. 3.1.2, 7.3.18).

§2. *glandis – inlinitur.*

Comparanda: Plin. 24.7.14 (burnt beech-nut and honey); Marc. 6.18.

This inclusion of Cyprian oil (henna oil) might have been the result of the
    author misreading his notes or Pliny, as the next passage from Pliny to
    which the text refers (29.34.106) was preceded with the phrase *cinis cum
    oleo cypro et melle* "ash with Cyprian oil and honey".

§2. *cinis – myrteo . . .*

Comparanda: Plin. 29.34.106; Marc. 6.19.

Burnt hooves applied with vinegar were more common (e.g. Diosc. *MM* 2.44.1,
    Eup. 1.89.3; Gal. K12.341; Alex. *Therap.* 1.443), although ass hooves were
    occasionally used (e.g. Gal. K12.341; Aët. 6.56).

§2. *. . . cinis – liquida.*

Comparanda: Plin. 29.34.107; Diosc. *MM* 2.2.1, *Eup.* 1.89.2; Aët. 2.172,
    6.55–6; Alex. *Therap.* 1.443; Paul. Aeg. 7.3.5; cf. Marc. 6.19.

Pliny described that either the whole hedgehog was burnt to ash and used with
    honey, or just its skin burnt to ash and mixed with liquid pitch; the *Medicina
    Plinii* lacks this nuance.

Burnt hedgehog material was recommended with other medicaments (e.g.
    Cyran. 2.13; Prom. *Coll.* 1.4, 3.12; Gal. K12.413; Ps-Gal. K14.329; Aët.
    6.56).

§3. *gallinacei – inlinitur.*

Comparanda: Plin. 29.34.109; Marc. 6.6.

Cyranides (3.34) recommended dried, smoothed chicken dung applied with
    soda and sweet unguent.

§3. *sandaraca – aceto.*
Comparanda: Plin. 34.55.177; Marc. 6.29.
Sandaraca, σανδαράκη: red arsenic sulphide, sometimes called realgar.
Galen (K12.403) included a mix of red arsenic sulphide, but with soda and material sourced from oaks. Dioscorides (*MM* 5.105.1, *Eup.* 1.89.1) recommended
its use with either pine or turpentine resin. One red arsenic sulphide-based
compound was recorded numerous times (Thessal. *De virtutibus herbarum*
1.12.4; *Cyran.* 2.38; Aët. 8.16; Harpocrat. in Boudreaux 1912, 150).

§3. *fluentem – myrteo.*
Comparanda: Plin. 28.46.166; Marc. 6.20.
Burnt hare belly was also specified with myrtle oil (Prom. *Coll.* 3.13; Plac.
3α.11, 3β.13) Burnt hares' heads were applied with bear fat (Gal. K12.331;
Aët. 2.155).

§3. *fel – inlinitur.*
Comparanda: Plin. 28.46.164; Marc. 6.20.

5. *capillis denigrandis*

Unlike the preceding chapter, this is completely cosmetic. This final discussion
relating to the scalp, might have been placed last to ensure readers understood the
author's medical credentials before reading this.
These treatments mostly worked by affecting how hair grew back. Compare
the logic of this process to the majority of advice provided in the *Medicina Plinii*
relating to depilatories (3.32).

§1. *potest – pertinent.*
Dying hair was rarely discussed for this reason (cf. Gal. K12.439–47).

§1. *sed – recusantium.*
Literary discussions of red hair predominantly related to Scythians and
Germans.

§§2–3. *quemadmodum – abluitur.*
Comparanda: Plin. 20.34.109; *Cyran.* 3.21; Ael. *NA* 1.48; Plac. 27.1; Marc. 7.7.

§3. *sextarius – est.*
Comparandum: Plin. 32.23.67–8 (applied in the sun); cf. Marc. 7.11.

§4. *siliquae – inlinuntur.*
Comparanda: Plin. 22.73.153; Marc. 7.12.
Pliny's use of the verb *inficio* "to stain or dye" implies that this was meant to
colour existing hair. The *Medicina Plinii* alone provides a measurement.

§4. *folia – renascantur*.

Comparanda: Plin. 24.10.15; Diosc. *MM* 1.74.2; Seren. 4 l. 46; Marc. 7.9.

The use of the verb *renascor* "to be reborn" by the author, along with Marcellus' references to grey hair, suggests that this was recommended for grey hair especially.

§4. *spondilio – fiunt*.

Comparanda: Plin. 24.16.26; Marc. 7.1.

Spondilium/spondylium, σφονδύλιον: *Heracleum sphondylium*. It is commonly known by various names including cow's parsnip, bear's-wort, spicknel, and hogweed.

§5. *operae – perunguant*.

Comparanda: Plin. 30.46.134 to prevent grey hair; Seren. 4 ll. 48–9; Marc. 7.8; Ps-Theod. *Ad.* I,2(6).

6. auriculis

The author explicitly acknowledged that this chapter reflected a topical shift in his opening sentence. He did not include anything similar in the following chapter relating to the parotid gland, but its additional subheading, "i.e. swelling which arise below the ears", illustrates that this was a change to focus on a new area of the head moving away from the scalp and hair discussed before.

§1. *proxima – offensam*.

Ear pain was considered to have the potential to cause insanity and thus lead to death (Cels. 6.7.1A).

§1. *scio – occurrerint*.

The suggestion that doctors charged excessively is a continuation of anti-doctor rhetoric. It should be noted that the author did not merely include every treatment in a given portion of Pliny's text; he appears to have used some curatorial process when collating his treatments.

§2. *gari – infunditur*.

Comparanda: Plin. 32.25.78; Marc. 9.14, 9.112. Cf. Marc. 9.36.

Garum: a popular sauce in antiquity made from fermented and salted fish guts.

Galen (K12.637) recommended a similar compound for a foul smell and spreading sore/ulcer within the ear which used the same proportions.

Garum was also used to treat ear pain and inflammation (e.g. Diosc. *Eup.* 1.54.4; *Cyran.* 4.50; Gal. K12.622; Orib. *CM* 10.35.2).

§3. *ad – sunt*.

Comparanda: Plin. 32.25.77; Marc. 9.14; Cassius 28.

Conchiliata/conchyliata, κογχυλιωτός: a rarely used adjective to describe something dyed purple.

§3. *ranarum – tollit.*
Comparanda: Plin. 32.25.78; Marc. 9.96.

§3. *si – prius.*
Comparanda: Plin. 32.25.78; Marc. 9.112.

§3. *sucus – instillatur.*
Comparanda: Plin. 24.47.77 for painful and purulent ears; Ps-Apul. 99.7.
Galen (K12.647) recommended its use for serous ulcerations.
Other ivy juice preparations were recommended by Dioscorides (*MM* 2.179.2,
   Eup. 1.54.1, 1.57.2) and Galen (K12.30).

§4. *mel – exsiccate.*
Comparandum: Plin. 22.50.108 (honey and rose oil alone).
When honey and rose oil were used together, it was often with additional
   medicaments, but not frankincense (e.g. Gal. K12.622; Aët. 5.125).

§4. *parum – gargarizant.*
Comparanda: Plin. 23.28.59 (squill-flavoured vinegar); Marc. 9.125.
See commentary on *Medicina Plinii* 1.13.3 for squill-flavoured vinegar.
Celsus recommended gargling for ear complaints (6.7.4A, 6.7.7C, 6.7.8B).

§4. *auricularum – soluti.*
Comparanda: Plin. 20.40.103–4; Ps-Theod. *Ad.* I,8(21).

§5. *foliorum – instillatur.*
Comparandum: Plin. 24.73.119.
Dioscorides (*Eup.* 1.57.2) recommended bramble leaf juice with oil for sores
   with a discharge.
Juice from bramble stems was more commonly recommended (e.g. Ps-Apul.
   88.1; Marc. 9.85; Ps-Theod. *Ad.* I,8(21)), and unspecified bramble juice was
   recommended for pain (Ps-Gal. K14.551, 404–5).

§5. *fel – purgat.*
Comparanda: Plin. 29.39.133; Ps-Theod. *Ad.* I,8(21).
Pecus: a vague term which can refer to sheep, cattle, or any agricultural livestock. This imprecise terminology likely indicates that the exact source was
   not terribly important; elsewhere both Pliny and the author used more specific language.
Dioscorides (*MM* 2.78.4) considered bull's bile to be stronger than sheep's, but
   they were used for the same treatments.
Bile and honey were used to address hearing difficulties (Ps-Gal. K14.493),
   pain (Gal. K12.634), and to cleanse (Aët. 3.139).

§5. *canini – dolorem* . . .
Comparanda: Plin. 29.39.133; Marc. 9.7; Ps-Theod. *Ad.* I,8(21).

§5. . . . *gravitatem – emendat.*

Comparanda: Plin. 29.30.133; Marc. 9.121.

Gravitas has numerous meanings within a medical context including "heaviness" which likely influenced Jones' decision to translate this as "hardness of hearing" (LCL: *Pliny Natural History VIII*, 267), but can also refer to "offensive" or "fetid-smelling"; terms used to describe some ear complaints. Marcellus understood *gravitas* to mean deafen, as he used *exsurdo* "to deafen" when describing the use of this treatment.

Wormwood was recommended for a range of hearing difficulties (Gal. K12.651, 659; Ps-Gal. K14.332, 405; Aët. 6.80; Alex. *Therap.* 2.95).

§5. *murium – dolorem.*

Comparandum: Plin. 29.39.134.

Cyranides (2.26) recommended mouse ash to treat ear-aches with other medicaments.

§5. *si – instillare.*

Comparanda: Plin. 29.39.134; Diosc. *Eup.* 1.64.1; Marc. 9.124.

§6. *si – inlinitur.*

Comparanda: Plin. 29.39.134; Seren. 12 ll. 178–9; Plac. 31.1; Marc. 9.79; Theod. 1.8.12; Aët. 6.76.

Dioscorides (*MM* 2.151.2) recommended chicken fat used with onion juice for this, or onion juice alone (*Eup.* 1.62.1; cf. Orib. *EM* 10.4).

§6. *deplorata – infunditur.*

Comparanda: Plin. 20.39.135; Marc. 9.125.

Dormice were only occasionally used to treat ears (Scribon. 30; Marc. 9.34).

Strigle: a misspelling of the ablative form of *strigilis*. Spencer (LCL: *Celsus II*, 228) described *strigilis* as a specialised instrument made of horn, but with no evidence; Langslow (1991, 790) suggests that there is no reason to suppose this was not an ad hoc use of the standard bath implement.

For the use of *strigiles* see Celsus (6.7.1C), Scribonius (39), Galen (K12.622–4 ξύστρα), Marcellus (9.1), and Pseudo-Theodorus (*Ad.* I,8(21)).

§6. *valde – instillati.*

Comparanda: Plin. 29.39.135; Diosc. *MM.* 2.67.1; Gal. K12.367; Seren. 12 ll. 171–3; Marc. 9.8, 9.64.

Earthworms were also boiled in rose oil (e.g. *Cyran.* 2.8; Aët. 2.168, 4.12, 6.81), or prepared in other ways (e.g. Gal. K12.367; Ps-Gal. K14.333; Orib. *CM* 10.35.2; Aët. 6.79; Alex. *Therap.* 2.79, 2.97; Paul. Aeg. 3.22.1).

§7. *verberatis – inlinuntur.*

Comparandum: Plin. 20.39.137 (honey with snails for fractured ears).

Snails were used to treat ear bruising (Aët. 6.88), sometimes with myrrh (Diosc. *MM* 1.64.4; *Eup.* 1.63.1), a combination also used for fractures (Gal. K12.664).

§§8–9. *senectus – habet.*

Comparandum: Plin. 29.39.137.

Linteolus: bandages or small linen cloths.

Various prepared unburnt snake's slough was more commonly used (e.g. Diosc. *MM* 2.17.1, *Eup.* 1.54.4; Gal. K12. 651, 622; Orib. *CM* 10.35.4; Marc. 9.102; Aët. 3.139, 6.80).

§9. *membrana – infunduntur.*

Comparanda: Plin. 20.39.139; Plac. 28.5; Marc. 9.95.

Venter: the digestive tracts of chickens include the crop and proventriculus which are composed of multiple layers; it is impossible to determine which was meant.

§9. *blattae – imponuntur.*

Comparandum: Plin. 20.39.139.

Blatta: identified here as cockroach (LCL: *Pliny Natural History III*, 493; LCL: *Pliny Natural History VIII*, 201) on account of its description as "fleeing the light" in Vergil's *Georgics* (4 1. 243, quoted in Columella 9.7.5; Plin. 29.10.28; Isid. *Etym.* 12.8), but this identification is not universal.

Cockroach is more likely in this instance as these were used by Greek doctors to treat ear complaints (Diosc. *MM* 2.36.1, *Eup.* 1.54.4; Gal. K12.632; Ps-Gal. K14.404; Orib. *CM* 10.35.2; Aët. 6.81).

§9. *nitrum – meditur.*

Comparanda: Plin. 31.46.117; Diosc. *MM* 5.113.3; Marc. 9.95.

Pseudo-Theodorus (*Ad.* I,8(21)) recommended this for noise and ringing in the ear.

§10. *sonitus – inmissum.*

Comparandum: Plin. 31.46.117.

The terms *tinnitus* "ringing" and *sonitus* "noise" were probably a differentiation between the natures of the sound heard by the tinnitus sufferer.

To treat tinnitus, soda was more often used with vinegar (e.g. Prom. *Coll.* 75.2; Gal. K12.645; Aët. 3.139), but this combination was also used to address accumulated filth (Plin. 31.46.117).

Galen (K12.645) described the use of soda, myrrh, rose oil, and vinegar to treat tinnitus.

§10. *purulentis – suco.*

Comparandum: Plin. 28.48.173.

§11. *si – sunt.*

Comparandum: Plin. 28.48.173–4.

Dioscorides (*MM* 2.78.3) recommended this to treat ruptured ears.

Other authors recommended sheep's bile rather than bull's (Marc. 9.25; Ps-Theod. *Ad.* I,8(21)). This is hardly surprising given the similarities between the two (Diosc. *MM* 2.78.4).

Galen (K12.648) recommended livestock (πρόβατον) bile with breast milk to treat ears that were ulcerated and discharging serous matter.

Breast milk was commonly used for various ear complaints with a variety of medicaments.

§11. *equini – instillatur*.
Comparanda: Plin. 28.48.174; Plac. 16.13.

§11. *sevem – suco*. . .
Comparanda: Plin. 28.48.175; Marc. 9.12.
Goose fat and basil juice were recommended for ruptured ears (Diosc. *Eup*. 1.55.1), inflammation (Gal. K12.663), and issues outside the ear canal (Aët. 6 .88).

§11. . . . *fel – inditur*.
Comparanda: Plin. 28.48.176; Ps-Gal. K14.334–5; Theod. 1.8.21; Ps-Theod. *Item ad* I,8(21).

§12. *omnibus – est*.
Comparanda: Plin. 28.48.174; Cels. 6.7.1C.
Most medical writers specified that each medicament be used warmed, so this was likely common practice.

§12. *urina – vase*.
Comparanda: Plin. 28.48.173; Plac. 7β.8; Marc. 9.9. Cf. Ps-Theod. *Ad*. I,8(21).

§12. *si – diverso*.
Comparanda: Plin. 28.17.60; Marc. 9.11; Aët. 6.76.
This worked on the principle that the water would be jarred out; Celsus (6.7.9B) also used this principle to remove foreign objects.

§12. *si – creditur*.
Comparanda: Plin. 28.7.37; Marc. 9.107; Ps-Theod. *Ad*. I,8(21)).

7. *parotidibus [id est farcimina quae sub auribus nascuntur]*

This chapter's placement following ear complaints reflects the author's view of the parotid gland in relation to the ear. He moved to the front of the face after this.

The parotid gland is the largest salivary gland and its inflammation is caused by a variety of medical conditions: salivary gland-stones blocking the duct, bacterial infections (including tuberculosis on rare occasions, which might account for similar treatments to those of *strumae* and other superficial abscess types), viral infections (including mumps), and tumours (benign and malignant).

Farcimen: derived from *farcio* "to stuff", this means "sausage". While the phrase "sausages which arise below the ears" certainly evokes a confronting image, it should be understood as "swellings" owing to the medical context.

§1. *raro – curatione*.

The use of surgical intervention generally was debated in antiquity, but the use of the scalpel to treat this was not discussed in extant literature. Celsus (5.28.7A) discussed the comparative results of incision and treatment with medicaments of *strumae*.

§1. *reprimit – inlitus*.

Comparandum: Plin. 20.36.95 (wild cabbage).

Marcellus (15.36) recommended using lower stems and roots of cabbage, either dried or burnt, with old axle-grease.

§2. *lupini – discutiunt*.

Comparanda: Plin. 22.74.154 (wild lupines); Marc. 15.37. Cf. *Med. Plin.* 3.5.2, 3.6.2.

Boiled bitter lupine meal was variously prepared and used (Gal. K12.675–6; Ps-Gal. K14.408; Orib. *Eun.* 4.44.6).

§2. *vitium – dessicant*.

Comparandum: Marc. 15.43.

§2. *apponitur – mulso*.

Comparanda: Plin. 32.25.78; Gal. K12.669, 672; Orib. *Eun.* 4.44.5; Marc. 15.75; Paul. Aeg. 3.23.13.

Cochylium, κογκύλιον: a small mussel or cockle. This shell was considered similar to *murex*. The slight difference between them might account for the variation, yet Dioscorides (*MM* 2.8.1) stated that cockle ash would accomplish the same outcomes as *murex*.

The Greek writers referred to above used old pork fat in place of honey.

§3. *sepiae – medentur*.

Comparandum: Plin. 32.28.88.

Marcellus (15.56) recommended this for *strumae*.

§3. *lini – mitigat*.

Comparandum: Plin. 20.92.249.

The use of linseed and honey was limited; Dioscorides (*Eup.* 1.139.1) recommended this with added goat fat, and Paulus Aegineta (3.23.13) recommended linseed meal with milk and honey.

§3. *ficus – adhibentur*.

Comparanda: Plin. 23.63.122; Garg. 49. Cf. *Med. Plin.* 3.5.2, 3.7.4.

Pliny's preceding explicit reference to figs described them as dried (23.63.121), but it is unclear whether this was how his subsequent advice was to be understood. The author assumed the wine used in Pliny's previous treatment was also used for this.

Variously boiled fig plasters were recommended (e.g. Diosc. *MM* 1.128.2, *Eup.* 1.139.2; Gal. K12.669, 672–3; Ps-Theod. *Ad.* I,9(24)).

§3. *comprimit – melle.*
Comparanda: Plin. 29.39.143 (without honey); Marc. 15.44.
Pigeon dung was used in other ways (Gal. K12.676; Ps-Gal. K14.408).

§4. *noctuae – auriculae.*
Comparandum: Plin. 29.39.143.
Noctua: variously translated as "little owl" or "night owl", this might be Athena's owl (γλαύξ); Dioscorides (*Eup.* 1.139.2) recommended smearing on the brain of that owl.
Marcellus (15.39) recommended the use of preserved "little owl" brain ground up with nard unguent.

§4. *parotidi – inlinuntur.*
Comparanda: Plin. 29.39.143; Marc. 15.72. Cf. *Med. Plin.* 3.6.8.
Multipeda: also called a centipede and millipede according to Pliny (29.39.136).

§4. *creta – siccat.*
Comparanda: Plin. 35.57.195 to stop fluxes; Diosc. *MM* 5.156.1; Gal. K12.669, 673.
Cimolian chalk was also recommended with other medicaments (e.g. Ps-Gal. K14.336; Theod. 1.9.24; Cassius 17; Alex. *Therap.* 2.123).

§5. *plantago – presanat.*
Comparandum: Ps-Apul. 1.20.
While this was likely based on Pliny (25.103.163), he recommended the use of axle-grease with a different herb.
Plantain was more commonly used with salt (e.g. Diosc. *MM* 2.126.2, *Eup.* 1.139.1; Gal. K12.668–70; Ps-Gal. K14.336; Marc. 15.38; Theod. 1.9.24; Cassius 17).

§5. *ursinus – cerae.*
Comparanda: Plin. 28.48.177; Marc. 15.45.
Cyranides (2.1) also recommended bear fat.

§5. *fimo – inlinuntur.*
Comparanda: Plin. 28.48.177; Marc. 15.76.
Axunga: axle-grease made from animal fat, most often pork.
Goat dung was also recommended with vinegar (Diosc. *MM* 2.80.2; Gal. K12.669, 671; Ps-Gal. K14.336, 408) and honey (Plac. 5a.9).

§5. *caput – sanat.*
Comparanda: Marc. 15.67; *Med. Plin.* 3.6.8.

8. epiphoris [hoc est ocularum umoribus]

This chapter shifts the text from the side of the head to the front of the face. Unlike the shift from the scalp to the ear region, the author did not accentuate this shift to chapters devoted to eye-related conditions.

Epiphora, ἐπιφορά: a persistent flow of tears or discharge from the eyes, hence the subheading "this is for humours of the eyes." Latin literature used *epiphora* to refer to multiple conditions featuring rheumy eyes whereas in Greek this was a specific condition. The *Medicina Plinii* sources most of the treatments from Pliny, but they reflect Greek approaches to similar eye conditions.

§1. *cochleae – prosunt.*
Comparanda: Plin. 29.38.118; Gal. K12.322 for rheum.
Snail flesh applied to the forehead dried rheum (Aët. 2.183, 7.98).

§1. *tumores – impositum.*
Comparandum: Plin. 31.47.124–5.
Penicillum: softest variety of sponge. It can also refer to a "roll of lint" (LCL: *Celsus II*, 200) or a "pad of wool" which Spencer (LCL: *Celsus II*, 193) used to translate an eye treatment. The use of *penicilla* in the treatment of eyes was also recommended by Theodorus (1.12.32) and Cassius (29).
Sponges were commonly recommended to treatment the eyes (e.g. Prom. *Coll.* 111.1–2; Orib. *CM* 9.23.14; Aëtius' *Book Seven* mentioned their use 30 times).

§1. *corticis – circumlinitur.*
Comparanda: Plin. 32.24.71 to soothe redness and swelling; Marc. 8. 158.
Ground cuttlefish shell/bone was used to treat various ophthalmic conditions (Diosc. *MM* 2.21.1; Prom. *Coll.* 97.3; Orib. *CM* 14.45.4; *Syn.* 2.31.1).
Breast milk was a common ingredient in eye salves (e.g. Cels. 6.6.8B, 6.6.14; Ps-Gal. K14.341; Orib. *Syn.* 3.122.3, *Eun.* 4.14.3; Alex. *Therap.* 2.7).

§2. *caro – refrigerat.*
Comparanda: Plin. 20.6.11; Garg. 15.
Pepon, πέπων: a type of melon, gourd, pumpkin, or cucumber (a member of the *Cucurbitaceae* family) that was eaten very ripe; its name derived from the Greek for "ripe".
Pliny stated that this was cooling (cucumbers are still used to cool eyes today) and that its flesh was used topically for *epiphora* and pain.
It was used as a plaster for inflammation (Diosc. *MM* 2.135.1, *Eup.* 1.30.1, 1.31.1; Aët. 7.98), and pain (Gal. K12.794).

§2. *alba – imponitur.*
Comparandum: Plin. 20.27.70.
Beet was little used elsewhere and in no manner similar to this (Diosc. *Eup.* 1.31.1; Marc. 8.32; Aët. 7.10).

§2. *eundem – impositi.*

Comparandum: Plin. 20.40.103.

Theodorus (1.12.33) recommended white *bulbus* and honey for ophthalmic
complaints.

§2. *apio – teguntur.*

Comparandum: Ps-Apul. 119.1.

Apium: named for the bees it attracted, this was either parsley or celery.

This appears to be the result of a misreading of Pliny (20.44.112) who recommended *apium* with honey along with fomentation with its juice for eye
conditions, but with bread for *epiphora* of the limbs. Gargilius (*Recensio
altera* 25 Rose 1875, 135)) recommended the use of *apium* leaves with
bread for undefined ophthalmic conditions.

Apium was recommended in other ways for eye conditions (Marc. 8.34;
Theod. 1.12.36). Celery was recommended for ophthalmic complaints (Gal.
K12.795; Ps-Gal. K14.347, 522).

Bread plasters were also common (e.g. Cels. 6.6.1K; Prom. *Coll.* 94.2–3; Gal.
K12.792; Ps-Gal. K14.341, 344; Theod. 1.12.35; Aët. 7.98; Paul. Aeg. 3.22.3).

§2. *ocimo – circumlinuntur.*

Comparanda: Plin. 20.48.121; Diosc. *Eup.* 1.35.1; Ps-Apul. 118.2.

Basil plasters were recommended to address rheumy eyes (Gal. K12.790, 793;
Ps-Gal. K14.345; Theod. 1.12.36). Basil was used in eye salves (*Cyran.*
1.24; Aët. 1.418).

§3. *ruta – dolorem.*

Comparanda: Plin. 20.51.135; Diosc. *MM* 3.45.3, *Eup.* 1.38.1; Ps-Apul. 90.5.

Dioscorides stated this helped severe pain and inflammation, but Pliny stated
that it relieved *epiphora*; perhaps *epiphora* should be understood as painful.

Rue was considered an appropriate medicament for ophthalmic conditions
(Orib. *CM* 14.45.4, *Syn.* 2.31.1), and its juice was used for incipient oph-
thalmia (Prom. *Coll.* 92.1; Ps-Gal. K14.408).

§3. *anethi – inlinitur.*

Comparandum: Plin. 20.74.196.

Dioscorides (*Eup.* 1.32.1) recommended dill root with water to sooth swelling
of the eyes. Promotus (*Coll.* 98.2–3) recommended it in some eye salves.

§3. *papaveris – imponitur.*

Comparanda: Plin. 20.80.209; Ps-Apul. 53.1.

Fructus: "fruit", but likely referred to poppy heads; Pliny recommended poppy
heads in this treatment and the *Medicina Plinii* uses *semen* to refer to poppy
seeds (3.19.4).

Poppy heads were used for rheumy eyes (Gal. K12.793; Ps-Gal. K14.345;
Garg. 19; Paul. Aeg. 7.16.14), and inflammation (Diosc. *Eup.* 1.30.2; Prom.
Coll. 94.5, 94.7; Orib. *Syn.* 8.40.3; Aët. 7.98).

Poppy stems were not commonly recommended; their only potential use without poppy heads was an unclear treatment for rheumy eyes (Theod. 1.12.36).

§3. *lini – circumlinitur.*

Comparandum: Plin. 20.92.249.

Dioscorides (*Eup.* 1.38.1) described this as a treatment for pain and severe inflammation. While frankincense was commonly used, linseed was not (Diosc. *Eup.* 1.32.1).

§4. *siliginis – circumlinuntur.*

Comparandum: Plin. 22.57.119.

Pliny did not specify that the grains be roasted on an iron plate for rheumy eyes. Theodorus (1.12.37) recommended wheat toasted in this manner for scaly ophthalmic eruptions.

Various grains and cereals were commonly used in plasters; see Alexander (*Therap.* 2.61) for their use to treat rheum.

§4. *item – adhibetur.*

Comparandum: Plin. 22.70.142.

Dioscorides (*MM* 2.107.3) recommended this for inflammation.

Lentils were used for various ophthalmic conditions (Gal. K12.798; Ps-Gal. K14.348; Orib. *Syn.* 8.45.1; Theod. 1.12.33; Aët. 7.90; Paul. Aeg. 3.22.26).

§4. *lentisci – suspendunt.*

Aëtius (7.95) included mastic (*Pistacia lentiscus*) in a forehead sticking plaster to address rheum.

Mastic leaves were also applied to the eyes to address inflammation (Diosc. *Eup.* 1.30.1; Plin, 24.28.43) or with other medicaments for rheum (e.g. Prom. *Coll.* 109.1, 109.5; Gal. K12.790–1; Ps-Gal. K14.344).

§4. *mandragorae – sedant.*

Comparandum: Plin. 25.94.147.

Mandrake root was little used for ophthalmic conditions (Gal. K12.795). Mandrake juice was a more common medicament for rheum (e.g. Cels. 6.6.1I; Prom. *Coll.* 96.1; Gal. K12.745), and in salves (Aët. 7.102, 7.106).

§5. *folia – tollunt.*

Comparanda: Plin. 25.95.153; Theod. 1.12.36.

Hemlock was used topically to treat rheumy eyes (Cels. 6.6.1I; Gal. K12.792; Ps-Gal. K14.344; Paul. Aeg. 3.22.5), pain (Gal. K12.748; Aët. 7.102), and to address incipient conditions (Ps-Gal. K14.345).

§5. *anacollima – applicatur.*

Comparanda: Plin. 29.11.39; Plac. 29.2.

Lana non curata: literally "not prepared wool". Pliny described it as not treated with fuller's weed, so was likely still naturally greasy. Most wool used for medicine was this type (*Med. Plin.* Prol. 7).

Anacollima/anacollema, ἀνακόλλημα: an adhesive patch or plaster. These were a common treatment for rheumy eyes, working by compressing the veins of the forehead which were believed to be the source of the discharge (Cels. 6.6.1H).

This treatment might have been a misreading of a popular treatment: a mixture of frankincense, fine wheaten flour, and egg white applied on either wool or fabric (Cels. 6.6.1H; Diosc. *Eup.* 1.34.1; Prom. *Coll.* 109.3; Gal. K12.796; Orib. *Eun.* 4.15.1; Paul. Aeg. 3.22.5). Pliny's and author's use of *pollen turis* "flour of frankincense" might have been a misreading of "frankincense and flour". This treatment was described as an ἀνακόλλημα by Dioscorides, Oribasius, Aëtius, and Paulus Aegineta. Other *anacollemata* were recommended to treat rheumy eyes (e.g. Gal. K12.322, K13.901; Orib. *Syn.* 3.146.1–2; Cassius 29; Aët. 2.183, 7.95; Paul. Aeg. 3.22.5, 7.16.58; Paul. Nic. 32).

Galen referred to another very similar treatment twice (K12.745, 795): myrrh was added and the frankincense, flour, and egg white were placed on linen and wool respectively.

§5. *ovi – praestat.*
Comparanda: Plin. 29.11.39; Diosc. *MM* 2.50.1; Plac. 29.1.
Egg whites were more often used with other medicaments.

§5. *lutea – imponitur.*
Comparandum: Plin. 29.11.42 (cooked yolks).
Celsus (6.6.1K-L) included a similar treatment comprised of an entire egg mixed with honeyed wine and applied on wool to provide a light, cooling, and soothing treatment; it checked rheum but did not dry, and thus prevented eyes from gumming up. Aëtius provided two similar applications: egg mixed with rose oil and wine applied on soft wool to treat inflammation (7.98); and whole beaten egg mixed with honeyed wine on soft wool placed on the eye for suppuration (7.30).

Both raw and cooked yolks were included in various treatments to address rheum (e.g. Gal. K12.745, 792, 796), pain (e.g. Gal. K12.793–4; Ps-Gal. K14.346), and inflammation (e.g. Cels. 6.6.9A; Diosc. *Eup.* 1.38.1; Ps-Gal. K14.341, 346; Theod. 1.12.32; Aët. 7.98; Alex. *Therap.* 2.7).

§6. *caseo – sedantur.*
Comparanda: Plin. 28.47.69; Plac. 5α.6, 5β.11; Marc. 8.40.
Elsewhere, fresh cheese was recommended with *apium* or celery (Diosc. *Eup.* 1.30.2; Gal. K12.792; Ps-Gal. K14.344; Theod. 1.12.35; Paul. Aeg. 3.22.5) and with other medicaments.

§6. *fimus – inlinitur.*
Comparandum: Plin. 28.47.172.

§6. *vulpinam – negant.*

Comparandum: Plin. 28.47.172.

Lippus: a condition of the eyes where they watered or were inflamed, similar to *epiphora*.

Marcellus (8.129) recommended a dried fox tongue amulet to remove white spots from the eyes.

9. oculis suffusis sanguine

This very short chapter continues the discussion of eye complaints. The author's decision to not give the preceding chapter a more generic title and incorporate this advice into it then move directly to nasal conditions is curious.

While this chapter's heading could be translated "for bloodshot eyes", the first treatment listed related to the result of a blow. Given that "bloodshot eyes" is not commonly used today to refer to the result of an injury, this phrase seems unsuitable, even though both "bloodshot eyes" and "eyes suffused with blood" are the result of a conjunctive haemorrhage.

§1. *sanguis – turturis.*

Comparanda: Plin. 29.38.126; Cels. 6.6.39A-B; Diosc. *MM* 2.79.1, *Eup.* 1.37.1; Orib. *Eun.* 4.19.1; Marc. 8.161; Aët. 2.85; Paul. Aeg. 3.22.7, 7.3.1.

In addition to these, the blood of a single bird was sometimes recommended: pigeon blood (Gal. K12.256, 796; Ps-Gal. K14.347; Plac. 30.2; Theod. 1.12.34); turtledove blood (*Cyran.* 3.43).

This treatment's logic was that the vision of these birds was restored following an injury (Cels. 6.6.39A-B).

§1. *superimponi – vino.*

Comparanda: Plin. 29.38.126; Plac. 30.2.

Splenium: a patch or plaster shaped like the spleen.

The use of a woollen pad over the eye following the use of blood is not as well attested (Marc. 8.168).

Celsus (6.6.39B) suggested that a plaster be used after the blood treatment to relieve any inflammation resulting from the injury. This was also recommended by Galen (K12.796) and Pseudo-Galen (K14.347), but after egg was poured in following the application of bird blood.

§1. *et – emendat.*

Comparanda: Plin. 20.51.142; Ps-Apul. 90.5; Marc. 8.165.

10. naribus

This chapter illustrates how the author progressed down the front of the face, moving from the eyes to the nose. This discussion addresses a number of nasal complaints, omitting runny noses, the subject of the subsequent chapter.

§1. *plerumque – saevienti.*

Comparandum: Marc. 10.1.

Apart from this and Marcellus, whose source was the *Medicina Plinii*, ancient
  writers did not consider nosebleeds to be frequently fatal.

§2. *in – obturantur.*

Comparanda: Plin. 20.21.44; Marc. 10.27.

Gargilius (21) recommended chive leaves with other medicaments. Chive juice
  was also recommended with vinegar (Diosc. *MM* 2.149.2; Theod. 1.14.44).

§2. *ruta – indita.*

Comparanda: Plin. 20.51.137; Diosc. *MM* 3.45.3, *Eup.* 1.200.2; Ps-Gal.
  K14.418; Ps-Apul. 90.1; Aët. 6.94; Ps-Theod. *Ad.* I,14(44).

The part of the rue plant and its preparation before placement within the nose
  was variously described.

§2. *eodem – est.*

Comparandum: Plin. 22.15.32.

Marcellus (10.39) recommended nettle root applied to the head.

Variously prepared nettle was also used inside the nostrils (Diosc. *MM* 4.93.1,
  Eup. 1.200.1; Orib. *EM* 86.1; Aët. 6.94).

§3. *semen – continetur.*

The *Medicina Plinii* seems to have erroneously combined three of Pliny's treatments: the application of nettle seed to check flow from the nose (22.15.32);
  wool with rose oil; and stoppering the ears with wool (29.9.31). It is unclear
  whether Pliny's "flow from the nose" was blood, but this treatment was
  separated from the use of nettle root, so it seems unlikely.

Marcellus (10.28) and Pseudo-Theodorus (*Ad.* I,14(44)) recommended this
  stoppering of the ears, and Marcellus (10.28) described stuffing the nostrils
  with wool and rose oil.

Wool was used in the nose in Greek medicine as a method of medicament
  application (e.g. Gal. K13.858; Ps-Gal. K14.418).

§4. *coagulum – infusum.*

Comparanda: Plin. 30.38.112; Marc. 10.29; Ps-Theod. *Ad.* I,14(44).

Rennet was recommended in other ways (e.g. Hippoc. *Acut. (Sp.)* 59; Diosc.
  Eup. 1.200.2).

§4. *adeps – pastillis.*

Comparanda: Plin. 30.38.112; Marc. 10.30.

§4. *prosunt – inlitae.*

Comparanda: Plin. 30.38.112; Marc. 10.24; Ps-Theod. *Ad.* I,14(44).

Variously prepared snails were recommended (Diosc. *Eup.* 1.200.2; *Cyran.*
  4.36; Aët. 6.94).

§5. *graveolentiae – subvenitur.*

Graveolentia: a fetid smell. Fetid smells of the nostrils were acknowledged as
   sometimes being the result of what was called ὄζαινα: a fetid nasal polyp
   (Scribon. 50; Cassius 31; Marc. 10.21).

§5. *sucus – infunditur* . . .

Comparanda: Plin. 24.47.76; Diosc. *MM* 2.179.3, *Eup.* 1.151.1; Ps-Gal.
   K14.402–3, 517; Marc. 10.63; Theod. 1.13.43.

Pliny recommended that the juice be sourced from white ivy.

§5. . . . *aristolochiae – cypero.*

Comparanda: Plin. 25.104.165 for ὄζαινα; Diosc. *Eup.* 1.151.1.

Cyperon: galingal or tumeric. Promotus (*Coll.* 113.1) included it in a compound treatment for ὄζαινα.

There was some confusion among later Latin authors regarding the precise
   nature of this treatment; see below.

Aristolochia was included in a nasal polyp treatment by Aëtius (6.90). See
   commentary on *Medicina Plinii* 2.26.14 for more details about *aristolochia*.

§5. *dracontei – emendat.*

Comparandum: Plin. 25.110.175.

Draconteum/dracontium: poisonous dragon arum, *Dracunculus vulgaris*.

Carcinoma: see commentary on *Medicina Plinii* 3.4.7.

Marcellus (10.62) recommended dragon arum seed, *aristolochia*, galingal, and
   melilot in equal measures to address both a fetid smell and nasal *carcinoma*.
   Pseudo-Apuleius (19.7) also combined dragon arum seed and honey with
   aristolochia and galingal to treat nasal *carcinoma* too. Theodorus (1.13.43)
   described the use of dragon arum juice instead of seed with honey to address
   a fetid small in the nose.

Dragon arum was also recommended to treat nasal polyps by Greek writers,
   using the root or its juice (e.g. Diosc. *Eup.* 1.150.1; Prom. *Coll.* 114.6; Orib.
   EM 12.1; Aët. 6.92).

§5. *dicitur – mularum.*

Comparandum: Marc. 10.60.

This advice was based on Pliny (30.11.31), but he recommended its use to treat
   gravedo "a head cold", not *gravelentia*.

11. destillationi

The author's decision to separate his preceding discussion of nasal complaints
from this chapter implies that he knew the root cause of a runny nose (most commonly a head cold) was different to those conditions outlined before this. Given
the movement of mucus downwards, it was logical to discuss this just prior to
mouth conditions.

Destillatio: commonly defined as rheum or catarrh, but it comes from the Latin verb *destillo* "to drip", and thus refers to a runny nose.

§1. *cinis – salis*.
Comparandum: Marc. 10.72.
Rose (1875, 24) and Önnerfors (1964, 19) state that Pliny 32.21.65 was the
    source of the *Medicina Plinii* for this treatment, but Pliny stated that this ash
    was used to treat uvula and tonsil conditions with honey.

§1. *porri – eduntur*.
Comparanda: Plin. 20.22.49 for *destillatio* related to the chest; Garg. 21; Marc.
    10.72; Ps-Theod. *Ad*. I,14(44).

§2. *caninum – circuligatur*.
Comparanda: Plin. 30.15.46; Marc. 10.73.
Corrigium: any leather thong or shoe-lace, but can also refer to a leash. Pliny's
    reference to *canina cutis* "dog skin" clearly indicated that was a dog-leather
    strap, but the readers of the *Medicina Plinii* could have been confused.
This is a magical treatment, perhaps a form of binding spell.

§2. *ostrea – dantur*.
Comparanda: Plin. 32.21.64; Marc. 10.75.

§3. *oleum – coicitur*.
Comparanda: Seren. 9 ll. 124–5; Marc. 10.74; Ps-Theod. *Ad*. I,14(44).

§3. *in – compescunt*.
Comparanda: Plin. 28.9.42; Marc. 10.71.

12. oris vitiis

Moving down the face from the nose, the author addressed a variety of health conditions under the title "Mouth Complaints": halitosis; complaints of the lips and gums; ulcers of the mouth, lips, and tongue; chapped and fissured lips, and a burnt mouth. After this, he worked his way inwards, addressing teeth, uvula, and throat.

§1. *oris – dentes*.
Comparandum: Plin. 30.9.27; cf. *Med. Plin*. 1.12.3.
Sapor: taste or smell.

§1. *admiscent – radices*.
Tamarix maritima: marine tamarisk. Beck (2017, 64) identifies this as *Tamarix
    tetandra*, a salt-tolerant plant that grows well in coastal conditions. *Maratima* might be a superfluous description, but its environment can affect it; it
    accumulates salt from its surrounding soil, so using tamarisk from a coastal
    location would have influenced its salt content (cf. Scribon. 128 advising
    the use of tamarisk by the sea).

§1. *mero – dicitur.*
Comparandum: Plin. 28.14.56.
Pliny recommended the use of cold water to prevent a toothache rather than halitosis.

§2. *folia – vitia.*
Comparanda: Plin. 24.9.14; Marc. 11.9.

§2. *aeque – nascuntur.*
Comparanda: Plin. 24.73.117; Diosc. *MM* 3.37.1, *Eup.* 1.74.1; Seren. 141. 232.
Pliny did not specify how or which part of bramble was to be used; Serenus and Dioscorides' *Euporista* described chewing an unspecified part and in *De Materia Medica*, Dioscorides described chewing bramble leaves to strengthen gums and to cure ἄφθα (for more on this disease see commentary on *Med. Plin.* 1.12.3).
Bramble leaves were recommended for ἄφθα and mouth ulcers (Orib. *Eun.* 2.1β.5; Aët. 1.62).

§2. *eiusdem – continetur.*
Comparanda: Plin. 24.9.14 (root, not shoot); Ps-Apul. 88.5.
All parts of the bramble were considered to be strongly astringent (Gal. K11.848), so swapping one part for another might not have greatly affected the treatment's effectiveness.

§3. *ulcera – commanducatae.*
Comparanda: Plin. 25.89.174; Diosc. *MM* 2.126.3; Ps-Apul. 1.21.
Dioscorides (*Eup.* 1.78.2) also recommended washing the mouth out with plantain juice for ἄφθα. While ἄφθα is commonly translated as oral thrush, it was defined as a superficial mouth ulcer suffered by children (Ps-Gal. K19.441).
Plantain was variously used with other medicaments (e.g. Diosc. *Eup.* 1.75.2; Soran. *Gyn.* 2.51.2; Ps-Theod. (*Ad.* I,15(45))).

§3. *membrana – medetur.*
Comparanda: Plin. 29.11.46; *Cyran.* 3.55; Prom. *Coll.* 79.3; Marc. 11.5; Aët. 8.19.

§3. *oris – infricatus.*
Comparanda: Plin. 30.9.27; Marc. 11.11; cf. *Med. Plin.* 1.12.1.

§4. *linguae – sanant.*
Comparanda: Plin. 30.9.27; Plac. 32.2.
Swallows, often chicks, were more commonly used burnt to ash (Gal. K12.938–9, 943; Orib. *CM* 10.34.4, *Syn.* 3.174.1; Aët. 8.49).

§5. *adversus – mandere. . .*
Comparanda: Plin. 25.90.175; Marc. 11.12.

Galla Syriaca: *galla* is oak-gall (also called oak-apples, gall-nuts, or gall-apples); a growth on oak trees which occurs when the gall wasp inserts her larvae into the tree's shoots or leaf buds. They contain large quantities of tannins. The description *Syriaca* is likely a synonym for *Commagena* which the author used to refer to the best quality oak-gall (see commentary on *Med. Plin.* 2.10.5). Oak-gall was often included in mouth treatments owing to its astringent properties, but not for halitosis.

Serenus (14 l. 233) recommended myrtle and mastic without oak-gall to treat halitosis.

Mastic resin was chewed to address halitosis (Diosc. *MM* 1.70.3), and mastic flower was recommended with wine and myrrh (Orib. *Eun.* 4.55.2).

§5. . . . *vel — vino*.
Comparandum: Plin. 25.90.175.
Myrrh was known to improve halitosis (Diosc. *MM* 1.64.4, *Eup.* 1.80.1), and was used with other medicaments to address this (Orib. *Eun.* 4.55.2; Aët. 8.56).

§6. *eadem – emendantur*.
The combination of ivy berries, cassia, myrrh, and wine is recorded nowhere else.

§§6–7. *hoc – accipit*.
Comparanda: Plin. 23.71.136; Garg. *Recensio altera* 79 (Rose 1875, 196).

Stomachum: the author of the *Medicina Plinii* or an early copyist seems to have mistakenly written *stomachum* "stomach" instead of *stomaticen*, "a specialist mouth drug". The described preparation relates in no way to the stomach, and Pliny described it as a stomatic.

The *Medicina Plinii* omits dried *omphacium*, unripe grape juice, which Pliny had included. This omission might have been deliberate; Gargilius replaced it with split alum.

Celsus (6.11.5) recorded a similar treatment for ἄφθα prepared from mulberry juice mixed with saffron, myrrh, alum, wine, and honey.

Stomatics featuring mulberries in Greek texts were not as common as those featuring bramble berries (mulberries: Gal. K12.901–2, 920, 949; Ps-Gal. K14.360; Orib. *Eun.* 4.68.11; bramble berries: Gal. K12.912–5, 920, 929, 948; Ps-Gal. K14.359; Orib. *Syn.* 3.173.1, *Eun.* 4.68.11); this might explain why a bramble option was added within the manuscript tradition.

§7. *item – accipiet*.
Comparanda: Plin. 23.71.136; Theod. 1.17.50.
The reference to the stomach was likely an error.

§8. *capitis – graveolentiam*.
Comparanda: Plin. 28.49.178; Marc. 11.13.

§8. *ulcera – emendat*.
Comparanda: Plin. 28.50.185; Marc. 11.8.

Goose fat was a common ingredient in compounds used to treat chapped or more severely fissured lips (e.g. *Cyran.* 3.51; Prom. *Coll.* 79.1, 79.6; Ps-Gal. K14.424; Orib. *EM* 24.1, *Syn.* 3.180.2, *Eun.* 4.56.2; Aët. 8.19; Paul. Aeg. 3.26.12). Fats derived from cattle were also recommended (Orib. *Syn.* 3.180.2, *Eun.* 4.56.2).

§8. *amurca – subvenit.*
Comparandum: Plin. 23.37.74 for mouth and gum ulcers.
Amurca, ἀμόργη: sometimes referred to as the watery substance pressed out of olives as part of the oil production process (Varro, *Rustica* 1.64), but also referred to as the sediment of pressed olives by Dioscorides (1.102.1; cf. Plin 23.37.74–5). Pliny (15.3.9) also described *amurca* as the bitter, watery fluid which came from pressed olives; this was probably what was understood by the author and his readers.
The author specified the *amurca* from black olives each time he referred to it (1.13.3, 3.24.3), but Pliny only recommended this type to treat chilblains and to foment infants.
Amurca was recommended for ulcerated gums (Diosc. *MM* 1.102.1); swollen gums (Ps-Gal. K14.433); mouth ulcers (Aët. 8.19, 8.42); and chapped lips (Diosc. *MM* 1.102.1; Paul. Aeg. 3.26.12). It was also used with various medicaments for other mouth complaints (e.g. Gal. K12.1000; Orib. *CM* 10.34.4; Paul. Aeg. 3.26.11).

13. dentibus

The text shifts from the mouth generally to the teeth here. With the exception of babies' teething, the topic of the following chapter, this starts the author's move inwards into the oral cavity.

Toothache was considered among the worst pains someone could experience (Cels. 6.9.1), therefore it is not surprising that a significant portion of the *Medicina Plinii* teeth discussion was devoted to it.

§1. *cucurbitae – compressus.*
Comparanda: Plin. 20.8.16; Marc. 12.26; Ps-Theod. *Ad.* I,16(18).
Cucurbita sativa: cultivated *cucurbita* commonly translated as gourd. There are many varieties to which this might refer.
Pliny stated that this treatment was derived from the cultivated *colocynthis* (κολοκυνθίς), a wild κολοκύνθη, round gourd (Diosc. *MM* 4.176.1). Gourds were variously used for toothache (Diosc. *MM* 4.176.2, *Eup.* 1.66.2; Gal. K12.857; Aët. 8.29).

§1. *inula – confirmat.*
Comparanda: Plin. 20.19.38; Ps-Apul. 96.2; Marc. 12.39.
Inula: elecampane, *Inula helenium*.
It was also used for toothache (Prom. *Coll.* 118.2; Aët. 8.30).

§2. *aqua – dentibus.*

Comparandum: Plin. 20.23.53.

Garlic was variously prepared as a mouthwash (Diosc. *MM* 2.152.3; Gal. K12.855, 857; Paul. Nic. 35; *Geopon.* 12.30.3).

§2. *asparagi – mobilitatem.*

Comparanda: Plin. 20.43.111; Marc. 12.39.

Pliny described the juice of the root boiled in wine as healing if it was held in the mouth.

Asparagus which "grew among stones", perhaps wild asparagus (Diosc. *MM* 2.125 RV), treated toothaches (e.g. Diosc. *MM* 2.125.1, *Eup.* 1.66.3; Gal. K11.841; Orib. *Eun.* 2.1α.76; Aët. 1.51; Paul. Aeg. 7.3.1).

§3. *acetum – continet.*

Comparanda: Plin. 23.48.59; Diosc. *MM* 5.17.2, *Eup.* 1.74.1; Marc. 12.27.

The *Medicina Plinii* fails to include that this vinegar was squill-flavoured. Squill-flavoured vinegar was significantly different; it took a minimum of one hundred days to make (Diosc. *MM* 5.17.1–2).

Squill-flavoured vinegar was recommended for inflamed teeth (Paul. Aeg. 3.26.2) and toothache (Ps-Gal. K14.432). Squills and vinegar were used for sore teeth (Gal. K12.856; Ps-Gal. K14.356).

§3. *olivae – stabilit.*

Comparandum: Plin. 23.37.74.

Muria: brine or pickle.

The author misunderstood Pliny's discussion of *amurca* in the same manner as he did at 1.12.8; the additional reference to brine appears nowhere else. It is worth noting that salt was used in the preservation of black olives. Columella (12.50.2) described placing salt over black olives and leaving them to sweat and allowing the *amurca* to drip out in this process. Perhaps the *muria* of black olive *amurca* referred to this material.

§3. *caprifici – dolorem.*

Comparanda: Plin. 23.64.129 (decocted root held in mouth only); Marc. 12.28.

There are few extant references to external applications for toothache: Celsus (6.9.1) recommended hot plasters applied to the jaw in cases of extreme pain.

Wild fig root decoctions were used to address pain prepared with vinegar (e.g. Diosc. *Eup.* 1.66.2; Gal. K12.855; Aët. 8.30; Paul. Aeg. 3.26.2).

§4. *mori – dolori.*

Comparanda: Plin. 23.7.140; Diosc. *MM* 1.126.2, *Eup.* 1.68.2; Marc. 12.57.

§4. *nucleus – medetur.*

Comparanda: Plin. 24.5.10; Diosc. *Eup.* 1.67.1; Marc. 12.58.

Oak-gall was recommended for a variety of dental conditions (Diosc. *MM* 1.107.1, *Eup.* 1.68.2; Gal. K12862; Ps-Gal. K14.356; Orib. *EM* 23.4).

§4. *taedae – continetur.*

Comparanda: Plin. 24.27.41; Diosc. *MM* 1.69.2; Gal. K12.855; Ps-Gal. K14.356; Marc. 12.9; Paul. Aeg. 7.3.4.

Taeda: a torch, but in this context was resinous pine which could be used as a torch.

Shavings were also boiled in wine (Theod. 1.16.46; Cassius 32), or oil (Aët. 8.30), and it was used with additional medicaments (Cels. 6.9.2; Scribon. 58; Gal. K12.857).

§5. *aqua – confirmat.*

Comparanda: Plin. 24.23.42; Diosc. *MM* 1.70.2; Marc. 12.39.

Galen (K12.873–4) recommended chewing Chian mastic.

§5. *ruborum – tenetur.*

Comparanda: Plin. 24.73.119; Marc. 12.63.

Unspecified parts of bramble were chewed to strengthen teeth and gums (Diosc. *Eup.* 1.74.1).

§6. *millefolium – imponitur.*

Comparandum: Marc. 12.7, cf. 12.59.

Millefolium: see commentary on *Medicina Plinii* 3.3.6 regarding the identity of this plant.

Rose (1875, 27) and Önnerfors (1964, 21) state that Pliny (24.95.152) was the source for this treatment, but the two passages have nothing in common except *millefolium* and tooth pain.

§6. *radix – commanducatur.*

Comparanda: Plin. 25.105.165; Cels. 6.9.2; Diosc. *MM* 4.68.5, *Eup.* 1.66.1; Gal. K12.857; Ps-Gal. K14.355; Orib. *Eun.* 4.66.3; Marc. 12.59.

Hyoscyamus ὑοσκύαμος: henbane, *Hyoscyamus niger*.

Henbane root and vinegar was a popular treatment, although Celsus mixed it with vinegar and water while Galen and Pseudo-Galen added honey. Not all authors specified that it be chewed like the author, Pliny, and Marcellus specified.

Henbane was commonly used in classical dental medicine (e.g. Gal. K12.855; Ps-Gal. K14.346; Orib. *Eun.* 4.59.2; Cassius 32; Aët. 8.29–30, 8.35), but the entire plant is toxic with some analgesic properties.

§6. *plantaginis – cohuuntur.*

Comparanda: Plin. 25.105.165; Marc. 12.60.

Decoctions of plantain root, often in vinegar, were recommended (Diosc. *Eup.* 1.66.1; Gal. K11.839; Orib. *Eun.* 2.1α.65; Aët. 1.46).

§7. *quinquefolium – fricare.*

Comparanda: Plin. 25.105.166; Cels. 6.9.2; Scribon. 53; Diosc. *MM* 4.42.2; Gal. K12.856, 879; Orib. *Eun.* 4.59.1.

Fragum: fruit of the strawberry, here describing the fruit of cinquefoil. The description that the plant produced "strawberries", was likely sourced from Pliny 25.62.109.

Quinquefolium: cinquefoil is usually identified as *Potentilla reptans*, creeping/ European cinquefoil. Herbals reference strawberry cinquefoil, also called mock strawberry, and identified as either *Potentilla* or *Duchesnea indica*. The fruit of this plant closely resembles the depiction of strawberries in medieval manuscripts and might be the plant referred to here.

Cinquefoil's preparation differed from author to author: Scribonius, Celsus, Galen, and Oribasius recommended its root decocted in wine; Dioscorides stated that it was decocted to one-third.

Cinquefoil root was also recommended decocted in vinegar (Diosc. *Eup.* 1.66.1; Ps-Gal. K14.523).

§7. *hysopo – conluuntur.*
Comparanda: Plin. 25.105.166; Diosc. *MM* 3.25.2; *Cyran.* 5.20; Gal. K12.856–7; Ps-Gal. K14.496; Orib. *Eun.* 4.59.1.

Hyssop was decocted in either vinegar or wine when its preparation was described.

§8. *cavis – inditur.*
Comparanda: Plin. 30.8.23; Seren. 14 l. 240; Marc. 12.21.

§§8–9. *vermes – testa.*
Comparanda: Plin. 30.8.23; Diosc. *MM* 2.67.1; Seren. 14 l. 243; Marc. 21.31.
Earthworms, their ash and themselves boiled in oil, were recommended by *Cyranides* (2.8), but used differently to the manner described here. Galen (K12.800) recommended sprinkling earthworm ash on food.

§9. *harenula – dolorem.*
Comparanda: Plin. 30.8.24; Marc. 12.34.
"Snails' horns" likely refers to the tentacles on which snail's eyes are positioned.

§10. *idem – alligatus.*
Comparandum: Plin. 30.8.26.
Marcellus (12.61) also recommended raven dung wrapped in wool, but crammed into the cavity.

§10. *inviolate – liquescat.*
Comparanda: Plin. 31.45.101; Marc. 12.21.
Salt prophylactics were recommended, but with other medicaments (Gal. K12.876–7; Orib. *Eun.* 4.64.1). Cassius (32) recorded a similar treatment featuring three grains of salt in the mouth before the sun rose, but it treated rather than prevented a toothache.

§10. *cervina – fricatur.*

Comparandum: Plin. 28.49.178 (burnt deer horn).

The author might have drawn upon a tradition using unburnt deer horn. Burnt or raw deer horn could have been used according to Dioscorides (*Eup.* 1.66.1), so burnt was not necessarily the unspecified standard despite its common usage (e.g. Scribon. 60; Diosc. *MM* 2.59.1, *Eup.* 1.66.1; Gal. K12.890; Seren. 14 l. 235; Plac. 1α.2, 1β.2; Marc. 12.8; Paul. Aeg. 3.27.7).

§11. *tali – est.*

Comparandum: Plin. 28.49.179.

§11. *ossa – praestat.*

Comparanda: Plin. 28.49.179; Seren. 14 ll. 235–6; Marc. 12.32.

Marcellus (13.10) also recommended its use as a toothpowder with nard. Aëtius (8.37) recommended cleaning the teeth with a burnt deer bone.

§11. *caprino – colluuntur.*

Comparanda: Plin. 28.49.182; Seren. 14 ll. 229–30.

Washing teeth with goat's milk was recommended to secure teeth following a blow (Plac. 5β.15; Marc. 12.32; Cassius 32).

§12. *ebulum – teneatur.*

Ebulum: *Sambucus ebulum*, known as danewort, dead-wort, and dwarf elder.

§12. *folia – teneat.*

Boxwood had a limited medicinal use in antiquity (see Plin. 34.35.133) and neither it nor dill (nor anise) appears among dental treatments.

14. dentium infantium

The separation of teething from other tooth-related conditions suggests that the treatments outlined in this and the previous chapter were likely not generic analgesics suitable for any pain, but specific treatments. Teething was rarely discussed in classical literature so while its inclusion might be surprising, the chapter's brevity is not. The positioning of this discussion following teeth was logical, but does not relate to the subsequent chapter devoted to the uvula.

§1. *Dentes – tangant.*

Comparanda: Plin. 28.78.258; Seren. 58 ll. 1031–2; Plac. 16.3; Ps-Theod. *Ad idem* I,16(49).

The use of deciduous horse teeth might have been a purely magical amulet. Tying this around the neck, as described by Serenus, Placitus, and Pseudo-Theodorus, could have allowed the infant to use it to cut their teeth; deciduous horse teeth are sharp enough to cut the inside of a foal's mouth unless they are filed, and there is no evidence for this practice in the Graeco-Roman world (Taylor *et al.* 2018, E6707–15). As an amulet, this used *similia simili-bus* magic; horses lose the first tooth to erupt first like humans.

Magical materials working better when they did not touch the ground were not unusual (see commentary on *Med. Plin.* 3.21.2).

§1. *lacte – perfricantur.*

Comparanda: Plin. 29.78.259; Seren. 58 ll. 1033–4. For hare brain alone: Soran. *Gyn.* 2.49.2, Latin translation 1.134; Gal. K12.874; Orib. *Eun.* 4.63.2; Plac. 3α.16, 3β.25; Paul. Aeg. 1.9.1.

Cerbello: this appears to be *cerebellum* misspelled.

Hare brain softened gums according to Oribasius and Paulus Aegineta.

§2. *delphini – caniculae.*

Comparandum: Plin. 32.48.137.

Canicula: variously translated as "dog-fish", shark, or little dog. This was sourced from Pliny's discussion of marine animal-based treatments so it was likely a type of fish. *Canicula* could endanger people at sea (Plin. 9.70.151–3, 13.50.139), so was likely fairly big. Dog teeth were also used in relation to teething (*Antidot. Brux.* 216).

Pliny's discussion of *canicula* teeth might not have related to teething (his Latin is not clear), so this might be a misunderstanding of how a *canicula*'s tooth was used.

Cyranides (4.15) described hanging a dolphin's tooth around the neck.

§2. *cerebrum – datur.*

Comparanda: Pliny (30.47.135) stated that this brain was extremely useful for teething; Pseudo-Theodorus (*Ad idem.* I,16(49)) recommended rubbing it on the gums like the *Medicina Plinii* recommends using hare brain.

15. *uvae*

This chapter continues the author's movement further inwards within the oral cavity from the teeth. This discussion is followed by chapters devoted to the tonsils and peritonsillar regions of the throat.

Uvula complaints described in classical texts relate to swelling and/or inflammation, or relaxation of the muscles of the soft palate. Inflammation and swelling is caused by viral (commonly colds or *mononucleosis* viruses) or bacterial (commonly strep throat, *Streptococcus pyogenes*) infections. In antiquity it was often thought to result from phlegm descending into it from the head (Hippoc. *Morb.* 2.10). The relaxation of the uvula and the surrounding muscles commonly causes snoring, but can result in blocking the airway, causing sleep apnoea.

§1. *cinis – inlinitur.*

Comparanda: Plin. 32.21.65; Seren. 15 ll. 276–7; Marc. 14.14.

§1. *garum – subicitur.*

Comparandum: Plin. 32.28.90.

While *garum* was not recommended by Greek writers, burnt pickled *mena* heads were (see commentary on *Med. Plin.* 1.17.1).

The use of a spoon to hold a medicament in position was recommended by numerous medical writers (e.g. Gal. K12.944, 962, 983; *Med. Plin.* 1.15.3–4; Orib. *Syn.* 3.176.3, *Eun.* 4.69.5; Aët. 8.43; Paul. Aeg. 3.26.16).

§1. *radicum – reprimit.*

Comparanda: Plin. 20.36.9 (wild cabbage); Seren. 15 ll. 276–7; Ps-Theod. *Ad.* I,17(53).

Cyranides (5.10) also recommended this ash mixed with fat to treat a relaxed uvula.

§1. *cines – levat.*

Comparanda: Plin. 20.73.196; Garg. 28; Seren. 15 ll. 276–7; Ps-Theod. *Ad.* I,17(53).

Levat could mean either "it relieves" or "it lifts". Jones (LCL: *Pliny Natural History VI*, 113) translates *levat* as "relieving an inflamed uvula", but Pliny made no reference to inflammation. If *levat* means "it lifts" the advice of the *Medicina Plinii* would agree with Galen's recommendation to use burnt dill to treat a relaxed uvula (K12.984–5).

§2. *sinape – melle.*

Comparandum: Plin. 20.82.237.

Gargling was a common treatment method (e.g. Hippoc. *Aff.* 4; Gal. K12.973; Ps-Gal. K14.361–2; Orib. *Syn.* 3.176.3, *Eun.* 4.69.5).

§2. *sucus – gargarizatur.*

Comparanda: Plin. 22.15.36; Diosc. *MM* 4.93.2, *Eup.* 1.82.1; Marc. 14.22; Ps-Theod. *Ad.* I,17(53).

§2. *rubi – remedio.*

Comparanda: Plin. 24.73.19; Marc. 14.15.

Other kinds of bramble decoctions were recommended (e.g. Cels. 6.14.1; Gal. K12.960–1, 974; Ps-Gal. K14.360–2; Orib. *Eun.* 4.69.3; Leo 4.8), but not always gargled.

§3. *eorundem – resilit.*

Comparanda: Plin. 24.73.119; Ps-Apul. 88.6; Marc. 14.16; Ps-Theod. *Ad.* I,17(53).

§3. *hirundinis – inlinitur.*

Comparanda: Plin. 30.11.31; Gal. K12.359, 977–8; Marc. 14.17; Aët. 2.195; Ps-Theod. *Ad.* I,17(53). Cf. *Med. Plin.* 1.16.4.

Swallow ash was also recommended without honey (e.g. Diosc. *MM* 2.56.1; Plac. 32.1).

§4. *laseris – cochleario.*

Laser: the juice obtained from the root and stalk of the *silphium* plant (often identified as *Ferula tingitana*) when it was tapped for this purpose (Diosc. *MM* 3.80.2).

The use of *laser* was recommended by Pliny (22.49.104), but its preparation bears no resemblance to the advice in the *Medicina Plinii*. Celsus (6.14.2) provided the closest, recommending that *laser* be pounded, cold water added to it, and the resulting liquid placed under the uvula in a spoon.

Dried medicaments were used in spoon treatments (e.g. Gal. K12.962; Orib. *Eun.* 4.69.5), and Aëtius (8.43) might have recommended the use of *laser* in this manner, but his text is not clear. *Laser* was also applied with honey (Diosc. *MM* 3.80.5, *Eup.* 1.82.1; possibly also Gal. K12.984 who included it under an incorrect heading).

§4. *si – est.*

Comparanda: Plin. 30.17.60; Marc. 14.11.

§4. *caesus – emendat.*

Comparandum: Plin. 28.34.132 for bruises.

The author of the *Medicina Plinii* might have thought that the darkening of a swollen uvula, as described by Hippocrates (*Morb.* 2.10), was a form of bruising.

16. tonsillis

Complaints of the tonsils are very similar to those of the uvula, the topic of the previous chapter, with the exception of muscular relaxation, and modern medicine attributes them to the same causes (see introductory commentary on *Med. Plin.* 1.15). This accounts for the comparable treatments included in this chapter and the previous one. In addition to this, some of these remedies were recommended by Pliny for *angina* which the author discussed in the following chapter. As a result, the identification of various throat conditions was fluid, and this explains why some medical writers described general throat treatments.

§1. *quae – prodest.*

Comparandum: Plin. 30.11.31.

Dioscorides (*MM* 2.70.5) and Aëtius (8.48) recommended gargling warm milk and cow's milk respectively for inflamed tonsils.

§§1–2. *fimus – destillationem.*

Comparanda: Plin. 30.11.32 (fig and soda with pigeon dung); Marc. 14.33.

Pliny wrote about the use of the pigeon dung and fig plaster and the use of snails (described at the end of §2, see below) in direct succession. The description of the treatment of "roughness of the throat and catarrh" was addressed by the snail remedy according to Pliny.

Soda was included in a number of treatments (e.g. Orib. *Eun.* 4.70.2; Alex. *Therap.* 2.139); Aretaeus (*CA* 1.7.7) described soda's use externally in a cerate for *angina*.

§2. *alium – gargarizatum.*

Comparanda: Plin. 20.23.52 for *angina*; Marc. 15.30. Cf. *Med. Plin.* 1.17.1.

Pusca: a misspelling of *posca*, a drink made of vinegar and water. This spelling is used consistently throughout the text.

Galen (K12.972) stated that gargling vinegar and water was a common treatment for the tonsils.

§2. *cochleae – potui.*

Comparanda: Plin. 30.11.32; Marc. 14.34.

Passum: commonly translated as raisin wine. Columella (12.39.1–4) described how it was made.

The decision by the author to separate this treatment from the dried fig plaster might indicate something about his process; he did not just write material down directly from his copy of Pliny, and likely took notes prior to composing his text.

§3. *si – levabit.*

Comparanda: Plin. 30.11.32; Seren. 15 ll. 287–8; Marc. 15.21.

Another example of the medico-magical use of crickets is *Medicina Plinii* 3.24.5.

§3. *lacte – gargarizatur.*

Comparanda: Plin. 28.51.189; Marc. 15.68.

The author misread *malva* (mallow) in Pliny as *myrrha* (myrrh).

§4. *tonsillis – inliti.*

Comparanda: Plin. 28.51.189; Plac. 2α.8, 2β.8; Marc. 15.22.

§4. *hirundininis – inlinitur.*

Comparanda: Plin. 30.11.31; Diosc. *MM* 2.56.1; Gal. K12.977; Marc. 15.26; Aët. 8.49; Ps-Theod. *Ad.* I,7(53). Cf. *Med. Plin.* 1.15.3.

Swallow ash also treated *angina* with honey (e.g. *Cyran.* 3.50; Aët. 8.50), and without (Plac. 32.1). For more about this ash see commentary on *Medicina Plinii* 1.17.4.

§5. *lini – gargarizatur.*

Comparanda: Plin. 20.92.249; Marc. 15.31. Cf. *Med. Plin.* 1.17.1.

Pliny described this anise (the author *anesum* as *anethum* as he did at 1.1.2) to treat *angina*. Pliny did not recommend gargling vinegar.

Dioscorides (*MM* 5.13.3) recommended gargling vinegar to check discharges in the throat and to treat *angina*.

Linseed plasters were recommended for inflamed tonsils (e.g. Aët. 8.48), and *angina* (Aret. *CA* 1.7.4; Aët. 8.50; Alex. *Therap.* 2.145).

§§5–6. *rubi – prodest.*
Comparanda: Plin. 24.73.118 for *angina*; Marc. 15.33.
Dioscorides (*MM* 4.37.1) described how to create this medicament, but did not recommend its use for tonsils or *angina*.
Bramble juice prepared differently was included in other treatments (e.g. Gal. K12.973).

§§6–7. *herba – prodest.*
Comparanda: Plin. 24.110.171, 30.12.35; Marc. 15.70.
These treatments appear to be the result of crasis or early corruption within the manuscript tradition. Pliny described the use of a plant which grew on a rural dung-heap with no reference to mice (24.110.171) for *angina*, and that a mouse boiled down with vervain was drunk (30.12.35). Combining the mouse with the dung-heap plant created a completely new treatment.
"A plant which grows on a rural dung-heap" might not have referred to a specific plant, but been similar to a "plant growing on a statue's head" (*Med. Plin.* 1.1.4); if it was meant to be similarly magical, the connection between *angina* or tonsils and rural dung-heaps is not apparent to a modern audience.
Verminaca: a misspelling of *verbenaca* (vervain). A similar misspelling, *verminacia*, appears in an appendix to a codex of Pseudo-Apuleius (*Ad III Herba Verbanaca* 13).
Vervain decoctions were used elsewhere to treat the tonsils (e.g. Diosc. *MM* 4.60.2, *Eup.* 1.81.1; Περί βοτανων των ζ´ ἀστερων in Boudreaux 1912, 161).

§7. *caninum – circumdatur.*
Comparanda: Plin. 30.12.35; Marc. 15.71.
Caninum corrigium might have meant dog leash (see commentary on *Med. Plin.* 1.11.2). The magical use of this might have related to a Greek name for *angina*, κυνάγχη, which also meant "dog collar" or "dog choker".

§7. *fimus – inlinuntur.*
Comparandum: Plin. 30.12.35.

17. angina [id est intra fauces farcimina qua nascuntur]

This chapter concludes the discussion of the oral cavity and throat. Following this, the author moved onto skin complaints originating on the face.
Angina: variously translated, most commonly as quinsy, it is not related to the modern disease called angina. *Angina* was an acute infection of the throat which could cause choking, whereas quinsy has a specific definition today: the collection of purulent material in the peritonsillar space that requires surgical incision and drainage. *Angina* can refer to peritonsillitis or abscesses within

the peritonsillar tissue resulting from failure to treat tonsil infections. Celsus (4.7.1–2) stated that *angina* was called συνάγχη, κυνάγχη, or παρασυνάγχη, depending on the severity of the symptoms, and the Greek terms have been most commonly translated as a sore throat. This crossover between treatments for the tonsils, uvula, and peritonsillar region suggests that doctors were aware of the similarity in their natures.

§1. *menarum – inlinitur.*
Comparanda: Plin. 32.18.90; Marc. 15.69.
Mena/maena, μαίνα: the fish *Spicara maena*.
These were recommended for the uvula by Greek writers (Aët. 2.155; Paul. Aeg. 7.3.10; cf. Gal. K12.333).

§1. *alium – gargarizatur.*
Comparanda: See *Med. Plin.* 1.16.2 and commentary.

§1. *lini – imponitur.*
Comparandum: *Med. Plin.* 1.16.2.
Boiling the material down to one-third was introduced by the author.

§1. *acetum – gargarizatur.*
Comparandum: Seren. 15 l. 278.
Dioscorides (*MM* 5.13.3) recommended gargling vinegar, but did not mention salt. Salt and vinegar were described together by Dioscorides (*MM* 5.109.3) applied with honey and oil.

§2. *nucis – imponitur.*
Comparanda: Plin. 23.77.148; Marc. 15.32.

§2. *pix – inlinitur.*
Comparandum: Plin. 24.23.38; cf. Diosc. *Eup.* 1.82.2.
Pix Bruttia: Bruttian pitch. A resin extracted from pitch-pines by heating, collected in bronze cauldrons, and thickened by mixing vinegar with it (Diosc. *MM* 1.72.5; Plin. 16.21.52–16.22.53).
Dioscorides (*MM* 1.72.1) also recommended pitch alone, while later Greek writers recommended liquid pitch smeared on with soda and old oil (Orib. *EM* 35.3; *DMAC* 6.3).

§2. *fel – succurritur.*
Comparandum: Plac. 31.2.
This treatment appears to be the result of the author partially combining Pliny's recommendation to use goose bile, *elaterium*, and honey (30.12.33) and the use of bull or goat bile with honey (28.51.189), a treatment he correctly included at 1.17.6. Placitus most probably copied this incorrect treatment from the *Medicina Plinii*.

§3. *pullus – facit.*

Comparanda: Plin. 30.12.33; Cels. 4.7.5; Marc. 15.34.

Riparia: sand martin.

Pliny's description of the *silvester* swallow indicates that it was a different
swallow to that which made its nest in homes, and should not be read as
merely referring to a different source location for the same bird.

Celsus included this prophylactic because it was commonly recommended (see
below).

§4. *eosdem – potione.*

Comparandum: Plin. 30.12.34 (swallow ash in bread).

Celsus (4.7.5) also recommended the ash of a burnt swallow which had previously been preserved in salt in a draught of honeyed water. He also stated
that he had not read of this or the swallow prophylactic in any medical
texts, but included it because it was harmless and a common folk remedy.
Strangely, there are numerous references to the use of swallow ash in contemporary or later Greek medical texts (see commentaries on *Med. Plin.*
1.15.3, 1.16.4), and the ash was also included in compounds to treat *angina*
(e.g. Gal. K12.938, 941–3; Orib. *Syn.* 3.174.1; Aët. 8.50).

One-*drachma* doses of dried swallows were also recommended drunk in water
(Diosc. *MM* 2.56.1; Gal. K12.359).

§4. *milipedae – imponitur.*

Aqua mulsa: while this can be translated as "honeyed water", this term was
used to refer to a mead-like beverage made from fermented honey and water
(see Columella 12.12 for details).

This treatment appears to be the result of the author combining Pliny's
recommendation to use millipedes in a one-*hemina* draught of mead to treat
angina (30.12.34) and his preparation of *misy* by cooking it with vinegar
and honey to treat tonsils and *angina* (34.31.121–2). This error explains
why the text failed to include vital details about how the millipede draught
was to be drunk, and why it was described as applied.

§5. *hyssopum – gargarizatur.*

Comparanda: Plin. 26.11.23; Diosc. *MM* 3.25.2, *Eup.* 1.83.1; Orib. *EM* 35.1–2;
Aët. 8.50.

The *Medicina Plinii* fails to include figs in this hyssop decoction as all other
records did. This error might not have rendered the remedy useless as hyssop
decoctions of various kinds were commonly recommended (e.g. Cels. 4.7.3;
Aret. *CA* 1.7.5–6; Ps-Gal. K14.437; Orib. *EM* 35.1–2, *Syn.* 3.174.1; Aët.
8.50; *DMAC* 6.3).

§5. *peucedanum – datur.*

Comparandum: Plin. 26.11.23.

§6. *fel – inliniutr.*

Comparanda: Plin. 28.51.189 (bull or goat bile); Diosc. *MM* 2.78.3, *Eup.* 1.83.1; Plac. 4α.6, 4β.6; Marc. 15.27.

Dioscorides (*MM* 2.78.4) described bear's bile as suitable for the same complaints as bull's, while also stating that bull's bile was more efficacious than that of goats of bears (*MM* 2.78.2).

§6. *ipsius – prodest.*

Comparanda: Plin. 28.10.43; Scribon. 67.

18. lichenis [id est inpetigones]

Having concluded his discussion of the oral cavity, this chapter commenced the author's exposition on dermatological conditions originating on the face. It starts with lichen and is followed by chapters devoted to *elephantiasis* and weeping sores on the face.

Lichen, λειχήν: a disease named for its similar appearance to lichen that grows on stones and trees. It has been identified variously as ringworm, psoriasis, or a form of eczema. Pliny claimed that it was introduced to Italy during the reign of Tiberius from Turkey, but lichen is recorded within the Hippocratic Corpus with remedies similar to those given by Pliny and later medical writers (Hippoc. *Morb. mul.* 2.82).

Inpetigo/impetigo: not the modern disease (see commentary on *Med. Plin.* 3.4.5). Celsus (5.27.17) described four kinds of *impetigo*, none of which closely resembled the description in Pliny or the *Medicina Plinii*.

§1. *graeco – immunibus.*

Comparanda: Plin. 26.2.2; Marc. 19.1; Cassius 11.

Mentagra: "chin gout", a pun on *mentum* "chin", where it first appears, and the Greek suffix – *agra* (compare with *podagra*). This term was used occasionally in Greek literature: four times in Galen (K12.839, 841–2) and three times in Aëtius (8.16).

§2. *descendit – furfure.*

Comparanda: Plin. 26.2.2; Marc. 19.1.

Comparisons with *furfur* "bran", was not uncommon for dermatological conditions. See commentary on *Medicina Plinii* 1.2.1.

§2. *Manlius – curandum.*

Comparanda: Plin. 26.3.4: Marc. 19.1.

Manlius Cornutus: *Prosopographia Imperii Romani*[2] 135.

§3. *huic – caprae.*

Comparandum: Plin. 29.30.93.

Uva taminea/taminia: a wild vine which bore grapes similar to the scarlet berry (Plin. 23.13.19). This grape was recommended by Pliny with blister beetles (28.45.161, 30.23.81), but Scribonius (249) recommended these grapes alone.

Cantharis: blister beetles, Spanish fly, or cantharides; extremely poisonous and skin irritants, which Dioscorides described as having ulcerative properties (Diosc. *MM* 2.61.2).

Blister beetles were recommended elsewhere, but mixed with other medicaments to offset the accompanying skin irritation (Gal. K12.839, 841–2, 847; Cassius 11; Paul. Nic. 111).

§3. *murinus – aceto. . .*
Comparanda: Plin. 30.10.29; Marc. 19.17.
Mouse dung was applied with other medicaments (*Cyran.* 2.26; Aët. 8.16).
Vinegar alone was considered helpful (Hippoc. *Morb. mul.* 2.82; Diosc. *MM* 5.13.1).

§3. *. . . cinis – praecipiunt.*
Comparandum: Plin. 30.10.29.
Marcellus (19.1) recommended washing the face with soda prior to using a blister beetle compound.

§4. *inliniunt – marini.*
Comparanda: Plin. 32.26.83; Marc. 19.2.

§4. *delphini – inliniunt.*
Comparandum: Plin. 32.26.83.
This appears to be a crasis of Pliny's recommendations of either stingray liver boiled in oil or the ash of a dolphin applied with water.

§4. *eos – est.*
Comparandum: Plin. 26.3.3.
The association between lichen and kissing was popularly understood (Martial *Epigrams*, 11.98 l. 5). Pliny described the disease as more prevalent within the upper classes because of kissing, and Tiberius tried to ban kissing as a result of it (Suetonius *Tiberius*, 34.2).

§4. *ficulni – inlinuntur.*
Comparanda: Plin. 26.10.21; Marc. 19.3.

§5. *hibisci – quartas.*
Comparanda: Plin. 26.10.21 (undefined glue); Marc. 19.4.
Gluten lupinum: either lupine- or wolf-glue. Glue can be made from both flour and animal skins. It has been translated as lupine-glue only because lupines were more readily available than wolf skins.
Hibiscum: marshmallow, *Althaea officinalis*.

§5. *flos – laudatur*.
Comparanda: Plin. 26.10.22; Marc. 19.4.
Flos: commonly meaning flower, *flos* can also refer to a glue-like substance found in flowers and berries. For this reason, Jones (LCL: *Pliny Natural History VII*, 280–1) chose to translate it as "scum". Kneading lime with a sticky fluid like that found in mistletoe berries seems more probable than trying to knead it with the small mistletoe flower.

§5. *tithymalli – adhibetur*.
Comparanda: Plin. 26.10.22, cf. 26.39.64; Ps-Apul. 109.4.
Tithymallus: a form of spurge. Beck (2017, 313) identifies it only as a member of the *Euphorbia* gens.
Pseudo-Theodorus (*Simp.* 125) stated that spurge cured *impetigo*.
Greek authors also recommended the use of spurge to treat lichen (Diosc. *MM* 4.164.4; Gal. K12.142; Orib. *Eun.* 2.1τ.11; Aët. 1.391). Dioscorides went so far as to describe the specific use of its "milky juice", a sticky latex common to *Euphorbiae*, and thus similar to the *flos* described above.

§6. *thapsiae – imponitur*.
Comparandum: Plin. 26.10.22.
Thapsia: *Thapsia garganica*, sometimes translated as "deadly carrot". *Thapsia* only appears once in a compound (Gal. K12.842).

§6. *glutinum – imponatur*.
Comparanda: Plin. 29.50.186; Marc. 19.13.
Glue made from genitals was considered to be of high quality, but was normally sourced from bulls (cf. Plin. 28.71.236).
Glue was also included in compounds with sulphur (Gal. K12.832–3; Aët. 8.16), dissolved in vinegar alone (Diosc. *MM* 3.87.1; Paul. Aeg. 7.3.19), and included in pastilles (Orib. *Syn.* 7.49.10, *Eun.* 3.60.1; Paul. Aeg. 4.3.2).
Sulphur was most commonly used with resin (Diosc. *MM* 5.10.7; Gal. K12.217; Orib. *Syn.* 7.49.4, *Eun.* 2.10.10, 3.59.4; Aët. 2.54), and was included in various compounds (e.g. Gal. K12.834; Orib. *EM* 77.2, 78.6, *Syn.* 3.100.1; Aët. 8.16).

§6. *lomentum – aqua*.
Lomentum: a skin-conditioning cosmetic made primarily from bean meal (Plin. 30.43.127; Martial *Epigrams*, 3.42, 14.60); a bean meal (Plin. 18.30.117; Veget. *Mulomed.* 2.127, 3.8.4; Pall. *Agric.* 11.14.9; *Antidot. Brux.* 35, 146); or a chemical lotion made from salt, *misy*, and a particular stone which was burnt with gold, excluding bean meal (Plin. 33.25.85). Bean meal *lomenta* might have included oil (see commentary on *Med. Plin.* 3.6.2).
Pliny (33.25.85) recommended using the chemical *lomentum*. Bean meal was used with various medicaments (Marc. 19.68; Aët. 8.16).

19. elephantiasi

This chapter continued the author's discussion of facial dermatological conditions. Like lichen, the topic of the preceding chapter, this was a specifically named disease, unlike the generic weeping facial sores which follows this.

Elephantiasis is thought to have been a virulent type of leprosy, and cannot be securely identified as lymphatic filariasis which is sometimes called elephantiasis today. Pliny (26.5.7) stated that *elephantiasis* did not occur in Italy prior to the time of Pompey the Great, so most likely in the second quarter of the first century BCE.

§1. *a – manibusque.*
Comparanda: Plin. 26.5.7; Marc. 19.18.
Scabies: see introductory commentary on *Medicina Plinii* 3.26.
Celsus (3.25.1–2) provided a similar description, but did not describe it beginning with the nose.

§2. *hic – populis.*
Comparanda: Plin. 26.5.8; Marc. 19.18.
Lucretius (6 ll. 114–5) and Galen (K11.142) also associated the disease with Egypt.

§2. *totus – temperatur.*
Comparanda: Plin. 26.5.8; Marc. 19.18.
It is impossible to determine Pliny's source. Only Pliny and those who used him as a source described the use of human blood, so it might be part of Pliny's anti-Egypt bias; compare his description of Egypt as the source of diseases like lichen and *elephantiasis*, and of unscrupulous Egyptian doctors who excessively charged to treat them (26.3.4).

§3. *his – inlinitur.*
Comparanda: Plin. 30.29.118; Seren. 10 l. 132; Plac. 20.1; cf. Marc. 19.18.

§3. *radix – apponitur.*
Comparanda: Plin. 20.42.109; Garg. 31; Marc. 19.20.

§3. *mentastri – adhibentur.*
Comparanda: Plin. 20.52.144; Seren. 10 l. 134; Ps-Apul. 91.2; Marc. 19.21.
Mentastrum: identified by Pseudo-Apuleius as καλαμίνθη, a member of the *Calamintha* genus and variety of catmint.
Variously prepared catmint applications were recommended (Gal. K12.5; Orib. *CM* 45.27.13, *Eun.* 2.1κ,4, 3.62.4; Aët. 1.175).

§3. *. . . cedro – inlinuntur.*
Comparanda: Plin. 24.11.19; Diosc. *MM* 1.77.3; Seren. 10 l. 131; Marc. 19.21.
Cedar oil/resin was included in two compound ointments (Orib. *CM* 45.29.75; *DMAC* 51.3), but elsewhere described as taken (Diosc. *MM* 1.77.3, *Eup.* 1.195.1; Orib. *EM* 76.8; Paul. Aeg. 4.1.3).

20. *ulceribus in facie manantibus*

This short chapter concluded the discussion of facial dermatological conditions. The only description of this is the chapter's title, "For weeping sores on the face", so it is impossible to determine why the author left this complaint for last; it has no determinable association with the neck, the topic of the next chapter. For that reason, *elephantiasis* which spread down the body would have been a more logical topic with which to conclude.

Ulcus has been translated here as "sore" because Pliny used the term *vulnus* to describe this complaint in the first treatment provided in the *Medicina Plinii* (see introductory commentary on 3.2).

§1. *bulbi – medentur*.
Comparandum: Plin. 20.40.102.
Serenus (10 l. 135) described this as a treatment of *elephantiasis*.

§1. *nitrum – succurrit*.
Comparanda: Plin. 31.46.120; Marc. 19.55.

§1. *faciem – cygni*.
Comparanda: Plin. 30.10.30; Ps-Theod. *Ad.* I,36(94).

21. *cervicibus et his quae mollienda sunt*

Unlike the preceding dermatological conditions, this chapter returns the text to specific parts of the body, the neck, and the "head-to-toe" approach, as the following chapter's title relates to the shoulder's and sides.

Pliny seems to have been ignorant of the connection between the neck and "those which need to be softened", whereas later Latin medical texts, including the *Medicina Plinii*, were not. Those treatments included by this author, which Pliny described as treating *duritia* which were derived from Dioscorides, were recommended for a specific complaint: σκλήρωμα. Oribasius (*CM* 45.7.1) described this as a fleshy, calloused, hard, sebaceous cyst or *struma* which arose on the neck; he went on to state that these could also appear elsewhere (*CM* 45.7.4; cf. Paul. Aeg. 3.68.1). Σκλήρωμα was a particular complaint in Greek medicine, but Pliny only recognised that its name literally meant "hard", and rather than understanding what it meant medically, he only translated the word as *duritia*, an "induration". This is a word he used to describe numerous conditions unrelated to the neck, glandular swellings, or sebaceous cysts, but some of his treatments addressed these conditions. The placement of these treatments under this heading illustrates that the author understood what this meant in Greek medicine.

§1. *tubera – adeps*.
Comparanda: Plin. 30.33.107; Seren. 15 l. 283; Plac. 25.1; Marc. 18.7.
With the exception of Pliny and Placitus, all texts refer to this treatment as explicitly treating the neck.

§1. *farina – temperatur.*
Comparanda: Plin. 20.92.250; Marc. 18.12.
Pliny did not include wine in his treatment, but he recognised this as treating
indurations of the neck. Pliny's text appears to have been at least partially
based on Dioscorides' treatment of *strumae* (*Eup.* 1.145.4) and was similar
to his treatment of parotid gland swellings (*MM* 2.103.1).
The addition of wine to the mix was likely what made it "emollient-like".

§2. *farina – tusa.*
Comparanda: Plin. 22.58.123; Marc. 18.13.
Pliny made no reference to the neck, and specified the use of dried fig.

§2. *lenticula – discocta.*
Comparanda: Plin. 22.70.144; Diosc. *MM* 2.107.2 for σκλήρωμα and *struma*;
Seren. 15 l. 284. Cf. *Med. Plin.* 3.6.2.

§2. *fici – contrita.*
Comparanda: Plin. 23.63.118 for *strumae*; Marc. 18.8 for neck; Ps-Theod. *Ad.*
I,10(26). Cf. *Med. Plin.* 3.6.3.

§2. *hammoniacum – impositum.*
Comparanda: Plin. 24.14.23; Diosc. *MM* 2.84.2 for σκλήρωμα.
Hammoniacum/Ammoniacum: the incense or gum derived from the latex of
the *Ferula marmarica* produced in the region of the oracle of Ammon, after
which it was named, at Siwah.
The author misread Pliny's text as using honey with the gum to treat indurations, and its use alone to treat calluses (cf. *Med. Plin.* 2.26.6) when it was
the other way around.

§2. *iuniperi – inlinitur.*
Comparanda: Plin. 24.36.54; Ps-Theod. *Ad.* I,10(26).
Pliny stated that juniper seeds matured indurations.

§3. *folio – tumori.*
Comparandum: Plin. 24.46.74.
Alnus: alder.
Aleum: a late spelling of *alium*, garlic.

§3. *ovorum – rosaceo.*
Comparanda: Plin. 20.11.45 (egg, not yolks); Marc. 18.15.

§3. *fel – inlinitur.*
There are no obvious comparanda for this. Pliny (28.51.190) described smearing warm wild boar or ox bile on *strumae*.

§4. *butyro – perfricantur*.
Comparanda: Plin. 28.52.192; Marc. 18.5.

§4. *opisthotoniam – infusa*.
Comparanda: Plin. 28.52.192; Prom. *Coll.* 50.11; Marc. 18.3.
Opisthotonia, ὀπισθοτονία: a rigor of the tendons that draws the head to the shoulder-blades (Cels. 4.6.1). This is a form of tetanus.

§4. *fimus – inlinitur*.
Comparanda: Plin. 28.52.192; Seren. 15 l. 285; Marc. 18.3.

§4. *opisthotonicis – dantur*.
Comparandum: Plin. 30.36.110.

§5. *adeps – dantur*.
Comparanda: Plin. 28.70.234 for indurations on the body; *Cyran.* 2.23.

§5. *in – est*.
Comparanda: Plin. 28.17.60; Seren. 15 ll. 280–2.

22. *umeris et lateribus*

The author's "head-to-toe" approach is continued here, moving from neck complaints to the "shoulders and sides", even though the majority of these ministrations treated pleurisy. This concentration on pleurisy made the subsequent chapter's focus on the breast a part of a logical progression.

Celsus (4.13.1) stated that a lot of side pains were what Greek medical writers called pleurisy (πλευρῖτις), often accompanied by fever, and associated with pneumonia, just as it is today. Some of these treatments might have related to other forms of side pain too, but most automatically translate *dolores laterium* as pleurisy.

§1. *doloribus – inlinitum*.
Comparanda: Plin. 30.13.41 (wax, not egg); Marc. 18.1.

§1. *sal – adicitur*.
Comparanda: Plin. 31.45.102; Marc. 18.2. Cf. *Med. Plin.* 3.30.6.
Dioscorides (*MM* 5.109.2) provided a similar treatment for pain generally.

§2. *haec – sequuntur*.
The salt treatment was also recommended for pleurisy (Aret. *CA* 1.10.11; Cassius 66; Paul. Aeg. 3.33.2; *DMAC* 8.3).

§2. *galbanum – impositum*.
Comparanda: Plin. 24.13.21; Diosc. *MM* 3.83.2.
Galbanum was included in compounds used to treat "sore sides" (e.g. Cels. 5.18.2; Gal. K13.1007; Aët. 8.76).

§2. *cochleae – prosunt.*
Comparandum: Marc. 24.10.

Tisana/ptisana, πτισάνη: either barley gruel or drink made from it that is often translated as "barley water", but is properly called "*ptisana* juice".

The author might have partially based this on Pliny (30.18.53), who recommended snail ash boiled down in *ptisana*.

Aretaeus (*CA* 1.10.8) recommended the consumption of turpentine resin, but with eggs, oil, pine resin, and sulphur.

§3. *cochleae – laudatur.*
Comparandum: Plin. 30.18.53 (hoopoe heart).

§3. *lanae – vetere.*
Rose (1875, 36) and Önnerfors (1964, 29) suggest that this was based on Pliny 29.9.32, but its contents bear no resemblance to this text except for the mention of greasy wool.

Marcellus (18.18) recommended this treatment for shoulder complaints.

Wool was occasionally recommended with oil but with other medicaments (e.g. Aret. *CA* 1.10.10; Orib. *EM* 34.1; Paul. Aeg. 3.33.2). Axle-grease/old fat was used on side pain, but with burnt cabbage stem ash (e.g. Orib. *Syn.* 9.8.2, *Eun.* 4.80.5; Paul. Aeg. 3.33.3).

§4. *vel – excalefaciunt.*
Rose (1875, 36) and Önnerfors (1964, 29) claim that this was based on Pliny 29.10.38, but there are significant differences between the two texts. Pliny stated that clean fleece, with or without sulphur, was used to treat *caeci dolores*, "blind pains", a phrase interpreted by Jones (LCL: *Pliny Natural History VIII*, 206) as a "pain of uncertain locality or origin", not the sides.

Wool and sulphur were recommended as a topical treatment of or fumigant for pleurisy (Cels. 4.13.2; Aret. *CA* 1.20.10; Aët. 8.76).

§4. *vel – excalefaciunt.*
Comparandum: Plin. 34.44.151.

23. *pectori*

While this continues the progression down the body from the preceding title, "For shoulders and sides", it also acts as in introduction for the subsequent chapters. Its list of chest- or lung-related conditions includes those which follow in Book One: coughs (including the expectoration of purulent matter) and bringing up blood; but then mentions tuberculosis, the first chapter of Book Two; and *synache*, a Greek name for *angina* which might have been accidentally listed in the place of *syntexis*, Book Two's second chapter. This list suggests that the separation of Book One from Book Two was introduced by later copyists early within the manuscript tradition, and was not the author's original intent.

24. tussi

The author addressed coughs first following his breast "introductory" chapter. He did not always specify the variety of cough with each treatment addressed. Some ministrations recommended were commonly used to treat coughs which were deemed discrete conditions as well as coughs which were considered symptomatic of other diseases discussed elsewhere, including pleurisy and tuberculosis.

§1. *sedatur – medetur.*
Comparanda: Plin. 20.23.56, 22.69.140; Seren. 16 1. 293; Marc. 16.48; Ps-Theod. *Ad.* II,21(62).
Pliny did not recommend boiled garlic and honey, but this was a remedy for children's coughs (Ps-Gal. K14.441); so the author might have taken this from a Greek source. Eating boiled and/or raw garlic was recommended (Diosc. *Eup.* 2.31.6; Ps-Gal. K14.504; *Geopon.* 12.30.4).

§2. *adversus – ieiunis.*
Comparandum: Plin. 23.30.35 for chronic cough.
Falernian wine: made from grapes grown at the base of Mount Falernus north of Capua. It was a high quality, Italian wine (Plin. 14.8.62; Gal. K6.275). Galen (K11.87) described it as a thin, white wine which was slightly astringent, and it had a high alcohol content (Plin. 14.8.63). Pliny described three varieties; a dry, a sweet, and a light, so perhaps the dry was preferred by Galen.

§2. *ficus – propinatur.*
Comparanda: Plin. 23.63.122 for chronic cough; Diosc. *MM* 1.128.1; Garg. 69.
While common cough medicaments, hyssop and figs were often accompanied by other medicaments when used together (e.g. Plin 26.15.29; Diosc. *Eup.* 2.31.2; Marc. 16.49; Paul. Aeg. 3.28.6; *DMAC* 8.3).

§3. *sunt – siccat.*
Comparanda: Plin. 30.15.46; Ps-Theod. *Ad.* II,21(62).
Pliny specified that they be dried or roasted.

§4. *testae – sorbentur.*
Comparanda: Plin. 30.15.46; Ps-Theod. *Ad.* II,21(62).
Pliny recommended drinking raw snails.

§4. *ad – eduntur.*
Comparandum: Plin. 30.16.49. Cf. *Med. Plin.* 1.25.3.
The *Medicina Plinii* replaces Pliny's first new wine (i.e. from grapes prior to pressing), with saffron.

§5. *sevum – medetur.*
Comparanda: Plin. 30.19.55 for old cough; Marc. 16.50.
Pseudo-Theodorus (*Ad.* II,21(62)) recommended adding old sheep's milk cheese.

§5. *ova – dantur.*
Comparanda: Plin. 29.11.47; Seren. 16 l. 297.

§5. *ova – bibuntur.*
Comparandum: Plin. 20.11.47.
Pliny included an equal measure of oil.

§6. *sandaraca – editur.*
Comparanda: Plin. 34.55.177 (red arsenic sulphide and resin in food); Marc.
    16.51.
The popular egg and sulphur treatment (e.g. Cels. 4.10.4; Diosc. *MM* 5.107.1;
    Ps-Gal. K14.505; Plac. 29.3) might have influenced the choice made by the
    author to give this with a supping egg.
Red arsenic sulphide was included in a number of cough remedies (e.g. Cassius
    33; Paul. Aeg. 3.28.13), but it only occasionally appeared with turpentine
    resin (Aët. 8.61; Alex. *Therap.* 2.179).
Turpentine resin was thought to help coughs (e.g. Diosc. *MM* 1.71.2; Ps-Gal.
    K14.440), but only Paulus Aegineta (2.47.1) advised its use with egg
    elsewhere.

§6. *ursinum – melle.*
Comparandum: Plin. 38.53.193.

§6. *salivae – sanant.*
Comparanda: Plin. 28.53.193; Plac. 16.1; Marc. 16.51; Ps-Theod. *Ad.* II,21(62);
    Antidot. Brux. 77.
This remedy was magical, possibly a transfer spell, as the horse from which the
    saliva was sourced was said to die.

§7. *pulmo – sumendus.*
Comparanda: Plin. 28.53.193; Marc. 16.61.
Pseudo-Galen (K14.444) recorded a very similar treatment for tuberculosis,
    but the dried deer lung and honey were drunk daily.

§7. *sorbitiunculam – dabis.* . .
Comparanda: Plin. 28.68.231 for coughs and tuberculosis; Ps-Theod. *Ad.* II,21
    (62).
Alica, χόνδρος: spelt, emmer groats, or a grain used to make gruel, but because
    of its association with the Greek term, it is often described as a gruel or
    porridge.
This kind of gruel was described by Aretaeus (*CA*. 1. 10.6) as good for pleurisy.

§7. . . . *picem – ovo.*
Comparandum: Plin. 24.24.40 for old coughs and frequent expectorations.
Pliny did not recommend this in egg. Liquid pitch with other medicaments is
    recorded twice (Diosc. *MM* 1.72.1; *Geopon.* 16.11.2).

§7. *iecur – datur*.

Comparandum: Plin. 29.53.193 with wine.

Marcellus (16.39) recommended wolf liver, but given dried or burnt in a specific draught.

Pliny (29.67.230) is recommending wolf liver and wine to treat tuberculosis.

25. *sanguinem reicientibus*

The author continued his discussion of the breast and coughing with this chapter. Spitting, coughing, vomiting, or ejecting blood were sometimes described as a symptom and at other times labelled a discrete condition in medical texts. The treatments included here sometimes addressed both. Tuberculosis and abscesses of the thoracic cavity, especially the pleural membrane (which is discussed in the next chapter), were two of the most common complaints whose symptoms include bringing up blood.

§1. *si – aceto*.

Comparanda: Marc. 16.34; Ps-Theod. *Ad.* II,22(65).

Rose (1875, 38) and Önnerfors (1964, 31) attribute Pliny 24.95.152 as the source for this treatment, but Pliny made no reference to falls or spitting blood.

Bringing up blood as a result of falling from a height was described by Galen (K10.338), perhaps as the result of a ruptured stomach as described by Marcellus.

§1. *cruenta – propinantur*.

Comparanda: Plin. 29.11.43; Plac. 29.15; Marc. 16.35.

§2. *si – hauritur*.

Comparanda: Plin. 20.11.47; Marc. 16.74.

Dioscorides (*MM* 2.50.1) and *Cyranides* (3.55) recommended sipping raw eggs, but with no additives.

§2. *ad – bibuntur*.

Comparanda: Plin. 30.15.44; Marc. 16.75.

Pliny specified that snails be removed from their shells and did not mention cooking them.

Cassius (39) recommended snails well boiled in a moderate amount of vinegar.

§3. *prodest – sunt*.

Comparanda: Plin. 23.54.101; Marc. 16.76; Alex. *Therap.* 2.193; *DMAC* 26.3.

Paulus Nicaeensis (42) added dates.

§3. *cochleae – devorantur*.

Comparanda: Plin. 30.16.49; Marc. 16.75; Ps-Theod. *Ad.* II,22(65).

§3. *cochleae – eduntur.*
Comparandum: Plin. 30.16.49; cf. *Med. Plin.* 1.24.4.

§4. *spongiae – sorbetur.*
Comparanda: Plin. 31.47.129; Marc. 16.77.
Ps-Galen (K14.513) recommended burnt sponge ash with honey and pepper.

§4. *porri – sorbetur.*
Comparanda: Plin. 20.22.48; Cels. 4.11.6; Garg. 21.
Frankincense was recognised as assisting (e.g. Diosc. *MM* 1.68.3; Gal. K12.60;
   Aët. 1.252; Paul. Aeg. 7.3.11).
Leek was recommended elsewhere with other medicaments (e.g. Ps-Gal.
   K14.533; Alex. *Therap.* 2.195).

§4. *farina – sumitur.*
Comparanda: Plin. 20.60.127; Diosc. *MM* 2.85.3, *Eup.* 2.30.1; Marc. 16.83.

§5. *aqua – propinatur.*
While these were used to treat the emission of blood, their use together like this
   is not recorded elsewhere. Rose was recommended (e.g. Diosc. *Eup.* 2.30.1;
   Theod. 2.22.63), as was rue (e.g. Ps-Gal. 14.533; Theod. 2.23.67; *DMAC*
   29.3), but hyssop was far more commonly used for *vomica* (e.g. Theod.
   2.23.67; Aët. 8.73; Alex. *Therap.* 2.223; Paul. Aeg. 3.32.2; *DMAC* 29.3).

§5. *maruvii – bibitur.*
Comparandum: Plin. 20.89.241.
Marruvium: a misspelling of *marrubium*, horehound, *Marrubium vulgare.*
Horehound was commonly used (e.g. Gal. K13.98; Orib. *EM* 30.1; Marc.
   16.69; Theod. 2.23.67).

§6. *uvae – sanguinem.*
Comparanda: Plin. 23.7.11; Diosc. *MM.* 5.3.1.
The method by which grapes were preserved in wine pressings was fully
   described by Columella (12.45.2–3).

§6. *oleastri – tria.*
Comparandum: Plin. 23.38.76.
Marcellus (16.92) described the use of a wild olive leaf decoction to treat
   vomica without honey or dosage advice.

§7. *palmae – eduntur.*
Comparandum: Plin. 23.51.97.
Palma Thebaica: Theban date (see Strabo 17.1.51). Date decoctions were also
   eaten (e.g. Aret. *CA* 2.2.14; Garg. *Recensio altera* 98 (Rose 1875, 206); Aët.
   8.70; *DMAC* 26.3).

§7. *cydonia – cruda.*

Comparanda: Plin. 23.54.100; Garg. 43; Marc. 16.76.

Eating quince was recommended with either its nature unspecified (Diosc. *MM* 1.115.1) or the option of raw or cooked given (*DMAC* 26.3).

§7. *nuclei – devorantur.*

Comparanda: Plin. 23.75.44; Diosc. *MM* 1.123.1, *Eup.* 2.30.2; Garg. 53; Orib. *CM* 11.α.44; Marc. 16.84.

Only the *Medicina Plinii* recommends the use of catmint instead of standard mint.

§7. *semen – bibitur.*

Comparandum: Plin. 23.81.159 (the myrtle seed/berry decoction only).

Variously prepared myrtle was recommended (Diosc. *Eup.* 2.30.1: Aët. 8.70; *DMAC* 26.3).

Nettle seeds were described by Aëtius (3.143) as suitable for cleansing the lungs and thoracic cavity, and included in a compound to treat *vomica* by Alexander (*Therap.* 2.225).

§8. *gummi – sit.*

Comparanda: Plin. 24.64.105; Diosc. *MM* 1.123.2, *Eup.* 2.30.2; Aret. *CA* 2.2.15; Garg. 53; Orib. *EM* 30.1; Marc. 16.79; Cassius 39.

§8. *ruborum – claudit.*

Comparanda: Plin. 24.73.118; Marc. 16.80. Cf. Ps-Theod. *Ad.* II,22(65).

Bramble was recommended in other ways (e.g. Diosc. *Eup.* 2.29.1; Gal. K11.848; Orib. *EM* 30.1, *Syn.* 9.2.1, *Eun.* 2.1β.7; Aët. 1.62; *DMAC* 26.3).

§9. *eorundem – potione.*

Comparanda: Plin. 24.73.19; Marc. 16.80.

Bramble branches and shoots prepared differently were recommended (Ps-Theod. *Ad.* II,22(65); *DMAC* 26.3).

§9. *cornus – potatur.*

Comparanda: Plin. 28.53.194; Diosc. *MM* 2.59.1, *Eup.* 2.30.3; Gal. K12.334–5; Marc. 16.81; Aët. 2.156; Ps-Theod. *Ad.* II,2(65); Paul. Aeg. 7.3.10.

What liquid this ash was given in varied.

§10. *bubulinus – sumptus.*

Comparanda: Plin. 28.53.195; Marc. 16.82.

Pliny made the point that this was specifically ox blood and different to bull's blood which was considered poisonous, but Aelian (*NA* 11.35) stated that a draught of bull's blood was a cure.

§10. *haedini – dantur.*

Comparanda: Plin. 28.54.196; *Cyran.* 2.4; Gal. K12.261; Marc. 16.82; Aët. 2.85.
The Greek writers recorded this using Greek measurement, resulting in a near
  identical result.

§10. *coagulum – modo.*

Rose (1875, 39) and Önnerfors (1964, 32) attribute this to Pliny, 28.53.194,
  but this passage makes no reference to deer rennet or vinegar. Pliny recommended either deer or hare rennet with vinegar but to treat bleeding and
  without stating whether it was applied or taken (28.73.239).
Hare or deer rennet were commonly recommended (e.g. Diosc. *MM* 2.75.1;
  Aret. *CA* 2.2.13; Gal. K12.274; Orib. *EM* 30.1, *Syn.* 9.2.6, *Eun.* 4.78.6;
  Marc. 16.81; Ps-Theod. *Ad.* II,22(65); Paul. Aeg. 7.3.16).

26. vomicae

This chapter continued the author's discussion of breast complaints. *Vomica* is
most likely what the author meant in his breast discussion as "purulent expectoration". There is no logical reason for this to be the final chapter of this work's first
book; conditions described in the breast "introductory" continue in Book Two.
Not only did the author fail to foreshadow the separation of Book One from Book
Two, this chapter lacks a conclusion like that included at 2.27.20.

§1. *vomicae – evomatur.*

Vomica: refers to any kind of abscess, but was most commonly used to refer
  to internal abscesses, and in the majority of cases, including this chapter,
  those of the upper thoracic cavity, especially on the pleural membrane.
  Celsus (2.7.33–5) stated that *vomicae* of this kind resulted from ongoing
  lung conditions, and while he did not give the Greek name, this kind of
  vomica can be identified as ἐμπύημα. Empyema is still used in medicine
  today to describe pus in the pleural space. This occurs most commonly as
  a complication of pneumonia or pleurisy, and thus is similar to the ancient
  disease; Celsus (3.4.1C) advised that this be strongly avoided. Hippocrates
  (*Aphor.* 5.8, 5.10) described this as the result of pleurisy or *angina*, and if a
  complication of pleurisy, it could lead to tuberculosis (5.15). Spitting blood
  was a symptom of *vomicae*.

§1. *vomicae – natas. . .*

Membranas supervacuas: while this phrase can be translated as "superfluous
  membranes", this makes no clinical sense. This Latin passage is quite similar to a description given by Oribasius (*EM* 32.1) and Aëtius (8.73) which
  describe an abscess "arising in the pleural membrane within the sides" (cf.
  Paul. Aeg. 3.33.1). They used the word ὑπεζωκότος with ὑμήν "membrane";
  ὑπεζωκότος as a noun refers to the pleural membrane, but as a participle can
  mean "surrounding", giving the sense of a "surrounding membrane" within

the sides or ribs. If the Latin *supervacuas* was read with *membranas* in a similar manner, perhaps understood as "*super vacuas*", it can be read as "the membranes surrounding the cavity in the sides" referring to the pleural cavity and mirroring the later Greek descriptions of this complaint.

§2. *eos – requies.*

Önnerfors (1964, 33) directs attention to Pliny 28.14.54 for a similar text. While Pliny (28.14.53–4) included references to anointing and walking, using similar vocabulary to this passage, it is in no way relevant to this.

Celsus (3.4.1) provided some similar advice for internal suppuration, including *vomicae* in his discussion; rubbing unaffected parts, gentle walks, and the consumption of various nuts with honey. A diet of fat birds was also recommended by Alexander (*Therap.* 2.219), with additional discussions about the consumption of baked goods (2.217) and desserts (2.223).

§3. *vomicae – demortuae.*

Comparandum: Plin. 30.16.50. Cf. *Med. Plin.* Prol. 7.

The description of this honey seems a superfluous addition; the author recommended this as the best honey for all medical conditions.

§§3–4. *ad – perducunt.*

Comparanda: Plin. 20.89.244; Seren. 39 ll. 750–4; Marc. 17.33.

Horehound was commonly used to treat *vomicae*, but prepared differently (e.g. Plin. 20.47.118; Orib. *EM* 32.3; Alex. *Therap.* 2.223–7; *DMAC* 29.3), and Aëtius listed it as suitable for cleansing the lungs and chest (3.143).

§5. *multi – credidisset.*

In addition to being described as a complication of other complaints, *vomicae* were especially seen as problematic to heal; a popular anecdote stated that Jason of Pherae suffered from this, was abandoned by his doctors because they could not heal it, and that he only got relief after being stabbed in the chest in battle (Cicero *De Natura Deorum*, 3.70; Valerius Maximus 1.8.6; Plin 7.50.166).

§6. *verum – tempore.*

This passage is interesting as the author stated that he had successfully treated patients; he used his own authority rather than that of unnamed sources here.

The description of winter being the worst time to acquire *vomicae* and that the time it took to heal gradually improved the closer one got to summer mirrors Aretaeus' description of the severity of pleurisy depending on the season (*SA* 1.10.5). This might have been because *vomicae* were often a complication of pleurisy.

Forty days was a significant length of time; Hippocrates (*Aphor.* 5.15) stated that when *vomicae* followed pleurisy, the lung needed to be cleared within 40 days from the abscess breaking or it developed into tuberculosis.

§§7–8. *mandragorae – curatio.*

Comparandum: Marc. 17.32.

Victoriatus: a coin half the weight of a *denarius* which featured the image of Victory.

The ingredients listed in the *Medicina Plinii* featured in a few compounds recorded by Galen (K13.87, 101), and closely resembles Galen's "mandrake pastille" (K13.100–1): four *drachmae* each of mandrake root bark and henbane seed; three *drachmae* each of frankincense, opium, saffron, and myrrh; formed into a pastille weighing three *oboli*, the same weight as a *victoriatus* (*Med. Plin.* Prol. 9). Galen provided no information relating to how it was administered.

Commentary on Book Two

As stated above, the separation of the text at this point into a second book does not seem to reflect the author's intended format. The only foreshadowed separation was the change from the *euporista* "head-to-toe" approach to the treatment of conditions which affected either multiple parts or the body as a whole (*Med. Plin.* Prol. 10) which were discussed in what has become entitled "Book Three".

1. pthisicis

If the reader considers this chapter as a continuation of the preceding chapters and ignore its placement in a separate book, this was a logical continuation of the author's discussion of breast-related conditions. The following chapter addressing *syntexis* also continued this.

Phthisis/pthisis, φθίσις: tuberculosis; a bacterial infection caused by *Mycobacterium tuberculosis*. Tuberculosis is often translated with the archaic term "consumption" and its sufferers, *phthisicus/pthisicus* as "consumptives". Tuberculosis was also called "wasting" (*tabes*, φθόη), relating to the symptomatic wasting of the body experienced by patients (Cels. 3.22.1). References to tuberculosis within classical literature are also identified by other symptoms, especially coughing blood, and its archetypal treatments, namely sea voyages.

For non-pulmonary tuberculosis, see the introductory commentaries of *Medicina Plinii* 2.3 and 3.6.

§1. *invenio – profuit.*

This treatment was offered only on the authority of the author. Milk was a common treatment (e.g. Cels. 3.22.10; Plin. 24.19.28, 28.33.125; Pliny the Younger *Epistles*, 5.19.7; Gal. K10.365–6), but pomegranate flowers were only included in compounds (Prom. *Coll.* 27.5; Gal. K13.64).

Scientific study has found pomegranates have anti-mycobacterial properties (Dey *et al.* 2015, 1474–80).

§2. *utilius – visitare.*

Comparanda: Plin. 24.19.28; Marc. 16.66.

Sea air and sailing, especially to Egypt, were well-known treatments (e.g. Cels. 3.22.8; Plin. 28.14.54, 31.33.62; Pliny the Younger, *Epistles*, 5.19.6; *DMAC* 27.3). Aretaeus stated that sea air acted as a desiccant on ulcerated lungs associated with tuberculosis (*CD* 1.8.1).

§3. *cancri – dantur.*
Comparanda: Plin. 32.39.118; Diosc. *MM* 2.10.1; Aët. 2.175.
Unspecified crab varieties were also recommended (Diosc. *Eup.* 2.40.2; *Cyran.* 4.28; Aët. 8.75).

§3. *lacerta – convalescat.*
Comparanda: Plin. 30.16.86; Marc. 16.62.

§4. *propinatur – austero.*
Comparandum: Plin. 30.26.86.
Various other snail preparations were recommended (Seren. 18 l. 342; Marc. 16.66; Ps-Theod. *Ad.* II,21(62)).

§4. *suis – sumptae.*
Comparandum: Plin. 28.62.230.
Laridum/lardum: bacon or bacon lard.

§4. *suis – propinatur.*
Comparandum: Plin. 28.62.231.

§5. *adipis – gluttitur.*
Comparanda: Plin. 28.37.137–8; Marc. 16.71.
Serenus (18 l. 343) recommended pills made from old grease.

2. syntexi

As a discussion of a condition related to tuberculosis, the topic of the previous chapter, this is a continuation of the author's exposition of breast-related maladies.

Syntexis, σύντηξις: the decline or wasting associated with tuberculosis. In Greek it was also a technical term (Gal. K10.203). Its use in Latin was extremely limited.

§1. *syntexis – est.*
The consideration of *syntexis* as a different disease to *phthisis* in the *Medicina Plinii* was contrary to most Greek medical writers who regarded it a symptom of *phthisis* (e.g. Hippoc. *Epid.* 3.13; Aret. *SD* 1.8.2; Ps-Gal. K19.419–20; Orib. *CM* 7.26.8; Paul. Nic. 44; Leo 4.17) or of other pulmonary diseases (e.g. Aret. *SD* 1.9.8, 1.16.6, 1.13.5, 2.2.1; Aët. 9.12).

§§1–2. *cui – adiciunt*.

Comparandum: Plin. 22.61.129 (without raisin wine).

Other gruel and gruel-like foods were recommended (Hippoc. *Acut. (Sp.)*. 32; Aët. 9.36; Paul. Nic. 44).

§2. *utillimum – lavari*.

This might have related to the beneficial nature of sea air (see commentary to *Med. Plin.* 2.1.2).

3. sciaticis

The positioning of this chapter, which is ostensibly devoted to the hip, following on from tuberculosis appears out of place within the format of *euporista* texts, but this might reflect the author's medical understanding; tuberculosis infections can enter the skeletal system and leave lesions on the bones. This is extremely painful, and hips are a site where these lesions occur. Tuberculosis-related bone lesions in the hips have been identified in at least one set of Pompeian remains. The "head-to-toe" approach is returned to by the author in the following chapter.

Sciaticus: later Latin spelling of *ischiadicus*/ἰσχιαδικός, the adjectival form used to describe sufferers of *ischias*/ἰσχιάς, a complaint variously translated as hip-gout, hip-disease, and even sciatica despite its modern use relating to the sciatic nerve. It has been translated as "hip-disease" to allow the broadest possible understanding.

§1. *vermis – bibitur*.

Comparanda: Plin. 28.18.54; Marc. 25.45.

§2. *cochleae – datur*.

Comparanda: Plin. 30.22.71; Seren. 36 l. 701; Marc. 25.7.

Aminnean wine: made from the Aminnean grape, an old Greek style of vine grown in southern Italy. Isidorus (*Etym.* 16.5.18) described it as a white wine.

The preparation of lizard to prevent nausea was similarly described by Pliny (30.27.90) and in the *Medicina Plinii* elsewhere (3.21.7).

§3. *rubiam – lau<a>ri*.

Comparanda: Plin. 24.56.94; Seren. 36 l. 300; Marc. 24.42.

Rubia: madder, *Rubia tinctorum*.

Drinking madder was a common treatment (Theophr. 9.13.6; Diosc. *MM* 3.143.2, *Eup.* 1.230.1; Gal. K11.878; Aët. 1.148, 12.1).

§3. *genestae – datur*.

Comparanda: Plin. 24.40.66; Diosc. *MM*. 4.154.1, *Eup.* 1.232.2; Seren. 36 ll. 698–9; Marc. 25.43.

Genesta: Spanish broom, *Spartium junceum*, or greenweed, *Genista tinctoria*. Pliny (24.40.65) identified this as the Greek plant *sparton*. Paulus Aegineta (7.3.18) also recommended its use.

§4. *fimus – inponitur*.

Comparanda: Plin. 28.56.198 (in leaves); Diosc. *MM* 2.80.1, *Eup*. 1.234.1; cf. Marc. 25.44.

Holus: a synonym for *brassica* in later Latin especially, but it was used as such as early as Varro (compare his *Rustica*, 1.16.6, with Theophr. 4.16.6). It can also refer to vegetables, pot-herbs, colewort, and turnips.

4. Praecordiorum dolori

The author returned to the "head-to-toe" format here by discussing the internal organs below the breast. While the complaints of the breast could be generally categorised as "lung complaints", this chapter addressed numerous internal organs below the lungs which did not relate to defecation or the urinary tract.

Praecordia: relates to diaphragm, hypochondria, or viscera generally. It is also defined as the parts of the body immediately below the heart, the lower chest in front of the heart, the region over the diaphragm, or the upper abdomen below the ribs.

In addition to the stomach and liver, some of these treatments related to the spleen and intestines, despite these having chapters devoted to them below.

§*1. in – ingerunt*.
Comparandum: Plin. 30.14.42.

§2. *his – est*.

Comparanda: Plin. 30.14.42; Seren. 23 ll. 439–41; Marc. 21.1.

Galen (K10.502) recommended applying puppies to the stomach as a non-magical treatment for dryness of the stomach.

§2 *bulbi – mollunt*.

Comparanda: Plin. 20.40.104; Seren. 23 l. 437; Marc. 21.12; Ps-Theod. *Ad*. II,29(91).

Dalby (2003, 64) suggests that *bulbus* might be a transliteration of βολβός, purse-tassels/grape hyacinth (*Muscari comosum*). Dioscorides (*MM* 2.170, *Eup*. 2.4.2) recommended purse-tassels (βολβός) plastered on to treat stomach conditions (see also Aët. 9.2).

§3. *et – prodest*.

Comparanda: Plin. 20.48.122; Seren. 23 l. 437; Marc. 21.12.

Basil was considered dispersive (Aët. 1.418; Paul. Aeg. 7.3.24), and therefore an appropriate application.

§3. *sextarius – saepius*.

Comparanda: Plin. 20.92.25 for the stomach; Seren. 23 l. 432–4; Marc. 21.9, 20.131; Cassius 42.

The use of linseed and fenugreek together was recommended for the liver (e.g. Diosc. *Eup*. 2.61.1; Orib. *EM* 48.15; Paul. Aeg. 3.46.4), and when expressly referring to the *praecordia*, they were more commonly given as options (e.g. Diosc. *Eup.* 2.16.1; Orib. *CM* 9.29.2, 9.31.3). These were considered to have the same properties when used as a plaster: dispersive and softening (Diosc. *MM* 2.102.1, 2.103.1).

§3. *aliqui – imponere.*
Comparanda: Marc. 21.13; Ps-Theod. *Ad.* II,29(91).
Önnerfors (1964, 38) claims that Pliny 24.120.187 was the source for this treatment, but the text does not closely match Pliny's advice which related to fenugreek not fennel. There is confusion between the two throughout the *Medicina Plinii* (see commentary to 1.2.1), but this is not necessarily another example.

§4. *cydonia – imponuntur.*
Comparanda: Plin. 23.54.101; Diosc. *MM* 1.115.2; Gal. K10.503; Seren. 23 ll. 435–6.
Quince was included in plasters for the stomach and *praecordia* (e.g. Orib. *EM* 38.3; Paul. Aeg. 3.37.1).

§5. *acori – prodest.*
Comparandum: Plin. 26.48.77.
Acorus: yellow or sweet flag. It was more commonly used for liver problems (e.g. Diosc. *MM* 1.2.2, *Eup.* 2.60.1; *Pap. Oxy.* 8.1088, ll. 48–55; Orib. *Eun.* 4.96.2), and splenic conditions (e.g. Diosc. *MM* 1.2.2, *Eup.* 2.62.1; Plin. 26.48.77; Gal. K11.820; Orib. *Eun.* 2.1α.19; Aët.1.17; Paul. Aeg. 7.3.1).

§§5–6. *his – tollentur.*
Comparanda: Plin. 30.16.48; Marc. 20.132.
Dizziness was a symptom associated with conditions of the liver, spleen, or viscera in the middle of the body (Aret. *CD* 1.3.2).

§7. *in – est.*
Comparanda: Plin. 31.33.66; Seren. 23.l. 438.

§7. *iocineri – inassata.*
Comparanda: Plin. 30.16.47; Marc. 22.3.

§§7–8. *stomach – medentur.*
Comparanda: Plin. 30.15.44; Seren. 17. 315–7; Marc. 20.35, 20.111.
Celsus (2.24.3) recognised the usefulness of snails for the stomach. Snails with *garum*, oil, and wine were recommended by Oribasius (*CM* 2.29.2, 3.29.7), but with *garum*, oil, anise, and water by Aëtius (2.183).

§8. *prosunt – devoratae.*
Comparanda: Plin. 30.15.45; Diosc. *MM.* 2.9.3.
Cyranides (4.32) recommended eating sea-snails to soften a hardened abdomen.

§9. aestimo – dicuntur.

The inability to keep food down was included as an element of stomach diseases (e.g. Cels. 4.12.7; Gal. K2.158–9, K11.45).

§9. *horum – sumitur.*

Comparanda: Plin. 30.20.59–60; Marc. 20.55, 20.85.

Ossifragus: a bird of prey whose name was literally "bone-breaker". It has been variously identified as a bearded vulture, osprey, or sea-eagle.

This treatment might have utilised sympathetic magic; Pliny (30.20.63) described the bird's digestive capabilities as marvellous and recommended its use magically to treat colic.

§10. *non – celerrime.*

Comparandum: Marc. 20.84.

§§11–12. *in – vitreo.*

Comparanda: Plin. 24.79.129; Scribon. 111; Columella 12.42: Garg. 41; Marc. 20.84 (cf. 27.2); Ps-Theod. *Ad.* II,27(77).

Ros Syriacus: sumach, members of the *Rhus* genus. Forster and Heffner's (LCL: *Columella III*, 271) translation of *ros* as rosemary is incorrect; this was either a dialectic difference in or mistaken spelling of *rhus* (Coromines 1939, 218–21). Sumach was a common ingredient in all copies of this recipe, but the *Medicina Plinii*, Columella, and Gargilius spelled it *ros*.

Lingula: a misspelling of *ligula*. *Ligulae* were long handled, tiny bowled spoons used to empty *unguentaria* found in medical and toiletry collections (Gibson 1983, 393); spoons without the pointed handle of a *cochlear*; or units of measurement, amounting to a quarter of a *cyathus* (Daremberg, Saglio, & Pottier 1904, 1253–4). *Ligula* was used as the dosage measure by Pliny, Scribonius, and Pseudo-Theodorus, but it cannot be determined which definition was meant.

This compound was called διὰ ὀπώρας by Columella and *oporice* by Gargilius. Extant Greek recipes (Gal. K13.142–3, K13.143, K13.289; Orib. *Syn.* 3.191; Alex. *Therap.* 2.269, 2.431; Metrod. 98) display more variety in the choice of fruit: quinces and sumach were common ingredients among all the recipes, with sorbs, pomegranates, and must was included in the majority of recipes. Fig was included in no other recipe.

§13–14. *fit – duae.*

Comparanda: Marc. 20.133; Ps-Theod. *Ad.* II,27(77).

Schoenus, σχοῖνος: rush or aromatic camel-hay, *Cymbopogon schoenanthus* (Beck 2017, 17).

Petroselinum, πετροσέλινον: literally "rock celery", often translated as parsley.

5. *ventri molliendo*

While the last treatments outlined in the previous chapter address problems of the stomach, this chapter is the first of many which relate to what was called *venter*, a term which could refer to various parts of the abdomen, including the stomach, belly, paunch, or the excretory system. This chapter's particular title could be understood as "for softening the stomach", but the phrase "*ventri molliendo*" was also used by Celsus (2.12.1C) when addressing the need to purge the bowel. For that reason it has been translated as "for opening the bowels". Most of the remedies provided in this chapter treat constipation, but a distinction must be made between this chapter's title which focused on the effects of ministrations, rather than the condition or its cause, and the topic of *Medicina Plinii* 2.8 which addressed constipation (*tenesmos*). The author did not choose to immediately follow this chapter with that particular discussion, and instead addressed diarrhoea treatments possibly owing to the similarity of each chapter's titles.

§1. *Menae – inlinuntur.*
Comparandum: Plin. 23.31.101.
Smearing bull's bile on the navel alone was recommended (Ps-Gal. K14.472; Plac. 11α.4, 11β.4), and Marcellus (30.25) recommended this with *elaterium* (see commentary to *Med. Plin.* 2.5.3).

§1. *lac – melle.*
Comparanda: Plin. 28.58.203; Seren. 27 l. 524; Plac. 5α.12, 5β.22; Marc. 20.137.
Goat milk and salt was described by Celsus (2.12.1A) as a purgative, but Dioscorides (*MM* 2.70.1) described goat's milk as binding the bowel. Salty drinks were considered helpful for constipation in popular culture (e.g. Plautus *Rudens*, ll. 588–9).

§1. *ventriculis – sit.*
Sarda: a salted fish (Plin. 32.17.46) described as the same size as Atlantic mackerel and whose "salt and sweet juices" loosened the bowels (Athenaeus 3.121).
This preparation is similar to Dioscorides' (*MM* 2.30.1) advice to use the liquid from a goby sewn in pig's tripe and boiled to move the bowels.

§2. *porri – sumuntur.*
Comparandum: Garg. 21; cf. Marc. 20.134.
Dioscorides (*MM* 2.149.1) described headed-leek as easing the bowel.

§2. *urticae – colligitur.*
Comparanda: Plin. 22.15.33; Marc. 20.135.
Nettles, not specifically their seeds, were used to soften the bowel (Diosc. *MM* 4.93.2; Orib. *CM* 2.58.46), but this use of nettle *semen* is restricted to Pliny and those who, like the author, used him as their source.

Pliny's description of how this was taken in bread is very similar to Theophrastus' method of taking Cnidian berries, *Daphne oleides* fruit, in bread
to prevent them from burning the throat (9.20.2). A common Greek word for
nettle was κνίδη, and κνίδιος κόκκος "Cnidian berry" could easily have been
misunderstood as "nettle seed" (κόκκος and σπέρμα were used interchangeably); in addition to this Pliny cited Theophrastus as a source for this book.

§2. *lens – sorbetur.*
Comparandum: Plin. 22.70.142.
Dioscorides (*MM* 2.107.1) stated that lentils cooked with their hulls softened
the bowel, but Hippocrates (*Reg.* 2.45) stated that lentils troubled the bowels and were not a laxative.

§2. *myrobalanus – citat.*
Comparandum: Plin. 23.52.98. Mayhoff 1897, 31 reads *ciet* ("moves the bow-
els"), LCL: *Pliny Natural History VI*, 478 *sistit* ("checks the bowels").
Behen-nut was used to clear the bowels (Diosc. *MM* 4.157.2; Aët. 1.107), but
Pliny might have misidentified it (see commentary to *Med. Plin.* 3.3.4).

§3. *fel – inlinitur.*
Comparandum: Plin. 28.58.203.
Elaterium: a strong purgative made from the seeds of wild/squirting cucumber
(Theophr. 9.9.4; Diosc. *MM* 4.150.3).

§3. *cydonia – ieiunis.*
Comparanda: Plin. 23.54.102; Marc. 20.135.
Quinces were not easily passed (Hippoc. *Reg.* 2.55) and were recommended
for diseases which needed the bowels checked (Diosc. *MM* 1.115.1–2).
Columella (12.47.2–3) and Pliny (15.18.60) described the process of preserv-
ing quinces in honey.

§3. *pruna – eduntur.*
Comparanda: Plin. 23.66.132; Diosc. *MM* 1.121.1; Gal. K6.353–4, K12.32;
Garg. 46; Seren. 27 l. 517.
Martial (*Epigrams*, 13.29) also referred to the laxative effect of plums.

§4. *mororum – datur.*
Comparanda: Plin. 23.70.135; Diocl. *Fr.* 154; Diosc. *MM* 1.126.1; Orib. *CM*
8.41.5.
Hippocrates (*Reg.* 2.55) described mulberries as easily passed.
Similar nomenclature used for mulberries and bramble berries make it difficult
to ascertain whether there are additional references.

§4. *ammoniacum – additur.*
Comparanda: Plin. 24.14.23; Diosc. *MM* 3.84.1.
It was also included in a compound (Aët. 9.28).

§4. *ulmi – purgat.*
Comparandum: Plin. 24.33.48.

§4. *aqua – suppositus.*
Comparandum: Plin. 30.21.68.

§5. *salicis – potatus.*
Marcellus (29.20) recommended a willow leaf-based potion to address bowel
pain.

§§5–6. *thalassomeli – picato.*
Comparanda: Plin. 31.35.68; Diosc. *MM* 5.12.1; Seren. 271. 533; Marc. 20.136.
Thalassomeli, θαλασσόμελι: literally "sea honey". Sea water was likely the
active ingredient (Diosc. *MM* 5.11.3; Athenaeus 1.32d; *Med. Plin.* 2.5.1 and
commentary).

6. ventri sistendo

Following a chapter devoted to its opposite, *"ventri molliendo"*, this chapter
addressed diarrhoea. The treatments offered here, or very similar ones, were commonly given for numerous diseases which feature diarrhoea as a symptom, especially dysentery and bowel disease (*coeliacus*), conditions addressed a little later
in the text, after *cholera* (the next chapter), colic, and constipation.

§1. *cancri – bibuntur.*
Comparandum: Plin. 32.31.101.

§1. *sativi – potatur.*
Comparandum: Plin. 20.17.35.
Goat milk was thought to bind the bowel (Diosc. *MM* 2.70.1).

§1. *ocimum – inlinitur.*
Comparandum: Plin. 20.48.122; cf. Garg. 22.

§1. *panicum – sumitur.*
Comparandum: Plin. 22.63.131.
Panicum, Italian millet, was described as less binding than standard millet
(Diosc. *MM* 2.98.1) which was used in gruel to check the bowel (Diosc.
MM 2.97.1). A similar treatment was described by Marcellus (27.100)
which might have confused this treatment and the next in the *Medicina
Plinii*, as he replaced *panicum* with *panis anticus* (very old bread).

§2. *vetus – bibitur.*
Comparandum: Plin. 22.68.138 (sailor's or old bread).
Panis nauticus: sailor's bread, possibly "ship's biscuit". The use of this
phrase by Pliny and in the *Medicina Plinii* are the only two examples.

De Grandsagne (1832, 192) suggests that sailor's bread was no different to soldier's bread, *panis militaris*. The author combined Pliny's options to form one treatment.

Dioscorides (*MM* 2.85.3) recommended old, dry bread to control diarrhoea, and Hippocrates (*Reg. Health* 7) recommended well-baked bread crumbled in wine to treat athletes' diarrhoea.

§2. *in – prosunt.*

Comparanda: Plin. 22.69.141; Marc. 27.101.

Dioscorides (*MM* 2.105.1) recommended eating Greek beans with their husks boiled in sour wine.

§2. *lens – sorbitur.*

Comparanda: Plin. 22.70.142; Diosc. *MM* 2.107.1; Orib. *Syn.* 9.15.2, *Eun.* 4.88.1; Paul. Aeg. 3.40.5; Paul. Nic. 65 for dysentery.

Dioscorides stated that its effectiveness was owed to lentils' astringent nature.

§2. *acetum – sorbetur.*

Pliny's use of vinegar was as an enema (23.27.56). Dioscorides (*MM* 5.13.1) recommended vinegar boiled with food for abdominal diarrhoea.

§3. *mala – eduntur.*

Comparanda: Plin. 23.55.104; Diosc. *MM* 1.115.4.

Beck (2017, 83) identifies "wild apples" as crab-apples. Dioscorides ascribed their efficacy to their astringency; as a result using the least ripe fruit was recommended.

§3. *aqua – bibitur.*

The use of ripened, dried wild plums boiled with concentrated must is the only similar treatment (Diosc. *MM* 1.121.1).

§3. *silvestrum – die.*

Comparanda: Plin. 23.68.133; Marc. 27.92; Ps-Theod. *Ad.* II,31(102) for dysentery.

§4. *mororum – bibitur.*

Comparandum: Plin. 23.70.135.

Dried unripe mulberries were also recommended for diarrhoea (Orib *Eun.* 4.88.4; Aët. 9.35) and dysentery (Orib. *Syn.* 9.15.5; Aët. 9.33; Paul. Aeg. 3.42.2).

§4. *sorbetur – myrti.*

Comparanda: Plin. 23.81.160; Ps-Theod. *Ad.* II,31(102) for dysentery.

Myrtle was used for its astringency (Aret. *CD* 2.7.4) for diarrhoea (Gal. K13.169–70) and dysentery (Prom. *Coll.* 130.8; Paul. Nic. 65).

§4. *palumbus – datur.*

Comparanda: Plin. 30.20.60; Theod. 2.31.101 for dysentery; Ps-Theod. *Ad.* II,31(102) for dysentery. Cf. *Med. Plin* 2.8.5 for colic.

Marcellus (27.60) recommended wild wood-pigeon boiled in raisin wine for bowel disease. Cassius (47) outlined a Greek *cholera* treatment of wood-pigeons called φάσσα (wild wood-pigeons) decocted in *posca*. Hippocrates (*Reg.* 81) recommended boiled doves and wild pigeons for watery stools.

§4. *fimus – inlinitur.*

Comparanda: Plin. 30.20.60; Ps-Theod. *Ad.* II,31(102) for dysentery.

Hot plasters applied to the stomach were used to assist colon conditions (Aret. *CD* 2.7.2), and pigeon dung was considered strongly warming (Diosc. *MM* 2.80.4).

§5. *bibitur – sanguis.*

Comparandum: Plin.30.20.61.

§5. *flores – propinantur.*

Avellana: later spelling of *Abellana* "hazel"; named after its place of origin, Abella in Campania (Plin. 15.24.88).

Cincinnus: a lock or curl, usually relating to hair. There is nothing obviously resembling this on hazel trees.

§6. *iuniperi – potantur.*

Comparanda: Plin. 24.36.55; Marc. 27.126; Ps-Theod. *Ad.* II,31(102) for dysentery.

Juniper berries were included in compounds (e.g. Gal. K13.169–70).

§6. *flos – die.*

Comparanda: Plin. 24.42.79 for looseness of bowels and dysentery; Diosc. *MM* 2.179.1, *Eup.* 2.50.2 for dysentery; Marc. 27.75 for bowel disease.

Tribus digitis sumptus: literally "taken in three fingers".

§6. *baca – potantur.*

Comparandum: Plin. 24.72.116 (*aquifolium*). Cf. *Med. Plin.* 2.7.3 for *cholera*.

The use of *acrifolium* in the *Medicina Plinii* is identical to Pliny's *aquifolium*, and thus they are assumed to be the same: holly. The difference in spelling cannot be attributed to evolution over time as *acrifolium* was described as a tree of ill omen in Tarquitius Priscus' *Portents Derived from Trees* (fr. 6, in Macrobius *Saturnalia*, 3.20.3).

§7. *ruborum – dantur.*

Comparandum: Plin. 24.73.119.

Decoctions of bramble branches, shoots, leaves, and fruit were also drunk (e.g. Diosc. *MM* 4.37.1; Ps-Gal. K14.495; Seren. 28 l. 556; Marc. 27.90).

Bramble was also recommended for dysentery (*Med. Plin.* 2.10.6 and commentary).

All parts of the bramble have been scientifically proved to contain anti-diarrhoeal properties (Verma *et al.* 2014, 103).

§7. *cochlearum – inspargitur.*
Comparandum: Plin. 30.20.59. Cf. *Med. Plin.* 2.11.8 and commentary for dysentery and bowel disease.

§8. *plantago – cocta.*
Comparanda: Plin. 26.28.44; Ps-Apul. 1.7; *Antidot. Brux.* 191 for dysentery; Paul. Nic. 65 for dysentery.
It was also variously prepared to address diarrhoea and related diseases (Diosc. *MM* 2.126.2, 2.126.4; Orib. *EM* 53.6; Marc. 27.15; Theod. 2.31.101; Aët. 9.35).

§8. *symphyti – bibitur.*
Comparandum: Plin. 26.28.45.
Comfrey was also recommended for dysentery (Theod. 2.31.101).

§8. *gallinacei – sumitur.*
Comparandum: Plin. 30.20.59.
Specially prepared beef and goat liver was recommended for dysentery (Marc. 27.106; Ps-Theod. *Ad.* II,31(102)).

7. cholorae

The author likely placed this discussion of *cholera* following on from the previous two chapters because his opening sentence referred to is as a complaint of the *venter*. The following chapters continue to address similar conditions, especially those of the excretory system, but *venter* was not used to describe their nature.

Cholera does not refer to the modern disease properly called "Asiatic cholera". Ancient *cholera*, called *cholera nostra* or "summer cholera" in early modern medical texts, was more likely food poisoning (Biraben 1998, 325–6). Its description as an epidemic disease can be accounted for by communal eating practices. The correlation between food and *cholera* was acknowledged: eating meat, especially undercooked pork, was identified as a potential cause, and its prevalence in summer, when meat was most likely to spoil, was noted (Hippoc. *Epid.* 7.1.82).

§1. *cholera – exhauriat.*
Per sedem exhauriat: literally "it exhausts through the seat".
Celsus (4.18.1) described it as also affecting intestines and added flatulence as a symptom.

§1. *adversus – eduntur.*

Comparanda: Plin. 20.26.67; Garg. 11; Seren. 16 ll. 290–1; cf. Marc. 30.64.

Hippocrates (*Epid.* 7.1.82) described boiled lettuce as a cause of *cholera*, but late Greek writers recommended lettuce boiled in various liquids (e.g. Alex. *Therap.* 2.329; Paul. Aeg. 3.39.1; *Geopon.* 12.13.4).

§2. *cydonia – sumuntur.*

Comparanda: Plin. 23.54.100; Diosc. *MM* 1.115.1; Marc. 30.65.

Greek writers also recommended quince without describing its preparation (e.g. Aret. *CA* 2.4.4; Alex. *Therap.* 2.327; Paul. Aeg. 3.39.2).

§2. *optime – exposuimus.*

Brodersen (2015, 87) identifies this as the compound described at *Medicina Plinii* 2.4.13; this fits with the identification within the *Medicina Plinii* of *praecordia* as including the stomach.

§3. *bacae – datae.*

Comparanda: Plin. 24.72.116; Marc. 30.65. See *Med. Plin.* 2.6.6. for diarrhoea.

§3. *mororum – bibitur.*

Comparanda: Plin. 24.73.120; Marc. 30.64.

The only Greek reference to bramble to treat *cholera* is Paulus Nicaeensis (67) who made no use of the berry.

§3. *aqua – infunditur.*

Comparandum: Plin. 31.33.66.

§§3–4. *mirifice – abstinere.*

The only vaguely similar treatment recorded was used to cleanse bile from horses with *cholera* (*Hippiatr. Cant.* 63).

Triblas: a misspelling of *tribulas* which appeared in some manuscripts instead. It likely relates to *tribulus*, either the act of pressing or a kind of threshing sledge.

8. torminibus

The precise definition of *tormina*/*tormen* is uncertain. The closest Greek terms for it are κωλικός, from which the translation "colic" is derived, and στρόφος, but these were referred to separately in numerous Greek medical texts. Celsus (4.22.1) stated *tormina* was the Greek δυσεντερία; but the transliteration of this was used to discuss a separate disease (e.g. *Med. Plin.* 2.10, 2.11). This illustrates one of the problems relating to the identification of and differentiation between gastrointestinal conditions: there was no consensus in terminology and definitions, and this problematic nomenclature is likely why treatments were recommended for multiple diseases. This chapter continued the author's long discussion of gastrointestinal conditions which started at the end of his chapter devoted to visceral pain (*Med. Plin.* 2.5.9 onwards).

§1. *lactuca – sinapi*.

There are variations of this: Marcellus (27.113–4) recommended decocted lettuce with cumin and oil, and misplaced mustard in the following treatment; Cato (*De agricultura,* 156.5–6, 157.9) and Pliny (20.33.82) described something similar, but used cabbage instead of lettuce without mustard.

Lettuce was variously recommended (*Cyran.* 5.8; Ps-Gal. K14.467, 470; Aët. 9.30), but examples of it failing to help were also recorded (Gal. K10.858–9).

Cumin was frequently recommended as a simple and in compounds (e.g. Diosc. *Eup.* 2.42.2; Ps-Gal. K14.464, 494; Cassius 51; Aët. 9.30, 9.31; Paul. Aeg. 3.43.3; Paul. Nic. 69), and wild cumin in water was also recommended (Diosc. *MM* 3.60.2; Plin. 20.57.159).

§§1–2. *ovum – bibitur*.

Comparanda: Plin. 29.11.50 for dysentery; Marc. 27.114.

Hippocrates (*Acut. (Sp.)* 53) included egg in his treatment of colic, but prepared medium fried.

§2. *holera – eduntur*.

Comparandum Plin. 20.34.86 for dysentery and bowel disease. Cf. *Med Plin.* 2.9.3, 2.10.1.

Pliny described "twice cooked", not "decocted", cabbage.

Cabbage and salt prepared with other medicaments were recommended (Cato *De agricultura* 156.5–6, 157.9; Plin. 20.33.82; Ps-Gal. K14.545).

§2. *ruta – miscetur*.

Comparanda: Plin. 20.51.136; Scribon. 121; Marc. 27.115.

Rue was often used to treat colic (see *Med. Plin.* 2.8.3 and commentary), but these are the only examples of humans taking hyssop with rue for this.

§3. *panis – sorbitionis*.

Rose (1875, 50) and Önnerfors (1964, 43) mistakenly identify Pliny 28.48.206 as the source of this treatment. While there is some correlation between the vocabularies – *tormina, panis, lac caprinum,* and *sorbeo/sorbitio* – the treatment outlined by Pliny bears little resemblance to that described in the *Medicina Plinii*. Önnerfors' theory (1964, 165) that this passage also related to Marcellus 27.100 which correlates with *Medicina Plinii* 2.6.2 illustrates that his approach to recognising comparanda is very broad.

For other uses of bread see Galen (K10.858–9) and Aëtius (9.30).

§3. *in – bibitur*.

Comparandum: Plin. 23.40.81 (using wild grape-flower oil); cf. Diosc. *Eup.* 2.47.2.

Rue was more commonly eaten (e.g. Arist. [*Pr.*] 20.34; Diosc. *MM* 3.45.2; Aët. 1.321; Paul. Nic. 69; Leo 5.15).

§3. *malum – emendat.*
Comparandum: Plin. 23.58.109; cf. Cato *De agricultura*, 126.

§4. *malum – discutit.*
Comparanda: Plin. 23.58.109; Marc. 27.116.

§4. *ruborum – prodest.*
Comparandum Plin. 24.74.118 for bowel disease. Cf. *Med. Plin.* 2.6.6–7, 2.7.3.
The inclusion of this under "colic" by the author illustrates the conflation of
  gastrointestinal complaints.

§5. *lien – bibitur.*
Comparandum: Plin. 30.20.61.

§5. *palumbus – pusca.*
Comparandum Plin. 30.20.61; cf. *Med. Plin.* 2.6.4 for diarrhoea.
Aëtius (9.30) recommended eating these birds, while Galen (K10.858–9)
  recommended any bird broth made from wine.

§6. *anas – moritur.*
Comparanda: Plin. 30.20.61; Marc. 27.33.
Frogs were used for similar acts of transfer magic (Marc. 27.123).
This might indicate a Latin tradition relating to ducks; Columella (6.7) stated
  seeing a duck eased oxen's stomach pain.

§6. *aqua – infunditur.*
Comparanda: Plin. 31.33.66; Diosc. *MM* 5.11.1; Marc. 27.125; *Geopon.* 16.9.1.
Enemas of all kinds were common treatments (Diosc. *MM* 3.45.2; Prom. *Coll.*
  119.8; Gal. K10.857; Aët. 3.79).

§6. *vinum – efficacissimum.*
Comparanda: Plin. 28.58.206; Diosc. *MM* 2.75.1 for bowel disease; Ps-Gal.
  K14.481 for bowel disease and dysentery; Seren. 30 l. 576; Marc. 27.57;
  Antidot. Brux. 141.
Galen (K12.274) recommended horse rennet.

9. Tenesmo

This chapter is one of the few for which the author provided a description of the
condition. The author's placement of *tenesmos* within the broader discussion of
gastrointestinal conditions was perfectly logical, but why he decided to place it
between chapters devoted to colic and dysentery rather than closer to his discussion of how to open the bowels cannot be determined.

§1. *tenesmo – eicit.*
Comparanda: Plin. 28.59.211; Scribon. 142; Marc. 28.3, 28.58.

Tenesmus/tenesmos, τεινεσμός: it would be easy to define this as constipation, but it would not convey the difference between this and the need to move the bowels (see *Med. Plin.* 2.5).

According to Hippocrates (*Aff.* 26), *tenesmos* arose from the same cause as dysentery, but was milder, shorter in duration, and not fatal.

Tenesmus has been used historically in modern medicine to describe both straining to defecate and urinate.

§1. *senectus – inlinitur.*
Comparanda: Plin. 30.19.57; Marc. 28.61. Cf. *Med. Plin.* 2.11.8 for bowel disease.

Stagnum: an alloy of silver and lead created as a part of the smelting process (Plin. 34.48.159–60). *Stagnum* vessels were known to affect their contents, likely owing to the sweetening effect of lead. Despite, or perhaps because of, this *stagnum* vessels were commonly recommended (e.g. Scribon. 30, 230, 269, 271; Plin. 29.10.35; Apuleius *Metamorphosis*, 10.21; *Med. Plin.* 2.11.8, 3.6.7; *Mulomed. Chiron.* 3.197; Marc. 8.9, 27.80, 29.50, 35.7, 35.9, 35.23; Veget. *Mulomed.* 1.15.4).

§2. *et – eduntur.*
Comparanda: Plin. 32.21.64; Marc. 28.59; Theod. 2.31.104.

§2. *lac – prodest.*
Comparanda: Plin. 28.59.211; Diosc. *MM* 2.70.5; Marc. 28.58; Theod. 2.31.104.

§2. *ius – colligitur.*
Comparanda: Plin. 32.31.101; Marc. 28.62.
Only the *Medicina Plinii* adds bread.
Fish soups were recommended for gastrointestinal conditions (Gal. K10.575; Aët. 2.141).

§3. *holus – sale.*
Comparanda: Plin. 20.34.86; Marc. 28.59; Theod. 2.31.104. Cf. *Med. Plin.* 2.8.1, 2.10.1 and commentaries.

§3–4. *aqua – vomitur.*
Comparanda: Plin. 31.33.64; Marc. 28.63.

§4. *pulticulam – dabis.*
Oribasius (*EM* 54.5) and Aëtius (9.42) recommended "wheaten barley gruel" πυρίνη πτισάνη (Paul. Aeg. 3.42.4 recommended gruel) to treat *tenesmos*-related to dysentery, without oil and salt.

10. Dysenteriae

This chapter continued the author's discussion of gastrointestinal conditions. Its placement following *tenesmos* might have been his acknowledgment that one of the symptoms of *dysenteria* was an inability to defecate despite a desire to do so. The positioning of this chapter immediately prior to the chapter devoted to bowel disease was logical given that these chapters refer to each other's complaints.

Dysenteria, δυσεντερία: could relate to numerous modern diseases; even in antiquity there was some debate about what exactly was meant by the term (see introductory commentary to *Med. Plin.* 2.8). For the most part, *dysenteria* was identified as a gastrointestinal problem, primarily associated with blood presenting in the stool on account of ulceration of the bowel, difficulty defecating, or excreting a watery stool (Aret. *SD* 2.9.1; Orib. *EM* 54.1). These symptoms match those of modern dysentery: the result of bacterial, viral, and parasitic infections. Research conducted on a Roman-era latrine indicates that the same causes of dysentery were commonly present in antiquity (Williams *et al.* 2017, 37–42).

§1. *holera – eduntur*
Comparandum: Plin. 20.34.86 for dysentery and bowel disease. Cf. *Med. Plin* 2.8.2, 3.93 and commentary.
Twice boiled cabbage without salt was also recommended (Diosc. *Eup.* 2.51.6; Orib. *CM* 4.4.4, *EM* 54.3).

§1. *per – aqua.*
Comparanda: Plin. 20.40.104; Seren. 25 ll. 491–2 for bowel disease.

§1. *coctum – datur.*
Comparandum: Plin. 20.47.122.

§2. *ruta – editur.*
Comparandum: Plin. 20.51.140.
Moretum: an herb cheese spread; its recipe and how it was made were recorded by Columella (12.59.1–4) and the poem "*Moretum*" (ll. 85–116) in the *Appendix Vergiliam.*
By comparing this to *moretum*, the author used popular culture as a short-hand to provide a description of its preparation; his audience would have understood the need to grind rue in a mortar, use a hard cheese, and add wine like they would oil or vinegar. Rue and cheese were ingredients of *moretum*, but wine was not.

§2. *cera – infunditur.*
Comparanda: Plin. 22.55.116; Diosc. *MM* 2.83.3, *Eup.* 2.51.6; Marc. 27.72.
Hippocrates (*Aff.* 23) recommended eating gruel.

§3. *sarmenta – aspergitur.*
Comparandum: Plin. 23.8–9.13.

The *Medicina Plinii* does not convey Pliny's advice well, and fails to state what the ash was sprinkled over. Pliny recommended roasted grape seeds after describing them as having the same properties as vine twigs, sprinkled into a draught (cf. Diosc. *MM* 5.3.2).

The use of grape seeds was commonly recommended (e.g. Aret. *CD* 2.7.4; Orib. *EM* 54.4, *Syn.* 9.15.5, *Eun.* 4.87.5; Aët. 2.134; Alex. *Therap.* 2.429; Paul. Aeg. 3.42.2).

§3. *sucus – inmittitur.*
Comparandum: Plin. 23.3.3.

§4. *cydonia – inmittitur.*
Comparanda: Plin. 23.54.100; Diosc. *MM* 1.115.1; Garg. 43.

§4. *myrti – propinatur.*
Comparanda: Plin. 23.81.159; Diosc. *Eup.* 2.50.3.
See commentary to *Medicina Plinii* 2.6.4 on their use in treating the bowel.

§4. *vinum – datur.*
Comparandum: Plin. 23.81.162.
Various myrtle decoctions were recommended (Gal. K13.151–2; Alex. *Therap.* 2.307; Metrod. 125), and vague references were made to myrtle's suitability (Orib. *Syn.* 9.15.5, *Eun.* 4.82.5; Aët. 2.134; Alex. *Therap.* 2.429).

§5. *galla – facit.*
Comparanda: Plin. 24.5.9; Marc. 27.73.
Galla Cammagena: galla is oak-gall (see commentary to *Med. Plin.* 1.12.5). Commagene, the northern province in Syria, was thought to produce the best oak-gall according to Pliny (24.5.9).
Oribasius described oak-gall as suitable (*Syn.* 9.15.5, *Eun.* 4.87.5), but it was normally taken (e.g. Diosc *MM* 1.107.2; Ps-Gal. K14.466; Orib. *EM* 54.15; Metrod. 70).

§5. *flos – bibitur.*
Comparanda: Plin. 24.47.79; Diosc. *MM* 2.179.1, *Eup.* 2.50.2; Marc. 27.74.

§6. *ruborum – eduntur.*
Comparanda: Plin. 24.73.119; Diosc. *Eup.* 2.50.2. Cf. *Med. Plin.* 2.6.7.
Bramble was variously used including root decoctions (e.g. Prom. *Coll.* 127.6; Orib. *EM* 54.15) and its fruit consumed (Orib. *Syn.* 9.15.9, *Eun.* 4.87.9; Aët. 9.33, 9.35; Alex. *Therap.* 2.429; Paul. Aeg. 3.42.2).

§7. *lutea – datur.*
Comparanda: Plin. 29.11.43; Marc. 27.76.

The use of egg yolks was described by Promotus (*Coll.* 124.4, 125.8) and Galen (K13.302), but in no way similar to this. For more on their use for gastrointestinal conditions see commentary on *Medicina Plinii* 2.11.4.

11. Coeliacis [id est torturae vel commissioni intestinorum]

By directly referring to dysentery, the topic of the previous chapter, this continues to reflect the conflation between gastrointestinal diseases. This also accurately reflects how these two complaints were often addressed together Greek medical texts. This is the penultimate chapter devoted to organs which might be described as *venter*, with the following chapter addressing parasitic worms.

Coeliacus should not be confused with the modern "coeliac" which refers to a disease of the small intestine caused by an allergy to gluten. It has been translated as "bowel disease".

The addition of the subheading "i.e. for the onset of agony or torment of the intestines" suggests that a copyist thought that *coeliacus* required some explanation.

§1. *bacae – propinantur*.
Comparandum: Marc. 27.120.
Dioscorides (*Eup.* 2.51.1) recommended ripe olives to treat both dysentery and bowel disease.

§1. *membranae – oportet*.
Comparandum: Plin. 30.19.58.
Frux: literally "fruit", but also "fruit of the earth" (any kind of grain or crop).
Neither Pliny nor the author referred to any internal organs of hens, yet Jones (LCL: *Pliny Natural History VIII*, 315) translates this as a membrane of hens' crops (cf. *Med. Plin.* 1.6.9). Jones' translation makes this similar to advice recorded by other writers (Diosc. *MM* 2.49.1; Orib. *EM* 53.6; Marc. 27.70; Aët. 9.35), but there is nothing in the text to legitimise this.

§2. *fimus – propinatur*.
Comparanda: Plin. 30.19.58; Ps-Theod. *Ad.* II,31(102).
Galen (K12.303) recommended dried pigeon dung without describing how.

§2. *plumbi – medentur*.
Comparandum: Plin. 30. 19.58.
Wild wood-pigeon was more commonly cooked in *posca* for gastrointestinal conditions (*Med. Plin.* 2.6.4, 2.8.5 and commentaries).

§3. *dysentericos – sumitur*.
Comparanda: Plin. 30.19.58; Ps-Theod. *Ad.* II,31(102).
Thrush was recommended for *cholera* (Orib. *EM* 52.9) and softening the bowels (*Cyran.* 4.38).

§4. *gravissimum – ventri.*

Comparanda: Plin. 30.20.59; Marc. 27.83.

Ileos, εἰλεός/ἰλιός: an intestinal obstruction, severe colic, or a generic "iliac pains".

§4. *dysentericis – devorantur.*

Comparandum: Plin. 29.11.44 (whole egg).

Marcellus (27.77) used eggs steeped in vinegar as an element of treatment.

Eggs prepared with vinegar were used in Greek treatments for bowel disease (Paul. Nic. 64), but more often boiled in vinegar for dysentery (e.g. Gal. K12.352; Orib. *Syn.* 9.15.4, *Eun.* 4.87.4; Aët. 2.134; Paul. Aeg. 3.42.2).

§5. *ova – cibo.*

Comparanda: Plin. 29.1149; Seren. 25 ll. 488–90; Marc. 27.71.

Ps-Galen (K14.466) recommended the consumption of bread made with eggs which had been steeped in vinegar for both dysentery and bowel disease. Dioscorides (*Eup.* 2.51.1) recommended eating bread made with egg yolks.

§5. *caseus – prodest.*

Comparanda: Plin. 30.19.55 for dysentery; Marc. 27.78.

§6. *sevum – medetur.*

Comparanda: Plin. 30.19.55 for dysentery; Marc. 27.75; Ps-Theod. *Ad.* II,31(102) for dysentery.

§7. *cochleae – bibiter.*

Comparanda: Plin. 30.19.55; Marc. 27.79.

The *Medicina Plinii* simplifies Pliny's advice.

§8. *cochlearum – bibitur.*

Comparandum: Plin. 30.19.56.

Snail ash was included in treatments for dysentery and bowel disease (Ps-Gal. K14.380; Orib. *Syn.* 9.15.5 6, *Eun.* 4.87.5–6; Alex. *Therap.* 2.429; Paul. Aeg. 3.42.2).

§8 *senectus – inlinitur.*

Comparanda: Plin. 30.19.57; Marc. 27.80; Ps-Theod. *Ad.* II,31(102). Cf. *Med. Plin.* 2.9.1 and commentary.

Rose cerate alone was also used (Aret. *CD* 2.7.2).

§9. *dysentericis – debent.*

Comparanda: Plin. 34.44.151; Marc. 27.81.

The nature of the drink warmed this way varied (Diosc. *MM* 5.80.2; Alex. *Therap.* 2.427; Paul. Aeg. 7.3.18).

§9. *caseus – inmittitur*.
Comparandum: Plin. 28.58.205 for dysentery and *tormina*.

§9. *ad – iubent*. . .
Comparanda: Plin. 29.59.207 (cheese application) for dysentery and bowel disease; Marc. 27.81.

§9. . . . *veterem – devorari*.
Comparandum: Plin. 29.59.207 for dysentery and bowel disease.
Vinum cibarium: a thin table wine normally served with meat (Rider 1589, "*vinum*").
Pseudo-Galen (K14.560) recommended shaved, aged cheese in sharp vinegar. Marcellus (27.66) recommended a different preparation of cheese and wine.

§10. *lac – decoctum*.
Comparanda: Plin. 28.58.206 for dysentery and *tormina*; Diosc. *Eup.* 2.50.2 for dysentery and bowel disease.
Boiled milk was a common treatment for bowel complaints (e.g. Diosc. *MM* 2.70.3; Gal. K12.291; Orib. *EM* 54.2; Alex. *Therap.* 2.427; Paul. Aeg. 3.40.5; Paul. Nic. 64; *DMAC* 42.3).

§10. *infunditur – decoctus*.
Comparanda: Plin. 28.58.209; Marc. 27.82.
The language is not explicit, but *infundo* here might mean "to clyster". It is translated here as "administer" to reflect this vagueness.
A topical use of bull glue was recommended by Paul. Aeg. (3.42.5).
Glue made from bull's hides was considered best (Diosc. *MM* 3.87.1).

§11. *frequenter – leporis*.
Comparanda: Plin. 28.51.199; Marc. 27.84, 28.21, 28.48.

12. *tineis*

This chapter concludes the author's ongoing discussion of gastrointestinal complaints which started at 2.4; it is included here likely because he described tapeworms as a complaint of the *venter*. Following this he addressed conditions of other organs within the lower part of the torso, continuing the "head-to-toe" approach.

Tinea: a late spelling of *taenia* (Rose 1894, 544), tapeworm.

While Pliny and the author wrote of either *taenia* or "animals in the belly or intestines", Greek medical writers recognised three kinds of parasitic intestinal worms: flat worm, round worm, both using an adjective with ἕλμινς, and ἀσαρίς. Peck (LCL: *Aristotle IX*, 172) suggests these are trematodes (flukes), nematodes (which includes hookworm, threadworm, and whipworm), and cestodes (tapeworms) respectively. That does not match Spencer's (LCL: *Celsus I*,

436) identification of Celsus' worms (4.24.1): flattened worms (tapeworm, *Taenia solium*), and rounded worms (giant roundworm, *Ascaris lumbricodes*).

§1. *tineae – cinere.*
Comparanda: Plin. 28.59.211; Plac. 1α.5, 1β.5; Marc. 28.26.
Serenus (29 l. 564) and Pseudo-Theodorus (*Ad.* II,30(98)) also recommended this for worms generally.
Burnt deer horn with other medicaments was recommended, but the variety of worm it treated differed between authors (Diosc. *Eup.* 2.68.1; Archig. 17; Paul. Aeg. 4.57.7).
Raw deer horn shavings were recommended to treat a variety of worms (e.g. Scribon. 141; Diosc. *Eup.* 2.69.3; Gal. K14.241; Ps-Gal. K14.549; Orib. *EM* 57.3; Cassius 72; *Antidot. Brux.* 43; Paul. Aeg. 4.57.5; Paul. Nic. 73).

§1. *raphani – miscetur.*
Comparandum: Marc. 28.27.
Pliny (20.13.26) recommended this for intestinal hernia and recommended radish with honey and vinegar for worms.
Eating radish and salt was recommended (Ps-Theod. *Ad.* II,30(98)).

§2. *radix – tangere.*
Comparanda: Plin. 20.19.38; Marc. 28.28; Ps-Theod. *Ad.* II,30(98).
Pseudo-Apuleius (96.3) recommended elecampane leaves. Elecampane was also included in compound treatments (Archig. 17; Orib. *EM* 57.3; Paul. Aeg. 4.57.8, 4.57.12).

§2. *alium – devoratur. . .*
Comparanda: Plin. 20.23.54; Seren. 29 l. 570.
Celsus (4.24.2) recommended eating garlic to treat children's worms.
Eating garlic was included as a partial treatment for various worms (e.g. Cels. 4.24.1; Scribon. 140; Diosc. *Eup.* 2.68.1; Ps-Gal. K14.574–5; Orib. *EM* 57.6; Alex. *Lumbric.* 2.599; Paul. Aeg. 4.57.11; *Geopon.* 12.30.1).

§2. . . . *betae – crudo.*
Comparanda: Plin. 20.27.69; Ps-Theod. *Ad.* II,30(98).
Cooked beets were recommended with mustard (Athenaeus 9.371b).

§3 *aqua – bibitur*
Comparanda: Plin. 22.74.155; Diosc. *MM* 2.109.1, *Eup.* 2.69.1; Marc. 28.29; Ps-Theod. *Ad.* II,30(98); Paul. Aeg. 7.3.8.
Various decoctions of lupines were commonly recommended most commonly for rounded worms (e.g. Cels. 4.24.1–2; Orib. *EM* 57.8; Paul. Aeg. 4.57.5; Paul. Nic. 73).

§4. *bulbi – bibitur.*
Comparandum: Plin. 20.39.99.

The only other reference to squills was the use of squill-flavoured vinegar (Archig. 17; Paul. Aeg. 4.57.7).

§4. *malum – potum.*
Comparanda: Plin. 23.58.109; Ps-Theod. *Ad.* II,30(98).
Cato (*De agricultura*, 126) recommended steeping pomegranates in wine and drinking for tapeworms, but pomegranate root decoctions were also used (e.g. Cels. 4.24.1; Diosc. *MM* 1.110.3, *Eup.* 2.67.1; Orib. *EM* 57.3).

§5. *acini – inlini.*
Comparanda: Plin. 24.47.77; Marc. 28.30; Ps-Theod. *Ad.* II,30(98).

13. lieni sive spleni

Here the author shifted from gastrointestinal complaints to splenic conditions, naming the organ in both Latin and transliterated Greek. Why he placed it following worms is not clear given that the spleen has more in common with the *praecordia* than the *venter* and its parasites, and has nothing in common with the lower back, the focus of the following chapter.

§1. *solea – remittitur.*
Comparanda: Plin. 32.32.102 (returning all fish to the water); *Cyran.* 4.6; Marc. 23.44.
This used transfer magic, both the disease to the fish and the flatness of the fish to the spleen.

§2. *aqua – sale.*
Comparandum: Seren. 22 l. 406.
Eating variously prepared cabbage was recommended (Cato *De agricultura*, 157; Diosc. *MM* 2.120.3, *Eup.* 2.63.3; Plin. 20.34.87).

§2. eius – est.
Comparanda: Plin. 22.73.151; Seren. 22 ll. 414–5; Ps-Theod. *Ad.* II,28(82).

§3. *sarmentorum – debebit.*
Comparanda: Plin. 23.3.5 (vine twig ash); Marc. 23.46.
Sarmentum: literally "twig"; commonly refers to vine twigs.
Vine twig ash and vinegar was also used topically (Diosc. *MM* 5.1.2, *Eup.* 2.64.1; Aët. 2.3).

§3. *acetum – bibitur. . .*
Comparandum: Cels. 4.16.2.

§3. *et – apponitur.*
Comparanda: Plin. 31.47.128 (*posca*); Gal. K13.256; Theod. 2.28.80; Paul. Nic. 60.

Hippocrates (*Liq.* 6) recommended cooling applications to reduce splenic swelling, and vinegar was considered cooling.

§3. *corymbi – prosunt.*
Comparanda: Plin. 24.47.76; Seren. 22 l. 409.
Ivy was thought to have same properties as vinegar (Plin. 24.47.75); this might account for its use internally and topically (e.g. Gal. K13.242; Ps-Gal. K14.377; Orib. *EM* 49.3; Ps-Apul. 99.3; Ps-Theod. *Ad.* II,28(82); *Geopon.* 11.30.4).

§4. *hederaceis – est.*
Comparanda: Plin. 24.47.79; Seren. 22 ll. 404–5; Ps-Theod. *Ad.* II,28(82).

§4. *lien – dicentur.*
Comparandum: Plin. 30.17.51.
This was a *similia similibus* magical application. Pliny described it as "Magian", perhaps relating to the sealing ritual.
Marcellus (23.47) described a near identical ritual using a dog's spleen, but that might have drawn upon a tradition of magically applying dog spleens (*Cyran.* 2.20, 2.21).

§5. *caninus – aceto.*
Comparanda: Plin. 30.17.51, 30.17.52; Plac. 9α.13, 9β.17; Marc. 23.48.
The noun "spleen" has been lost from the text but assumed in the translation.
Dog's spleens are the same shape as human's Aristotle (*Part. an.* 3.2), so an element of *similia similibus* magic was included; the magical nature is also supported by Pseudo-Galen's (K14.459) recommendation that patients unwittingly consume a puppy's spleen.

§6. *idem – praestat.*
Comparanda: Plin. 30.17.52; Marc. 23.62.

§6. *cochlearum – persanetur.*
Comparanda: Plin. 30.17.52; Marc. 23.64.
Nettle leaves were used in topical treatments (Diosc. *MM* 4.93.1, *Eup.* 2.64.1). Linseed was included in some plasters (e.g. Prom. *Coll.* 13.8–9; Gal. K10.796; *DMAC* 36.3).

§7. *lacerta – tangat.*
Comparanda: Plin. 30.17.52; Marc. 23.50.

§7. *sedat – potum. . .*
Comparandum: Plin. 28.57.200.

§7. *. . . cervini – aceto.*
Comparanda: Plin. 28.57.200; Plac. 1α.8.

Galen (K13.377) included burnt deer horn in a compound; deer horn filings
were also used (Hippoc. *Int*. 30; *Cyran*. 2.11; Gal. K14.241).

§7. *equi – bibitur.*
Comparanda: Plin. 28.57.200; Plac. 14.5; Marc. 23.30.
Oribasius (*EM* 49.1) described having a dry tongue as a symptom of spleen
disease; this might have been a magical response.

§8. *praesentaneo – imponuntur.*
Comparandum: Plin. 28.57.200.
The consumption of ox or cattle spleen was also recommended (Cels. 4.16.3;
Plin. 28.78.259).

§9. *haedi – praestat.*
Comparanda: Plin. 28.57.201; Ps-Gal. K14.460; Marc. 23.33.

§9. *radices – inlinuntur.*
Comparanda: Plin. 21.76.131; Marc. 23.48.
Lotae (washed) might have been a misspelling of *lutae* (yellow); Pliny and
Marcellus specified yellow, not washed, violet roots.

§9. *agarici – lienem.*
Comparanda: Plin. 26.68.75; Diosc. *MM* 3.1.3; *Eup*. 2.62.1.

14. lumborum dolori

While the previous chapter devoted to the spleen seems out of place, the author
securely returned to his "head-to-toe" format here as anal conditions and complaints of lower torso organs follow this.

"Lower back pain", "lumbago", or "pain of the loins" are all equally valid
translations of *lumborum dolor*. "Lower back pain" was rarely addressed as a
discrete complaint; Aëtius 5.130 provided one other exception.

§1. *acinorum – sanat.*
The *Medicina Plinii* omits the noun *strychnus*, "nightshade", the juice of which
berry Pliny (27.44.68) recommended. *Acinus* was used to refer to various
berries and grapes, so this omission would have confused his audience.

§1. *itemque – emendant.*
The author conflated Pliny's advice relating to taking elecampane for worms
and coughs with the application of its leaves with wine for the back
(20.19.38, cf. Ps-Theod. *Ad*. I,(XXXVII)).

§2. *pastinacae – emendant.*
Comparandum: Garg. 33.

Pliny (30.15.31) specified the use of *staphylinus* or *pastinaca erratica*, "stray parsnip", a kind of parsnip or carrot.

§2. *item – sanat.*
Comparanda: Plin. 20.21.46; Marc. 25.16; Ps-Theod. *Ad.* I,(XXXVII).
The text recommends taking chive juice in significantly less wine than Pliny advised.

§3. *itemque – emendat.*
Comparandum: Plin. 20.42.108.
Pseudo-Theodorus (*Ad.* I,(XXXVI)) recommended asparagus seeds.

§3. *apii – prodest.*
Comparanda: Plin. 20.44.115; Marc. 25.16.
Pliny did not provide doses.

§4. *holusatri – datur.*
Comparanda: Plin. 20.46.117; Garg. 27.
Holusatrum: alexanders, *Smyrnum olustrum*. Pliny did not provide doses.

§4. *radix – medetur.*
Comparanda: Plin. 20.42.109 (white wine); Garg. 31; Marc. 25.26; cf. Ps-Theod. *Ad* I,(XXXVII).
Serenus (24 ll. 454–5) also recommended asparagus.

§5. *item – imponitur.*
Comparanda: Plin. 20.50.130 (cress, *polenta*, and vinegar); Marc. 25.28; Ps-Theod. *Ad.* I,(XXXVII).
Gargilius (13) recommended this for hip-disease.

§5. *itemque – sanant.*
Giant fennel was recommended nowhere else.

§6. *lana – imponitur.*
Comparanda: Plin. 29.9.32; Seren. 24 ll. 451–4; Marc. 25.10; Ps-Theod. *Ad.* I,(XXXVII).
Nitrum Atticum: Attic soda; this is its only reference.

§7. *item – dolverint.*
This treatment is recorded nowhere else, and grammatical errors and incon-sistencies make it difficult to fully understand. The *Medicina Plinii* uses the masculine *ipsos* to refer to what was "carefully ground"; this can only refer to the feminine cypress cones, *pilularum*, or the neuter seeds, *granis*. The cypress tree is described as green, but cypresses are evergreens. It makes

logical sense, but not grammatical, to read *viridis* "green" with the cones; Pliny (17.14.73) described how brown cypress cones burst open to release their seeds. The author might have been specifying the use of unripe green cones which still contained their seeds.

§8. *item – adipe.*
Comparanda: Plin. 35.50.176; Seren. 24 1. 456.

15. sedis vitiis

The author here began to work from the lower back (his previous chapter) to the front of the lower torso. It is odd, however, that he addressed colon pain in the subsequent chapter.

Sedis vitium: literally "complaint of the seat"; a euphemism.

§1. *medicamentum – inflationes.*
Rhagadia/ragadia, ῥαγάς: "chap" or "crack"; Celsus (6.18.7A) described it as a fissure in the skin of the anus.
Condyloma, κονδύλωμα: a "callous lump", but other descriptions include Hippocrates' (*Haem.* 4) knob shaped like a mulberry which grows next to blood vessels of the anus, which, if it was especially protuberant, flesh grows around, and Celsus' (6.18.8A) small protuberance formed as the result of inflammation.

§§1–2. *ammoniaci – uteris.*
Lituematis: translated as haematite by Stoll (1992, 175), but without an explanation for his identification. He might have done this on the basis of a similar compound recorded by Galen (K13.309): it featured haematite, all the other ingredients of this compound, though in different quantities, and the addition of round alum. This compound treated *condyloma*, inflammation of the anus, and *ragadia*.
Önnerfors (1964, 50) incorporated this passage from a manuscript of the *Plinii Physica* (*Codex Bambergensis Medicus 1*, folio 29v) which measured the quantities in *scripuli* instead of *denarii*.
Elements of this compound were used to treat anal complaints with other medicaments (Cels. 6.18.7B; Scribon. 220; Plin. 24.5.9).

§3. *item – uteris.*
Another use of hyssop was a softening emollient made with animal-sourced lipids for *condyloma* (Prom. *Coll.* 72.8). See Aëtius (16.83) and Paul. Aeg. (3.59.2) for the only other uses.

§3. *item – aspergito.*
Marcellus (31.24) recommended horehound to treat fistulas of the anus.

§4. *item – sanat.*

Comparanda: Plin. 24.73.119; Cels. 6.18.8A; Diosc. *MM* 4.37.1, *Eup.* 1.208.1; *Med. Plin.* 2.17.1; Marc. 32.30; Paul. Aeg. 3.59.2.

§5. *item – imponitur.*

Comparanda: Plin. 30.22.70 to prevent stinging from "acrid humours", presumably in faeces; *Med. Plin.* 2.17.2; Marc. 32.31.

The *Medicina Plinii* omits swan grease from the recipe.

The use of white lead to treat *condyloma* was described elsewhere (e.g. Plin. 34.50.169; Orib. *EM* 82.4–8), and in similar combinations, but with additional medicaments by Galen (K13.309, 311–2, 532–3).

16. coli dolori

While the shift inwards to address colon pain after a chapter on anal conditions is logical, it is odd that the author did not include these treatments among his discussion of gastrointestinal complaints above. The reason for its omission might be because he did not use the term *colum* "colon" anywhere within those chapters. After this he returned to address an external anal condition which was addressed within the chapter prior to this.

§1. *ad – bibere.*

There was a tradition of using chickens' κοιλία (this might refer to any part of the digestive tract) to treat gastrointestinal conditions (*Cyran.*3.3; Orib. *EM* 53.6; Aët. 9.35; Paul. Aeg. 3.40.2). Theodorus (2.31.102; cf. *Med. Plin.* 1.6.9; 1.24.3) used similar language to describe the use of a burnt membrane from the bellies of capons and other birds used to treat dysentery.

§2. *sunt – oportet.*

Comparanda: Plin. 30.20.64; Marc. 27.132.

For a similar use of puppies see *Medicina Plinii* 2.4.2 and commentary.

§3. *vespertilionis – interaneorum.*

Comparanda: Plin. 30.20.64; Marc. 28.45.

Pliny attributed this prophylactic to the Magi.

§3. *cornu – vini.*

Comparandum: Plin. 28.59.211 for *tenesmos.*

Snails, deer horn ash, and other medicaments were recommended for colon pain (Scribon. 122), colic (Gal. K 13.280, 284), and dysentery (Paul. Aeg. 7.12.12).

§4. *facit – opera.*

Önnerfors (1964, 51) and Brodersen (2015, 103) state that this relates to *Medicina Plinii* 2.4.13–4.

§4. *hederae – datur.*

Pseudo-Apuleius (79.3) recommended sword-lily (*gladiolus*) berries for *praecordia* pain, but sword-lilies have no berry.

17. condilomatis

This chapter includes treatments which the author already provided in his discussion of anal conditions two chapters prior to this. He continued to move forward within the lower torso after this, and addressed the bladder next.

   Condiloma/condyloma: see commentary to *Medicina Plinii* 2.15.1.

§1. *oleum – imponere.*
Comparanda: Plin. 22.60.127; Marc. 31.42.

§1. *folia – sanant.*
Comparanda: Plin. 24.73.119; Cels. 6.18.8A; Diosc. *MM* 4.37.1, *Eup.* 1.208.1; *Med. Plin.* 2.15.4; Marc. 32.30; Paul. Aeg. 3.59.2.

§1. *radices – sedis.*
Comparanda: Plin. 24.73.120; Ps-Apul. 88.8; Marc. 31.43.

§2. *araneus – condylomata.*
The treatment is repeated from *Medicina Plinii* 2.15.5 (see commentary for comparanda).

§2. *adeps – imponitur*
Comparanda: Plin. 30.22.70; *Med. Plin.* 2.15.5.

§2. *adeps – sedat*
Comparanda: Plin. 30.22.70 for haemorrhoids; Marc. 31.28.

18. vesicae dolori et calculo

Moving from back to front in the lower torso, the author here addressed two common bladder conditions: pain and bladder-stones. It is curious that the author did not include urinary incontinence, the title of the following chapter, within this chapter under a more generic heading.

§1. *amyli – dolorem*
Comparanda: Plin. 22.67.137; Marc. 26.78.
Drinking starch simmered in water and drunk with sweetened wine was recommended (Cassius 46).
Starch was included in compounds for bladder ulceration (e.g. Prom. *Coll.* 18.5; Gal. K13.324; Orib. *EM* 63.7; Aët. 11.29; Paul. Aeg. 3.45.6); the simplest was drinking starch, linseed, and water (Ps-Gal. K14.383).

§2. *cicer – triduum*.

Comparanda: Plin. 22.72.150; Marc. 26.79.

Cicer arietinum: literally "ram's-head chickpea". This is also the scientific name for standard chickpeas.

Dioscorides (*Eup.* 2.119.4) recommended a chickpea decoction to address difficult urination and bladder-stones. They were included in compounds for difficult urination (Gal. K13.328).

§2. *cariotae – imponuntur*.

Comparandum: Plin. 23.51.97.

Date plasters were recommended for urinary irritation (Aët. 3.151), as were date-palm plasters for pain (Diosc. *Eup.* 2.110.1).

§3. *adversus – bibitur*.

Comparanda: Plin. 24.95.152; Ps-Apul. 89.4.

Millefolium with water and honey treated difficult urination and bladder-stones (Marc. 26.27).

Other uses of *millefolium* (see commentary to *Med. Plin.* 3.3.6 regarding Greek names for *millefolium*) were for blood present in urine (Diosc. *Eup.* 2.108.1) or difficult urination (Diosc. *Eup.* 2.113.5).

§3. *murino – prodest*.

Comparandum: Plin. 30.21.65 for bladder stone.

Marcellus (26.14) recommended this for difficult urination.

§3. *vermos – passo*.

Comparandum: Plin. 30.21.66 for bladder-stones.

Drinking earthworms was recommended for breaking up bladder-stones and difficult urination (*Cyran.* 2.8; Gal. K14.242; Aët. 2.168, 11.22, 11.23).

§4. *ad – pellit*.

Comparanda: Plin. 30.21.66; Marc. 26.91.

§4. *lapilli – inspargitur*.

Comparanda: Plin. 30.21.67; Marc. 26.12.

§5. *fimus – bibitur*.

Comparanda: Plin. 30.21.67; Marc. 26.80.

§5. *turturum – imponitur*.

Comparanda: Plin. 30.21.68; Seren. 31. ll.599–600; Marc. 26.81.

Unspecified preparations of turtledove dung were recommended for bladder-stones (Prom. *Coll.* 16.8; Ps-Gal. K14.576).

§6. *cicadas – bibere.*
Comparanda: Plin. 30.21.68; Diosc. *MM* 2.51.1; Ruf. 14.5; Aret. *CA* 2.9.4; Gal. K12.360; Aët. 2.193, 11.22; Paul. Aeg. 7.3.19.

§6. *contra – bibitur.*
Comparandum: Plin. 30.21.67.

§6. *de – bibitur.*
Comparanda: Plin. 30.21.67; Marc. 26.12.

§7. *turdorum – myrteis.*
Comparandum: Plin. 30.21.68.

§7. *aqua – datur.*
Comparanda: Plin. 30.21.68; Marc. 26.75.

§§7–8. *scorpio – bibitur.*
Comparandum: Plin. 32.32.102.
The *Medicina Plinii* alone specifies the consumption of both the animal and wine.
Killing a sea-scorpion in wine was not limited to bladder complaints (Orib. *CM* 14.50.1, *Syn.* 2.36). Sea-scorpion ash was used to break bladder-stones (Ps-Gal. K14.573).

§8. *lapillus – potatur.*
Comparanda: Plin. 32.32.102; Marc. 26.84; Ps-Theod. *Simp.* I,80.

§9. *inveniuntur – medentur.*
Comparandum: Plin. 32.32.102.
Bacchus fish were also called *myxon*/μύξων (grey mullet) according to Pliny (1.32).

§9. *echini – bibuntur.*
Comparanda: Plin. 32.32.103; Arist. *Hist. an.* 4.5, *Gen. an.* 5.3; Diosc. *Eup.* 2.119.4; Ruf. 14.5; Marc. 26.25; Aët. 2.171, 11.22.

§9. *difficultatibus – prodest.*
Comparanda: Plin. 37.12.51; Ps-Diosc. *Lapid.* 10; Marc. 26.17; Aët. 2.35.
Sucinum: an unusual name for amber. Some varieties of amber were thought to have been formed from lynx urine (Plin. 37.11.34).

§10. *plantaginis – prodest.*
Comparanda: Plin. 26.49.78; Diosc. *MM* 2.126.4; Ps-Apul. 1.24.

§10. *vesica – sumitur.*
Comparanda: Plin. 28.60.212; Marc. 26.102.

§10. *leporis – pellunt.*
Comparanda: Plin. 28.60.213; Plac. 3α.9, 3β.10; Marc. 26.19.

§10. *ungulae – bibitur.*
Comparanda: Plin. 28.60.213; Marc. 26.92.

19. incontinentiae urinae

While the title says "urinary incontinence", the comparanda for these treatments address bed-wetting, which received more attention in classical literature, whereas what is today called incontinence was only addressed in relation to spinal injuries. The positioning of this following the treatment of bladder-stones and pain was perfectly logical, as is the shift following this to the genitals.

§1. *verrini – cubili.*
Comparanda: Plin. 28.60.215; Marc. 26.128–9.
Pliny attributed this spell to the Magi.

§2. *ungulae – inspargitur.*
Comparanda: Plin. 28.60.215; Marc. 26.126.
Dioscorides (*Eup.* 2.106.1) recommended smoothed wild boar hoof.

§2. *leporis – bibitur. . .*
Comparanda: Plin. 28.60.215; Diosc. *Eup.* 2.106.1; *Cyran.* 2.24; Prom. *Coll.*
    23.5; Ps-Gal. 14.577; Seren. 31 ll. 387–9; Plac. 3α.1, 3β.1; Marc. 26.125;
    Aët. 11.25; Ps-Theod. *Ad.* I,27(78).

§2. *. . . et – eduntur.*
Comparanda: Plin. 28.60.215; Prom. *Coll.* 23.3; Gal. K13.319; Ps-Gal.
    K14.474, 577; Orib. *Eun.* 4.108.3; Plac. 3β.26; Marc. 26.125; Aët. 11.25;
    Paul. Aeg. 3.45.13.

§3. *anserum – sumuntur.*
Comparanda: Plin. 30.22.74; Marc. 26.123; Aët. 11.25.

§3. *cochleae – bibitur.*
Comparanda: Plin. 30.22.74; Ps-Gal. K14.572; Marc. 26.122.

20. verendorum vitiis

The author's shift from urinary conditions to genitalia was a logical progression. It should be noted that this chapter most likely addressed penile conditions only because the author did not discuss female complaints and he addressed testicular conditions in the subsequent chapter.

Latin medical writers had limited terminology with which to refer to genitalia, because the available vocabulary was not considered appropriate for "modest discussion" (Cels. 6.18.1). Medical texts tend to utilise euphemisms as a result; the choice of *verenda* (derived from the verb *vereor* "to revere") fits this trend.

§1. *si – inlinitur*.
Comparanda: Plin. 30.22.72 (sanies of cooked ram's lung); Plac. 4.β3; Marc. 33.39.
Formicatio: μυρμηκία, "ant-hill wart" (see introductory commentary to *Med. Plin.* 3.29). Μυρμηκία was rarely described as occurring on the genitals (Aët. 16.120), whereas θύμιον, the "thyme-coloured wart" was (e.g. Ps-Gal. K19.444; Orib. *CM* 50.8, *EM* 114.6; Aët. 16.121; Paul. Aeg. 3.59.2; Paul. Nic. 114).
Celsus (5.28.14B-C) described genital warts as the worst kind.

§1. *ceteris – aqua. . .*
Comparanda: Plin. 30.22.72; Marc. 33.56.

§1. *. . . sevum – frigida*.
Comparanda: Plin. 30.22.72; Marc. 33.55.

§2. *caro – frigida*.
Comparandum: Plin. 30.22.72.

§2. *mularum – inspargitur*.
Comparanda: Plin. 30.22.72; Marc. 33.38, 33.57; Ps-Theod. *Ad.* I,27(78).

§2. *ulceribus – scobis*.
Comparandum: Plin. 30.33.107.

§3. *muricum – singulariter*.
Comparanda: Plin. 32.34.108; Marc. 33.58.
Salsamentum, τάριχος: fish-pickle, salted fish, or brine pickle. Oribasius (*Syn.* 9.35.5, *Eun.* 4.102.5) described how salted fish heads were used to treat genital warts.
See introductory commentary to *Medicina Plinii* 3.8 for the nature of *carbunculus*.

§4. *cerebrum – suis*.
Comparanda: Plin. 28.60.213 (brain and blood) for genital *carbunculi*; Plac. 7α.2, 7β.2; Marc. 33.37.

§4. *sanat – imponitur*.
Comparanda: Plin. 28.60.214; Marc. 33.59.
Promotus (*Coll.* 19.15), recommended beets and mallow for inflamed genitals.

21. testiculis et ramicibus

The author's move from genital conditions to address testicular complaints and hernias in this chapter again reflects his logical approach to the body. A common hernia type which was the topic of ancient medical writers was that which occurs in the groin (inguinal), and the author shifted to groin complaints following this.

Latin terminology for hernia was simple: *ramex*; Greek terminology, which was occasionally adopted by Latin writers, was more precise. Greek used κήλη to refer to a hernia rarely, instead attaching it as a suffix to adjectives to define types of hernias. The more common varieties which shared some of the treatments outlined here were ἐντεροκήλη "intestinal hernia", and βουβωνοκήλη "inguinal hernia"; ὑδροκήλη, transliterated as *hydrocele*, was a collection of fluid in the scrotum (see *Med. Plin.* 2.21.6).

§1. *holus – apponitur.*
Comparanda: Plin. 20.34.89 (crushed beans); Garg. 30.

§1. *bulbi – medentur.*
Comparanda: Plin. 20.40.103–4 (applied for at least four days); Seren. 35 l. 681; Marc. 33.19; Ps-Theod. *Ad.* I,26(76).

§2. *rutam – imponunt. . .*
Comparanda: Plin. 20.51.141; Diosc. *Eup.* 1.132.2; Marc. 33.20; Ps-Theod. *Ad.* I,26(76).

§2. *. . . cyminum – rosaceo. . .*
Comparanda: Plin. 20.57.161; Cels. 6.18.6A.
Cumin was a common treatment for inflamed testicles, often prepared with raisins (e.g. Scribon. 238; Orib. *EM* 84.10, *Syn.* 9.36.1, *Eun.* 4.103.1; Paul. Aeg. 3.54.2; Paul. Nic. 85), and with added bean meal (Diosc. *MM* 5.3.3; Prom. *Coll.* 22.3).
Cumin was also used to treat hernia (Prom. *Coll.* 20.7), and *hydrocele* (Prom. Coll. 20.2, 20.5; Paul. Aeg. 3.53.3).

§2. *. . . farinam – myrrha.*
Comparanda: Plin. 20.92.251 for testicular complaints and hernias; Orib. *Syn.* 9.35.1, *Eun.* 4.102.1; Marc. 30.21; Ps-Theod. *Ad.* I,26(76).
Boiled linseed was recommended for testicular conditions (e.g. Cels. 6.18.6A; Diosc. *Eup.* 1.123.2; Prom. *Coll.* 19.14, 21.7; Orib. *EM* 84.10; Paul. Aeg. 3.54.2; Paul. Nic. 85).

§3. *contra – adhibetur.*
Comparanda: Plin. 22.69.140; Seren. 35 l. 682.
Various bean preparations, especially meal, were recommended (e.g. Cels. 6.18.6A; Diosc. *MM* 5.3.3, *Eup.* 1.132.2; *Med. Plin.* 2.21.4; Orib. *CM*

9.24.17, 9.35.1; Marc. 33.52; Paul. Aeg. 3.54.2). Plasters made of bean meal were considered the best (Gal. K12.50; Orib. *Syn.* 9.9.5, *Eun.* 4.82.5).

§3. *inflammationi – melle.*
Compare the use of beets on genitals (*Med. Plin.* 2.20.4 and commentary).

§3. *ad – inlinitur.*
Comparanda: Plin. 23.31.63; Seren. 35 l. 679; Orib. *EM* 84.13.

§4. *cupressi – prosunt.*
Comparanda: Plin. 24.10.15 for sunburn; Seren. 35 ll. 683–4.
Whether Pliny recommended *polenta* for hernias is open to interpretation.

§4. *pilulae – imponuntur.*
Comparanda: Plin. 24.10.15; Marc. 33.30; Theod. 1.28.79.
Cypress cones without axle-grease or bean meal were recommended to treat intestinal hernias (Prom. *Coll.* 21.4; Orib. *Syn.* 3.28.7, *Eun.* 3.1κ.101; Aët. 1.236; Paul. Aeg. 3.53.1, 7.3.10).

§4. *sucus – imponitur.*
Comparandum: Plin. 24.10.16.

§5. *farina – omnia.*
Comparandum: Plin. 24.120.188; cf. Ps-Theod. *Ad.* I,26(76).
Hydromeli, ὑδρόμελι: often translated as "*hydromel*" and literally means "honey-water" in Greek. Pliny (14.20.113) recognised it as a form of wine, but how, or if, it differed to *aqua mulsa* (see commentary on *Med. Plin.* 1.17.4 and Plin. 22.51.110) is unclear.
Önnerfors (1964, 55) incorrectly attributes Pliny 20.96.257 as the source of this. The author repeatedly mistook Pliny's use of fenugreek for fennel (cf. 1.2.1, 3.5.3), and Pliny's description of fenugreek meal decocted in *hydromel* with added axle-grease for genital conditions correlates with this treatment far better. This explains why fenugreek was more frequently recommended for testicular conditions (e.g. Cels. 6.18.6A; Orib. *EM* 84.10; Paul. Aeg. 3.54.2).

§5. *si – inlinitur.*
Comparanda: Plin. 30.22.72; Marc. 33.5.

§6. *taetris – aceto.*
Comparanda: Plin. 30.22.74; Marc. 33.40.

§6. *hydrocelis – dantur.*
Comparandum: Plin. 30.22.74.
Stellio/stelio: lizard, gecko, or newt named for its star-like spots on its back (Isid. *Etym.* 12.4.38).

Stelliones were described as different in Greece compared to Italy and Sicily (*De mirabilibus auscultationibus* 148; Plin. 8.49.111).

Other lizards (*Med. Plin.* 2.3.2, 3.21.7 and commentaries) and animals (*Med. Plin.* 3.21.6, 3.22.8) were prepared this way.

§7. *tumores – foventur.*
Comparanda: Plin. 31.33.65; Marc. 33.22.

§7. *si – imponitur.*
Comparanda: Plin. 31.47.129; Marc. 33.17.

22. inguinibus

While the inclusion of inguinal hernias in the previous chapters illustrates the author's intent to move down from the torso following the "head-to-toe" approach common to *euporista* texts, this was his first chapter dedicated to the legs alone. He discussed an array of groin and thigh conditions, before addressing leg ulcers in the following chapter.

§1. *negantur – tactum.*
Comparanda: Plin. 23.81.163; Marc. 32.20.
This magical prophylactic might have been extraordinarily old as taboos against iron suggest a pre-iron age origin (Luck 2006, 35).
Pliny stated that potential swellings occurred because of an ulcer/sore; this is now understood to be a serious infection affecting the lymphatic system.

§1. *cochleae – inlinuntur.*
Comparanda: Plin. 30.22.74; Seren. 35 ll. 686–7; Marc. 32.4.

§2. *inguina – genu.*
Comparanda: Plin. 28.12.48; Marc. 32.21.
Licium: any kind of thread or lace, but also a specific thread in weaving. Pliny stated that the thread should come from a loom.
Variations of this spell were provided by Pliny and Marcellus. Pliny stated that the knotted thread must be attached to the groin, a difficult place to secure an amulet, so the options within the *Medicina Plinii* of ankle, leg, or below the knee made this easier.
Another ritual of knotting a thread and speaking names was recorded in magical papyri (*PGM* 7 l. 210).

§3. *si – inlinitur.*
Comparanda: Plin. 28.61.218 (smeared on groin); Marc. 32.22.

§3. *inguinibus – oleo.*
Comparandum: Marc. 32.23; cf. Plin. 28.70.234 for general swelling. Cf. *Med. Plin.* 3.30.7 and commentary.

§4. *myrtea – circumligatur*.
Pliny 15.37.124 described myrtle twigs forming a ring for this treatment.
For the taboo on the use of iron see commentary on *Medicina Plinii* 2.22.1.

§4. *absinthium – prodest*.
Comparanda: Plin. 27.28.52; Ps-Apul. 101.4.

§4. *pollex – sedat*.
Comparanda: Plin. 28.9.42; Marc. 32.24.

23. ulceribus in crure vel in tibiis

This chapter continued the author's discussion of leg complaints by addressing ulcers
on the leg. Following this, the author shifted his focus further down to the ankle.
Crus: shank or entire leg.

Ulcus has been translated here as "ulcer" but it can refer to sore (see introductory
commentary on *Med. Plin.* 3.2). The *Medicina Plinii* provides a discussion of the
various types of ulcers recognised in antiquity at 3.4.1, but the inclusion of these
treatments in this separate chapter suggests that he considered these to be different.

Celsus (5.28.5) noted that "Chironean ulcers" chiefly occurred on the *crus* and
foot, but there is no correlation between his advice and that outlined here.

§1. *adeps – cerussa*.
Comparanda: Plin. 29.74.241; Marc. 34.4–5.
Rubrica: red ochre, red earth, or ruddle. *Rubrica* was a generic term for ochre;
    elsewhere Pliny recommended specific varieties, so this generic terminol-
    ogy indicates that any variety was suitable. Red ochre was noted for its
    drying properties and suitability for medicinal plasters (Plin. 35.13.31–
    35.16.35; cf. Vitruvius 7.7.2). Aëtius (2.4) recommended a specific variety
    (Lemnian earth) on ulcers.
White lead was used to treat various sores and ulcerative conditions (*Med.
    Plin.* 1.3.4–5, 2.25.2, 3.24.2 and commentaries).

§2. *maxillarum – inspargitur*.
Comparanda: Plin. 28.74.241; Marc. 34.6; Ps-Theod. *Ad.* I,(XL).

§3. *fimus – irino*.
Comparanda: Plin. 28.74.241 (Mayhoff 1897, 358 includes iris oil based solely
    on its inclusion in the *Medicina Plinii*); Marc. 34.7; Ps-Theod. *Ad.* I,(XL).
Butter was considered capable of filling ulcers (Diosc. *Eup.* 1.178.1).

24. talorum dolori et tumori

The shortness of this chapter devoted to the ankles, moving down the body from the
legs, likely reflects the limited problems which could be identified as occurring to
the ankles separate from the feet which the author addressed in the rest of this book.

§1. *muscus – imponitur.*
Comparanda: Plin. 31.38.72; Marc. 34.11.
Celsus (2.33.2) described moss as simultaneously repressive and cooling, so it
  likely felt nice while reducing swelling.

§1. *limus – prodest.*
Comparanda: Plin. 26.66.104; Marc. 34.12; Ps-Theod. *Ad.* I,(XII).
Limus: muck, mud, or slime.

§1. *fimus – melle.*
Comparandum: Ps-Theod. *Ad.* I,(XLII).
Pliny (28.62.223) recommended this to treat joint disease; joint diseases commonly include pain and swelling among their symptoms, so the author
  might have adopted this to address these symptoms.
Marcellus (34.13) provided a very similar treatment to this; featuring the identical use of wild boar (*aprunus*) dung instead of goat (*caprinus*) dung; this
  might be a copyist error.

25. pernionibus et vitiis pedum

This chapter begins the author's discussion of the feet, the final topic of *euporista*
texts. These conditions typically manifested on the upper part of the feet, and
are thus addressed separately to those which arise on the soles of the feet.
   This chapter's advice primarily treats chilblains and their complications, but
the text sometimes fails to state which treatment was meant for which condition.
This is not surprising as Pliny and later medical texts often did the same.

§1. *pulmo – imponitur.*
Comparanda: Plin. 32.36.111; Diosc. *MM* 2.37.1, *Eup.* 1.171.2.
Pulmo marinus: literally "sea-lung"; Pliny translated this from Dioscorides.
  Sea-lung cannot be positively identified but might be jellyfish or sea
  cucumber. Pliny (9.71.154) named it with *holothuria* (anemones or sea
  cucumber), and starfish. Aristotle (*Hist. an.* 5.15) claimed they were chiefly
  found around Caria.

§1. *cancri – imponitur.*
Comparanda: Plin. 32.36.111; Marc. 34.15; *Cyran.* 4.28.
Crab ash was used with other medicaments (e.g. Diosc. *MM* 2.10.1, *Eup.*
  1.171.1; cf. Paul. Nic. 131).

§1. *utiliter – est.*
Comparanda: Plin. 22.73.153; Marc. 34.15.
Bitter vetch decoctions were recommended for chilblains (e.g. Diosc. *Eup.*
  1.171.1; Orib. *Syn.* 7.45.1, *Eun.* 3.56.1; Paul. Aeg. 3.79.1; Paul. Nic. 131).

§2. *ficus – imponuntur*. . .

Comparanda: Plin. 23.63.123; Diosc. *Eup.* 1.171.4.

While Pliny failed to clearly specify whether the fig used was dried, his probable source, Dioscorides, did. Variously prepared figs were also recommended (e.g. Orib. *Syn.* 7.45.2; Paul. Aeg. 3.79.1; Paul. Nic. 131).

§2. . . . *ulceribus – alumina*.

Comparandum: Plin. 30.23.79.

Pliny recommended this for chilblains without reference to *ulcera*; perhaps the author recognised ulceration could be a complication.

Alum was included in preparations to treat chilblains themselves (Orib. *EM* 108.2, 108.5, *Syn.* 7.45.3; Paul. Aeg. 3.79.1), and ulcers or sores related to them (Diosc. *Eup.* 1.171.4).

§3. *si – imponitur*.

Comparandum: Plin. 30.23.79.

Understanding exactly how the author read Pliny's text is complicated by a lacuna in the middle of the relevant passage. Mouse dung was recommended for chilblains, but the lacuna in Pliny's discussion of wax on clean ulcers makes it impossible to discern whether these ulcers related to chilblains. His decision to swap Pliny's order of these treatments could be used to argue that they were.

§3. *vermium – imponitur*.

Comparanda: Plin. 30.23.79; Marc. 34.16.

§4. *cochlearum – sanantur*.

Comparanda: Plin. 30.23.79–80; Marc. 34.17.

Naked snails are slugs.

§4. *fimi – medetur*.

Comparanda: Plin. 30.23.80; Marc. 34.19.

It is impossible to determine whether these ulcers should be understood as related to chilblains, but unburnt hen's dung was a topical application for chilblains (*Cyran.* 3.34; Plac. 29.21; Ps-Theod. *Ad.* I,32(88)).

§5. *attritus – oleo*. . .

Comparanda: Plin. 28.62.222, 30.23.80; Diosc. *MM* 2.48.1, *Eup.* 1.164.1; Gal. K12.343; Orib. *Syn.* 7.5.5, *Eun.* 2.1δ.6, 3.19.2; Marc. 34.92; Aët. 2.162; Paul. Aeg. 3.79.7, 7.3.4.

§5. . . . *aeque – oleo*.

Comparanda: Plin. 28.62.22; Marc. 34.21; Ps-Theod. *Ad* 1, 32(88).

The author misread Pliny's text, reading *corium* (leather) as *cornus* (horn).

Pliny recommended burnt leather for chilblains and burnt goat-leather for rubbings made by shoes.

§6. *agninus – imponitur.*
Comparanda: Plin. 20.23.80; Diosc. *MM* 2.38.1, *Eup.* 1.164.1; Gal. K12.335;
    Orib. *Syn.* 7.5.4, *Eun.* 3.19.1; Aët. 2.154; Paul. Aeg. 3.79.7, 7.3.16.
Marcellus (34.18) recommended ram's lung on chilblains.

§6. *dentis – emendat.*
Comparandum: Plin. 30.23.80.
Subluvies: normally refers to a kind of foot-rot presenting in sheep, but Jones
    (LCL: *Pliny Natural History VIII*, 329) translated it as whitlow.
Horse-tooth powder was recommended for chilblains (Marc. 34.20; Ps-Theod.
    Ad. I,32(88)).

§6. *lacertae – sanat.*
Comparandum: Plin. 30.23.80. Cf. *Med. Plin.* 2.26.3.

§6. *tegumenti – medetur.*
Comparanda: Plin. 30.23.80 for sores and chaps; Marc. 34.22.
Testudo: tortoise or turtle; Latin does not differentiate between them.

§6. *adeps – sarcit.*
Comparanda: Plin. 28.62.221 for chilblains and cracks; Marc. 34.92.
Oribasius (*EM* 112.3) recommended the use of alum on cracks in the feet.

26. clavis et callis

This second chapter devoted to the feet addressed the sole rather than the upper
part of the foot like the preceding section. The author addressed the top and bottom
of the foot before shifting to an internal condition of the feet, *podagra.*

    Clavus can refer to a callus, wart, tumour, or other excrescences (see introductory
commentary on *Med. Plin.* 3.29). The Greek vocabulary for these complaints is
similar: ἧλος can refer to either wart or callus; τύλος to callus or risen knob; and
either can refer to a corn. Discussions of corns and calluses are complicated by
this. The potential confusion between hardened skin and warts was increased by
the similar treatments recommended for both.

§1. *plerumque – partibus.*
This description helped to differentiate *clavus* and *callus* from the author's
    discussion of warts (*verruca*) at 3.29.
Celsus (5.28.14C) provided a similar definition of *clavus.*

§2. *urina – tollit.*
Comparanda: Plin. 30.23.80; Marc. 34.49; Ps-Theod. *Ad.* I,32(88). Cf. *Med.*
    Plin. 3.29.1.

§2. *fimus – imponitur.*
Comparanda: Plin. 30.23.80; Marc. 34.50. Cf. *Med. Plin.* 3.29.1.

Sheep dung and vinegar were commonly applied to ἧλος, but it might refer
to warts (e.g. Diosc. *MM* 2.80.3; *Cyran.* 2.33; Gal. K12.301–2; Orib. *Syn.*
7.43.4, *Eun.* 3.55.3; Aët. 2.116; Paul. Aeg. 7.3.10).

§3. *iecur – medetur*.
Comparanda: Plin. 30.23.80; Diosc. *Eup.* 1.166.1; Seren. 63 l. 1095; Marc.
34.50, 34.105. Cf. *Med. Plin.* 3.29.1.
Lizard heads were also recommended (e.g. Diosc. *MM* 2.64.1, *Eup.* 1.166.1;
Gal. K12.344; Orib. *EM* 113.2; Paul. Aeg. 7.3.10).

§3. *vermes – oleo*.
Comparanda: Plin. 30.23.80; Marc. 34.106.

§3. *fimus – imponitur*.
Comparanda: Plin. 30.23.80; Marc. 34.51; Ps-Theod. *Ad.* I,35(93).
Oribasius (*EM* 113.2) recommended the use of generic bird dung to treat a
ἧλος.

§4. *fimus – prodest*.
Comparanda: Plin. 28.62.222; Marc. 34.52.

§4. *faba – alligata*.
Comparandum: Marc. 34.107.
While *silphium* or *laser* was used to treat corns and calluses (Diosc. *MM*
3.80.4, *Eup.* 1.166.1; Plin. 22.49.101, 22.49.103–4), only the author and
Marcellus included beans.

§5. *si – oleo*.
Lomentum's use as a skin-conditioner (see commentary on *Med. Plin.* 1.18.6)
might have made its use to soften hardened skin attractive. Paulus Aegineta
(3.80.1) recommended smearing a bean gruel made with vinegar to remove
both ἧλος and τύλος.

§5. *pollinem – enim*.
Comparandum: Plin 22.60.127.
Oribasius (*EM* 113.2) recommended the use of barley meal with vinegar for
ἧλος on the soles of the feet.

§6. *idem – hammoniacum*.
Comparanda: Plin. 24.14.23; Ps-Theod. *Ad.* I,32(88).
The author read Pliny's text on this as using *Ammoniacum* gum alone to treat
calluses, and with honey to treat indurations (cf. *Med. Plin.* 1.21.2) when it
was the other way around.
The use of *Ammoniacum* gum was recommended with various other medicaments (Diosc. *MM* 5.79.10; Gal. K12.736–7, 777–9), as an application after
they were softened (Diosc. *Eup.* 1.166.1; Orib. *EM* 113.2), and referred to

in passing when recommending better treatments (Orib. *EM* 113.2; Paul. Aeg. 3.80.1).

§6. *salicis – tollit.*
Comparanda: Plin. 24.37.56: Marc. 34.108.
Burnt willow bark was also recommended with vinegar (Diosc. *MM* 1.104.10, *Eup.* 1.166.1; Orib. *EM* 113.2, *Syn.* 7.43.2, *Eun.* 3.55.2; Paul. Aeg. 7.3.9).
Willow is a source of salicylic acid, the active ingredient in modern "corn caps" which remove corns by macerating their hardened skin.

§7. *utuntur – polline.*
Comparandum: Plin. 28.62.222.

§7. *urina – imponitur.*
Comparanda: Plin. 30.23.81; Seren. 63 l. 1096; Plac. 9α.18; Marc. 34.53; Ps-Theod. *Ad.* I,35(93). Cf. *Med. Plin.* 3.29.1.

27. podagrae dolori

This final chapter devoted to the foot condition *podagra* is the conclusion of the author's work following the "head-to-toe" approach common to *euporista* texts. This chapter forms a natural stopping point for this book before the author moved onto diseases and complaints not specific to a particular position in the body.

Podagra, ποδάγρα: most commonly translated as gout despite the fact that gout is now known to be the result of an excessive concentration of uric acid in the blood. This translation might be because they shared the stereotype that they were the result of a rich diet or lifestyle (e.g. Lucian *The Dream, or the Cock*, 23). The Latin spelling has been retained to provide accuracy.

Podagra literally translates as "foot-hunter" and its symptoms coincide with various arthritic and rheumatic conditions including gout. Variations of the name were used: *mentagra* described in the *Medicina Plinii* at 1.18.1; χειράγρα used for the same symptoms as *podagra*, but presenting in the hands. The placement of this discussion within the text following on from other feet complaints indicates that the author was focusing on the disease occurring in the feet.

The disease was rarely described as fatal, but occasionally deaths were recorded following complications (e.g. Hippoc. *Morb.* 1.3.144; Diogenes Laertius 5.4.68). Descriptions of famous cases outlined horrific pain and desperation among sufferers (Suetonius *Galba*, 21.1, *De grammaticis*, 3).

§1. *Muscus – prodest.*
Comparandum: Plin. 31.38.72. Cf. *Med. Plin.* 2.24.1.

§1. *farina – imponitur.*
Comparanda: Plin. 22.57.120; Seren. 41 l. 781; Marc. 36.64.
Frumentum: grains, most commonly wheat and barley.

If Pliny was his source, the author mistakenly recommended a treatment for contracting tendons. Dioscorides (*MM* 2.86.2) recommended applying barley boiled in vinegar, and barley meal was variously prepared in plasters (Prom. *Coll.* 54.1; Lucian, *Tragoedopodagra* [commonly translated as "Gout"], l. 159; Alex. *Therap.* 2.551).

§1. *utiliter – intestina.*
Comparanda: Plin. 32.36.110; Seren. 41 l. 782; Marc. 36.32.
See *Medicina Plinii* 2.26.2, 2.26.5 and commentaries for more.

§2. *ranae – vetere.*
Comparanda: Plin. 32.36.110; Marc. 36.32.
Lucian (*Tragoedopodagra*, l. 163) referenced boiled toads as a treatment. See commentary on *Medicina Plinii* 2.26.5.

§2. *in – polenta.*
Comparanda: Plin. 22.70.145; Diosc. *MM* 4.87.1; Marc. 36.63; Cassius 52.
Known as duckweed or water lentils, this plant was described rather than named. It was a popular treatment (Lucian *Tragoedopodagra*, l. 154; Orib. *EM* 75.1, 103.5; Alex. *Therap.* 2.513; Paul. Aeg. 3.78.7). Owing to its cooling properties it was especially recommended for "burning" *podagra* and generic fiery inflammations (Ps-Gal. K14.386).

§3. *adipe – perunguntur.*
Comparandum: Plin. 30.23.77.
Viper flesh was also recommended (Aët. 12.67).

§3. *sanguine – perunguntur.*
Comparandum: Plin. 30.23.78. Cf. Marc. 36.37.
This treatment might have used *similia similibus* magic as kites were thought to suffer from *podagra* (Plin. 10.12.28). Drinking dried, ground kite brain was also recommended (*Cyran.* 3.19).

§3. *hibisci – ponis.*
Comparandum: Ps-Apul. 38.1.
Marshmallow boiled in various liquids was commonly recommended (Cels. 4.31.4–5; Scribon. 160; Plin. 20.14.29; Marc. 36.45), especially for *podagra* without swelling, perhaps because it was described as warming.
Various parts of marshmallow were included in plasters (Orib. *EM* 75.15; Alex. *Therap.* 2.517–9, 2.537–9; Paul. Aeg. 7.17.7).

§4. *malvae – ponis.*
Malva erratica: stray or wild mallow. The only other references to its use, though not in this manner, are Greek (Orib. *EM* 75.7; Paul. Aeg. 3.78.7; *DMAC* 50.3).

§4. *lenticulum – imponis.*

Dioscorides (*MM* 2.107.2) described the use of lentils boiled with barley meal as a plaster, and Lucian (*Tragoedopodagra*, l. 158) listed lentils as a popular treatment.

§5. *urtica – apponitur.*

Comparanda: Plin. 30.23.78; Marc. 36.37.

Lucian's (*Tragoedopodagra*, l. 153) inclusion of crushed nettle implies it was a popular treatment, but it does not appear in other extant sources.

§5. *adipe – perunguntur. . .*

Comparandum: Plin. 32.36.110.

Cyranides (1.21) recommended the application of seal fat with cerate and resin.

§5. *. . . cuius – expedit.*

Comparanda: Plin. 32.36.110; *Cyran.* 1.21; Marc. 36.27; Alex. *Therap.* 2.581; Ps-Theod. *Ad.* I,(XLVI).

§5. *ranae – imponitur.*

Pliny (32.36.110) recommended this for joint disease, not *podagra*. Its inclusion in this chapter could be because the author recognised *podagra*'s association with joint disease (see 2.26.20).

Lucian listed frogs among his popular treatments (*Tragoedopodagra*, l. 164), and they were used in some compounds (e.g. Gal. K13.1026; Aët. 12.63).

§6. *lenit – axungia.*

Comparandum: Marc. 36.66.

Plantain was more commonly used with salt (Plin. 26.64.101; Ps-Apul. 1.13; Ps-Theod. *Ad.* I,38(97)).

Plantain features in Lucian's list of popular treatments (*Tragoedopodagra*, l. 150), and was recommended in other preparations (e.g. Aret. *CD* 2.12.2; Orib. *EM* 75.1, 103.4).

§6. *limus – prodest.*

Comparanda: Plin. 26.66.104 for swollen and painful ankles; Marc. 36.66. Cf. *Med. Plin.* 2.24.1.

§6. *ursine – utuntur.*

Comparanda: Plin. 28.62.219; Marc. 36.67.

§7. *bubulum – magificant.*

Comparanda: Plin. 28.62.220; Ps-Theod. *Ad.* I,(XLVI).

§7. *fimi – prodest.*

Goat dung was a common treatment (Lucian *Tragoedopodagra*, 1. 161), but Dioscorides (*MM* 2.80.2, *Eup.* 1.228.3) recommended its use unburnt with axle-grease.

§8. *cum – est.*

For examples of poultices associated with individuals see Galen (K13.355–6, 360).

§§9–13. *picis – molescit.*

Euphorbia/euphorbea: the milky juice or latex of *Euphorbium resinifera*, a member of the spurge family.

Opopanax: panax juice, especially of Heracles' woundwort (see commentary on *Med. Plin.* 1.1.4). Dioscorides (*MM* 3.48.4) recommended it in a plaster with raisins.

Aluta: an adhesive patch used in medical treatments.

Ammoniac salt: salt sourced from the desert near the Siwah Oasis and named for its oracle of Ammon. It is not *Sal Ammoniac*.

There were similar compound plasters. The closest Latin prescription included wax, roasted resin, pitch, *Ammoniacum* gum, frankincense, and *galbanum* (Scribon. 266). Celsus (4.31.6) described a much simpler mix of pitch, wax, and alum in equal parts to give relief.

Ammoniacum gum was recommended boiled with an equal weight of either pitch or wax and rose oil by Pliny (24.14.23) or used in a plaster with dry pitch by Dioscorides (*Eup.* 1.228.3).

The choice of vocabulary by the author (this is the only example of his use of the Greek word for alum, *stypteria*), and nature of this recipe suggests that it was Greek in origin. All of these ingredients feature in Greek plasters, although *euphorbea*, bull bile, and Ammoniac salt are rare. Comparable Greek prescriptions included a Neapolitan plaster (Gal. K13.1020); a pale green/yellow unguent (Aët. 12.63) which included *Ammoniacum* gum, split alum, *opopanax*, *galbanum*, wax, and frankincense; and Damocrates' "Dysrachitis plaster" (Gal. K13.797–9) which included round alum, *galbanum*, *Ammoniacum* gum, resin, and wax.

§13. *hoc – potest.*

The reference to a lack of staining implies that this was a common problem. Various plasters were named for their colour, and Aëtius' *About Hip Disease, Podagra, and Joint Disease* even included a chapter entitled "Other coloured unguents" (12.63).

The references to the loss of efficacy following, presumably, long-term use and its ability to be kept for long periods of time address problems which are common in modern pharmacology: the loss of pain relief provided by modern analgesics over time and the shelf life of some drugs.

§§14–18. *et – die.*

Comparandum: Marc. 36.68.

Camedria: the only use of this word in Latin literature. Pseudo-Apuleius (24.3) described the use of a *camedris* and Marcellus named the ingredient *chamaedryos* in his copy of this potion; it is most probably χαμαίδρυς, germander. Draughts of germander with centaury were recommended by Dioscorides (*Eup.* 1.227.1) and Paulus Nicaeensis (128).

Aristolochia: birthwort. Three varieties, all from the *Aristolochia* genus, were described in classical medicine: round or female; large, male, or δακτυλῖτις; and long or κληματῖτις (Diosc. *MM* 3.4.1–3). Round *aristolochia* is identified as *Aristolochia rotunda*. Drinking *aristolochia* was recommended (Gal. K11.836; Orib. *Syn.* 9.57.1, *Eun.* 2.1α.60; Aët. 1.43), but *aristolochia* is poisonous and has caused kidney damage when used in alternative medicine (Scarborough & Fernandes 2011, 3–21).

Stoechas, στοιχάς: French lavender. This did not commonly appear in treatments; its inclusion in a remedy recorded by Aëtius (12.67) is another rare exception.

Galingal appears in a number of remedies for joint disease, but only in one other treatment for *podagra* which was curiously described (Aët. 12.69).

Glass vessels: glass was described as "not smelling" (Petronius 50) and their use may have been a response to taint from reusing porous containers (Whitehouse 2001, 32), the caustic natures of some drugs, or adverse reactions with materials from which vessels were made. Glass *pyxides* thought to have contained *materia medica* have survived (Corning Museum of Glass, accession no. 44.1.68).

There were potential problems using the weight "silver *denarius*" at the time of composition (see commentary on *Medicina Plinii* Prol. 9).

Some similar draughts which include germander, centaury, *aristolochia*, tree fungus, and honey among other medicaments were recorded (Orib. *Syn.* 3.103.2; Aët. 12.67; Alex. *Therap.* 2.553–5, 2.571; Paul. Aeg. 7.11.59). Many more compound potions were recommended. Some of these potions were known for their number of ingredients: Lucian described how potions were drunk containing, four, eight, or "most popularly" seven ingredients (*Tragoedopodagra*, ll. 169–70).

§19. *radix – imponitur.*

Comparanda: Plin. 20.4.9; Diosc. *MM* 4.150.1, *Eup.* 1.228.6; Marc. 36.67.

Cucumis erraticus; also called *cucumis silvaticus* (Ps-Apul. 114), wild/ squirting cucumber, *Ecballium elaterium* (Beck 2017, 304).

Squirting cucumber root was recommended boiled in various other liquids (Cels. 4.31.6; Orib. *EM* 75.7; Ps-Apul. 114.1; *DMAC* 50.3).

§19. *mitigatur – abiscum.*

Comparanda: Plin. 28.62.220; *Cyran.* 2.24; Marc. 36.26.

Alexander (*Therap.* 2.581) provided a similar recommendation, but referenced the use of an ἀστράγαλος (the ball of a hare's ankle joint or a vertebra from its neck).

§20. *peractis – accidere. . .*

This passage is not especially clear, with the use of *inproviso* by the author which most commonly means "unexpected" seeming to be out of place with *solent* which relates to habitual or customary occurrences.

§20. . . . *percurremus – proxima.*

This segue to the next book gives a glimpse of the overall strategy of the author of the *Medicina Plinii* and his medical knowledge. His move from *podagra* to joint and tendon complaints was logical. In addition to his inclusion of a joint disease treatment (frogs in 2.27.5), *podagra* was often addressed in literature with joint complaints, and to a lesser degree tendon problems. Aretaeus (*SD* 2.12.1) made the point that ἀρθρῖτις (which he also considered related to tendons) was a general pain in joints, while *podagra* was its name when occurring in the feet. Paulus Nicaeensis (128) also stated that the only difference between ἀρθρῖτις and *podagra* was that *podagra* related to the feet alone. Cassius (52) addressed *podagra* and joint complaints together, and also noted a relationship between *podagra* and tendons. In addition to this, *podagra* and joint complaints were commonly addressed together in texts (Orib. *EM* 75, *Eun.* 4.116; Cassius 52; Aëtius *Book Twelve*; Paul. Aeg. 3.78). These examples do not even touch upon the multitude of topical treatments described as addressing both. Therefore, it is no surprise that the author moved from *podagra* to joint complaints when addressing "things as they come to mind".

Commentary on Book Three

Book Three is the point at which the author shifted from a typical *euporista* "head-to-toe" approach to medical writing to address conditions which affected the whole body or were not specific to a particular part thereof. Unlike the separation of Book One from Book Two, this partition appears to have been intended by the author as it was foreshadowed in the Prologue (Prol. 10) and followed on from concluding remarks at the end of the previous book.

1. Ad nervos et articulos

As stated above, the author's shift from *podagra* to joint and tendon conditions was a logical progression when moving from the *euporista* format to general conditions. The inclusion of injuries and strikes within this chapter (3.1.3 especially) seems to have influenced the author's decision to address wounds following this rather than moving directly to a discussion of cut tendons (3.3).

Nervus: tendon, sinew, or cords made from them. While the modern term "nerve" does derive from this, the author did not use this term to refer to nerves as they are understood now.

§1. *amphisbaena – imponitur.*
Comparanda: Plin. 30.36.110; *Cyran.* 3.9; Seren. 53 ll. 970–2; Plac. 23.6; Marc. 35.1; *Vulture Epistles* (Cumont 1926, 29).
Amphisbaena: a two-headed snake (Plin. 8.35.85; Ael. *NA* 9.23).

§1. *senectus – alligatur.*
Comparandum: Plin. 30.36.110.

§2. *beta – medetur.*
Comparanda: Marc. 34.109; Seren. 36 ll. 702–3.
Beet and fig were used more often separately (e.g. beet: Hippoc. *Epid.* 7.1.100; Orib. *EM* 75.7; Aët. 12.34; e.g. fig: Cels. 4.18.32; Plin. 22.75.159; Orib. *Syn.* 3.80.2; Aët. 3.179).

§2. *folia – imponuntur.*
Comparanda: Plin. 23.3.3; Marc. 34.63.
Barley was commonly recommended (Cels. 4.29.2; Diosc. *MM* 2.86.3, *Eup.* 1.228.2; Garg. 30; Orib. *EM* 75.7; Marc. 36.45).

§3. *acrifolium – prodest.*
Comparanda: Plin. 24.72.116 (holly and salt); Marc. 34.64.
Additions to Pliny's advice improved adherence to the skin.

§3. *incussos – curat.*
Comparanda: Plin. 30.23.78; Marc. 34.65.
Spider-webs were considered blood-staunching (Diosc. *MM* 2.63.1; Orib. *CM* 10.22.2).

§3. *articulis – capillorum.*
Comparanda: Plin. 30.23.79; Marc. 34.79.
Animal-sourced lipids were used frequently (e.g. Cels. 5.18.29; Scribon. 263; Gal. K13.696; *Cyran.* 2.23; Orib. *CM* 10.28.7; Marc. 35.23; Cassius 52; Aët. 12.49).

§4. *nervorum – melle. . .*
Comparanda: Plin. 30.36.110; Marc. 35.2, 35.29.
Cyprian oil/unguent was included in numerous tendon treatments (Scribon. 156, 206, 267; Gal. K12.635, K13.182–3, 696; Cassius 38), likely owing to its perceived heating and tendon-softening properties (Diosc. *MM* 1.55.3, 1.95.1; Plin. 23.46.90).

§4. *item – se.*

The author might have misread Pliny's advice regarding *galbanum* on "knots of the joints" (24.13.21).

Galbanum was likely included in numerous compounds (e.g. Cels. 5.18.28; Scribon. 255; Thessal. *De virtutibus herbarum* 1.8.4; Gal. K13.1013–16, 1050–2; Marc. 35.8) because of its warming, softening, and dispersive qualities (Diosc. *MM* 3.83.1; Orib. *Syn.* 2.27.1, *Eun.* 1.2χ.1; Paul. Aeg. 7.3.22).

§4. *stirax inlinitur.*

Comparandum: Plin. 24.15.24.

Stirax: storax, the gum of *Styrax officinalis.*

Storax was likely included in compounds (e.g. Scribon. 269; Gal. K13.967–8, 1036–7; Orib. *Syn.* 3.64.1; Marc. 35.24) owing to its heating and softening properties (Diosc. *MM* 1.66.2).

§4. *fimum – melle.*

Comparanda: Plin. 28.72.237; Marc. 35.20, 35.28.

§5. *tremulis – additum.*

Comparanda: Plin. 22.68.139, 32.41.120; Marc. 35.3. Cf. *Med. Plin.* 3.31.

Tremulus: trembling or shaking, or a person suffering from *paralysis* (involuntary tremors).

Castoreum: unctuous excretion from sacs situated in the groin of beavers.

The topical application of *castoreum* alone is well attested (Diosc. *MM* 2.24.1; Plin. 32.13.29; *Cyran.* 2.19; Aret. *CA* 1.2.12; Gal. K12.338–9; Marc. 20.6).

Vegetable, *"holus"* were added to Pliny's advice, but he recommended eating cabbage, *brassica* (see commentary on *Med. Plin.* 2.3.3), to treat *tremuli* (20.34.85).

Bathing was understood to relax tendons (Marc. 35.23).

§5. *articulorum – medetur.*

This treatment is repeated at *Medicina Plinii* 3.25.3 in a dedicated chapter (see commentary on *Med. Plin.* 3.25.3 for comparanda).

2. sanguine ex ulceribus sistendo

Here the author started a series of chapters relating to wounds, a topic he slightly touched upon in the preceding chapter. While the text addressed bleeding in particular here, the following chapters relate to different kinds of wounds.

While *ulcus* is most often translated as "ulcer", the injuries described here resemble wounds, its secondary definition. Isidorus (*De differentiis verborum*, 577) gave the impression that the difference between *ulcus* (a long-standing *vulnus*) and *vulnus* (a wound from a recent blow) was precise, but this does not reflect how these were used interchangeably.

§1. *fimus – sistit.*

Comparandum: Plin. 30.38.112.

Spathomele, σπαθομήλη: a flat, broad medical probe (Isid. *Etym.* 4.11.2–3).
Given its rarity and Greek etymology, this might reflect a Greek influence
on the approach by author to wound care.

The description for *spathomele* use could be read two ways: the ash and
honey might have been mixed with the *spathomele*, reading *mixto melle*
spathomele together, similar to Marcellus' description of its use (7.19,
14.44); or *spathomele* could be read with *imponitur plagae*, used to deliver
the medicament, similar to Galen's description (K10.889).

Horse dung was considered blood-staunching, but its preparation differed
among writers (Diosc. *MM* 2.80.3, *Eup.* 1.198; Plin. 28.73.239; *Cyran.*
2.17; Orib. *EM* 85.5; Marc. 10.26; Paul. Aeg. 4.53.5).

Egg shells were used to staunch blood (Orib. *EM* 15.1; Aët. 2.135; Paul. Aeg.
3.24.8).

§2. *polypus – adhibetur.*

Comparandum: Plin. 32.42.121.

Cephalopods were believed to bloodless (Plin. 11.49.133, 11.78.199; Ael. *NA*
11.37), so this might have utilised sympathetic magic.

§2. *cortex – glutinant.*

Comparanda: Plin. 23.3.4; cf. Diosc. *Eup.* 1.198.1; Orib. *EM* 85.5; Paul. Aeg.
4.53.5.

§3. *folia – sistunt.*

Comparanda: Plin. 23.67.132; Garg. 44.

§3. *pilulae – impositae.*

Comparandum: Plin. 24.29.44; cf. *Med. Plin.* 3.4.17.

§4. *ferulae cinis.*

Comparandum: Plin. 26.83.135.

Ferula: Giant fennel, *Ferula communis*; an acknowledged blood-staunching
medicament whose preparation varied (Orib. *CM* 46.1.111, *EM* 86.1; Aët.
6.94; Paul. Aeg. 4.53.5, 6.106.1).

§4. *hircini – sistit.*

Comparandum: Plin. 28.73.240.

3. recentibus vulneribus et nervis incisis

The shift from staunching blood in the previous chapter to addressing the wound
itself in this chapter illustrates a degree of common sense, and perhaps the author's
medical experience; no other first aid can be applied aid until bleeding is stopped.

While the author's discussion of cut tendons might have thematically followed on from his discussion of tendon and joint complaints, any wound which cut a tendon is considerably deep and would bleed profusely.

§1. *vermes – conglutinant*. . .
Comparanda: Plin. 30.39.115; Seren. 62 l. 1087.

§1. . . . *adeo – septimo*.
Comparanda: Plin. 30.39.115; Diosc. *MM* 2.67, *Eup*. 1.154.2; *Cyran*. 2.8; Gal.
    K12.363; Orib. *Syn*. 7.1.8, *Eun*. 3.13.8; Aët. 2.168; Paul. Aeg. 4.37, 7.3.3.

§1. *idem – solvuntur*.
Comparandum: Plin. 30.39.116.
Earthworms were variously prepared to treat sores, ulcers, wounds, and cut
    tendons (e.g. Plin. 30.23.79; Seren. 53 ll. 978–9; Marc. 4.38, 4.40, 35.22).
Vinegar is still used in modern medical practices as a desiccant.

§2. *cochleae – sanant*.
Comparanda: Plin. 30.39.116; Diosc. *MM* 2.9.3.
Snails were agglutinants (Cels. 5.2; Gal. K12.322–3; Orib. *EM* 84.4, *Syn*. 7.1.7,
    Eun. 3.13.7; Aët. 2.183), as were frankincense and myrrh (Cels. 5.2; Gal.
    K12.127; Orib. *CM* 11.λ.7, *Eun*. 2.1σ.36; Aët. 1.370; Paul. Aeg. 7.3.18).

§3. *efficaces – solvebat*.
Comparanda: Plin. 20.40.104; Ps-Theod. *Ad*. I,21(68).
Pliny and Pseudo-Theodorus described the use of *bulbus* with *mulsum*, "hon-
    eyed wine", rather than *muscum*, "moss", so *muscum* might have been writ-
    ten by error.
No *bulbus* candidate nominated by Jones (see commentary on *Med. Plin*.
    1.2.1) was a recognised agglutinant, but narcissus and white lily bulbs were
    (Diosc. *MM* 4.159; Gal. K12.85–6; Orib. *Eun*. 2.1v.4; Ps-Apul. 55.1; *Anti-
    dot. Brux*. 174; Paul. Aeg. 7.3.13).
If Dalby's (2003, 64) theory that *bulbus* was βολβός is correct (see commentary
    on *Med. Plin*. 2.4.2), Galen's βολβός ἥμερος was an agglutinant (K11.851),
    but Dioscorides' βολβός ἐδώδιμος was not (*MM* 2.170.1).
Damon was not referred to elsewhere.

§4. *myrobalanum – solidat*.
Comparandum: Plin. 23.52.98.
Jones (LCL: *Pliny Natural History VI*, 478–9) suggests Pliny confused *myrob-
    alanum*, the palm that bears behen-nuts, with the Egyptian date palm; the
    description of *myrobalanum* as a date here is a continuation of this error.
    This explains why only dates were recommended elsewhere (Gal. K13.375,
    Ps-Gal. K18a.808; Aët. 1.236, 7.45, 15.13). However, this does not explain
    the author's appropriate use of behen-nuts to open the bowels (see com-
    mentary on *Med. Plin*. 2.5.2).

§5. *et – imponuntur.*

Comparanda: Plin. 24.10.15; Diosc. *MM* 1.74.2, *Eup.* 1.154.2.

Cypress was used to treat wounds in other ways (Plin. 20.8.17; Gal. K12.52; Seren. 53 l. 975; Orib. *Eun.* 2.1κ.98; Aët. 1.236; Paul. Aeg. 4.37.1, 7.3.10).

§5. *rubi – sanant.*

Comparanda: Plin. 24.73.117; Ps-Apul. 88.7; Ps-Theod. *Ad.* I,21(68).

Different parts of bramble were recommended (Diosc. *Eup.* 1.154.1; Gal. K11.848, K12.577–8; Orib. *Eun.* 2.1β.5; Aët. 1.62; Paul. Aeg. 7.3.2).

§6. *et – imponitur.*

The use of *millefolium* alone is not recorded elsewhere, but there was a broader tradition for its use with axle-grease (Plin. 24.95.152; Seren. 43 ll. 813–4; Ps-Apul. 89.2).

There were numerous different types of *millefolium*, all acknowledged as suitable for wounds. Pliny described two varieties (24.95.152, 25.19.42). The first matches Dioscorides' μυριόφυλλον, water milfoil (*MM* 4.114.1), a recognised agglutinant (Diosc. *Eup.* 1.154.2; Paul. Aeg. 7.3.12). The second was known as *Achilleos, Heraclea panax* (Hercules' woundwort), *sideritis,* and *militaris* (Ps-Apul. 89). In Greek literature these were often different plants: Dioscorides (*MM* 4.36.1) recognised *Achilleos* (Achilles' woundwort) as *sideritis,* which was recommended for bleeding wounds (Gal. K12.121). *Militaris,* a translation of στρατιώτης, was also called χιλιόφυλλος (a literal translation of *millefolium*) according to Dioscorides (*MM* 4.102.1), was recommended for wounds too (e.g. Gal. K12.131; Paul. Aeg. 7.3.18), and is identified as yarrow.

It is impossible to deduce which *millefolium* the author meant, or if he was even aware of the multiple varieties.

§6. *centauriae – coquuntur.*

Comparandum: Plin. 25.30.67.

Large centaury's agglutinant properties were well known (e.g. Diosc. *Eup.* 1.154.2; Gal. K12.19; Orib. *Eun.* 2.1κ.40; Aët. 1.192; Paul. Aeg. 7.3.10), and specifically recommended (Diosc. *MM* 3.6.3; Ps-Apul. 34.5).

§7. *lana – imponitur.*

Comparandum: Plin. 29.9.31.

This appears to be the result of crasis between Pliny's advice for ulcers and wounds.

Pliny never specified the use of greasy wool, a known agglutinant (Cels. 5.2), but it was recommended as he described by others (Diosc. *MM* 2.73.1, 5.6.11: Gal. K13.752; Seren. 43 l. 815).

§7. *spongia – intumescere.*

Comparanda: Plin. 31.47.126; Diosc. *MM* 5.120.1.

Wet sponges were commonly used to close wounds (Cels. 5.2; Gal. K13.421; Orib. *Syn.* 7.1.5, *Eun* 2.1σ.21; Aët. 2.73; Paul. Aeg. 7.3.18).

§8. *et – tumorem.*
Comparandum: Plin. 28.74.242.

§8. *idem – praestat.*
Comparanda: Plin. 28.74.242; Ps-Theod. *Ad.* I,21(68).
Dioscorides (*MM* 2.80.1) recommended cattle dung (ἀπόπατος) applied to injuries.

§9. *recentes – iuvat.*
Comparandum: Plin. 28.74.243.
Glue's obvious agglutinant properties (Cels. 5.2) might account for how little it was recommended (Diosc. *MM* 3.87.1; Paul. Aeg. 7.3.19).

4. ad ulcera et ad cancer quod noma vocatur

While the preceding chapters addressed wounds and used the noun *ulcus*, this chapter addressed significantly different conditions: forms of ulcers. Despite the complications which surround their treatments, these are a type wound, which is likely why this large chapter was placed here. Given that following this chapter the author addressed a variety of abscesses, which if their treatment is mismanaged could result in ulceration, this positioning might again reflect his medical experience. In addition to this, the treatment of abscesses was also referred to within this chapter (3.4.9 and 3.4.12).

Cancer: a specific ulcer variety; named for its resemblance to crabs. It is not modern cancer.

Noma, νομή: a spreading ulcer named for its perceived "feeding" or "grazing" nature. Hippocrates (*Prorrh.* 2.13) considered it the most deadly ulcer.

§1. *scio – est.*
Various ulcers were recognised (Cels. 5.28; Gal. K10.385–6).
Ulcers and sores were called ἕλκος in Greek, and its meanings are similar to *ulcus* (see introductory commentary on *Med. Plin.* 3.2).

§2. *vermes – sistunt.*
Comparanda: Plin. 30.39.115; Marc. 4.38.
Cossus: a grub born in wood, perhaps specifically oak (Plin. 11.38.113, 17.37.220). Rackham (LCL: *Pliny Natural History III*, 503) translated this as goat-moth larvae, but only on account of it scientific name, *Cossus cossus*.
The author misread *anesum* (anise) as *anethum* (dill) as he did at 1.1.2, however burnt dill was used to treat ulcers (Gal. K10.381–2, K11.832; Orib. *Eun.* 2.1α.48; Aët. 1.37; Paul. Aeg. 4.44.6, 7.3.1).

§3. *fimo – sanantur.*

Comparandum: Plin. 30.39.114.

Fistula: an ulcer which forms a tunnel. In modern medicine it describes any abnormal tunnel within the body.

§3. *nomam – appositae.*

Comparandum: Plin. 30.39.116.

Small linen cloths with other medicaments (Gal. K13.733; Paul. Aeg. 4.44.1) and lint pledgets were recommended (Gal. K12.683; Orib. *EM* 83.3; Aët. 7.34; Paul. Aeg. 7.17.36).

§4. *cacoëthe – mel.*

Comparandum: Plin. 30.39.118; cf. Marc. 4.39.

Cacoëthes, κακοήθης: often translated as "malignant". In relation to ulcers it gives a sense of a chronic, intractable, or incurable nature (LCL: *Galen Method of Medicine I*, lxxxviii-ix).

§4. *eadem – debet.*

Comparanda: Plin. 32.44.126 (without cloths); Marc. 4.39.

Cyranides (4.50) recommended the use of young tuna.

§5. *vermes – tolluntur.*

Comparanda: Plin. 32.44.127; Marc. 4.40.

This complication was recognised as occurring in *noma* and putrid ulcers, and treated by drying (Gal. K13.733; Paul. Aeg. 4.42). Bile was a recognised desiccant (Gal. K12.277, 279–80).

§5. *quae – curantur.*

Comparanda: Plin. 32.44.127 (without specifying staleness); Marc. 4.40.

Salted fish products were used for numerous ulcerative conditions, helped by salt's desiccant nature (Diosc. *MM.* 2.32.1, 2.28.1; Gal. K13.732; Paul. Aeg. 4.44.1; Delatte 1939, 489).

§5. *radix – vocant,*

Comparanda: Plin. 20.6.11; Garg. 15; Marc. 4.41.

Favus: a direct translation of κηρίον, honeycomb. This refers to school sores (*Impetigo contagiosa*); the crust which forms after their blisters burst resembles honey (Beck 2017, 91). Pseudo-Galen (K14.324, 777) and Marcellus (4.41) described this as an affliction of the head, but school sores can present anywhere; the author's placement of this in Book Three suggests he knew this.

Dioscorides (*MM* 2.135.2) recommended this with honey.

§6. *semen – appellant.*

Comparanda: Plin. 20.13.27; Marc. 4.42.

Phagedaena, φαγέδαινα: a quickly spreading ulcer that eats flesh to the bone, with a viscous discharge, an intolerable smell, and inflamed flesh around the site (Cels. 5.28.3B). Its name derived from the verb "to eat", φαγεῖν.

§6. *porrus – purgat.*
Comparanda: Plin. 20.22.49; Garg. 21; Marc. 4.43.

§7. *alium – extrahit.*
Comparanda: Plin. 20.23.55; Marc. 4.44.
Garlic and resin were used in other ways (e.g. Hippoc. *Fist.* 7; Diosc. *Eup.* 1.183.1; Gal. K13.317; Orib. *Syn.* 9.35.6; Aët. 15.44).

§7. *vetera – die.*
Comparanda: Plin 20.33.81; Cato *De agricultura*, 157.3–5; Marc. 4.45.
Carcinoma, καρκίνωμα: this was often used interchangeably with *cancer*; they were not always differentiated between (Gal. K10.82–3). Celsus described it as an ulcer which afflicted the upper body, especially women's faces and breasts (Cels. 5.28.2A).
Pliny (from Cato) specified the use of *brassica*, cabbage (see commentary on *Med. Plin.* 2.3.4). The fomentation was independent from Pliny's advice.
Cabbage was variously used to treat ulcers (e.g. Diosc. *MM* 2.120.2; *Cyran.* 5.10; Gal. K12.42, K13.732; Orib. *Eun.* 2.1κ.80; Aët. 1.221; Paul. Aeg. 4.44.1).

§8. *sic – imponuntur.*
Comparanda: Plin. 20.33.82, 20.34.88.

§§8–9. *lini – emendat.*
Comparanda: Plin. 20.92.251; Diosc. *MM* 2.103; Marc. 4.46.
Dioscorides (Pliny's source) recommended this to cleanse ἥρπης, a term often translated as "shingles", but was derived from the verb "to creep", ἕρπω; therefore a "creeping ulcer".
While "creeping ulcer" can be read as a different condition to "eruptions of mucus" in Pliny, some ulcers have a mucus-like discharge, so the comprehension of the author of the entire passage relating to ulcers was clinically reasonable.

§9. *pustulas – imponitur.*
Comparanda: Plin. 22.70.142; Marc. 4.46.
Lentils were described as cleansing (Cels. 5.5.2; Diosc. *MM* 2.107.2).
Lentils were recommended for pustules which could potentially become ulcerated (Cels. 5.28.15; Aët. 4.21). They were also used to treat various ulcerative conditions (e.g. Diosc. *MM* 2.107.2; Gal. K13.734; Ps-Gal. K14.324; Orib. *EM* 89.15, 98.2; Aët. 7.32; Paul. Aeg. 4.20.3).

§10. *lenticulae – trito.*

The author misread Pliny 22.70.143, reading *sedem* as *sed*, and thus recommended lentil juice with rose oil and quince for ulcers instead of "complaints of the seat".

Lentils were commonly used for mouth and genital ulcers (e.g. Hippoc. *Epid.* 7.1.47; Cels. 6.18.2F, 7.3.3; Gal. K13.317; Orib. *CM* 43.42.4, 50.2.9; Marc. 4.46, 11.1; Aët. 8.49). Quince and quince oil were recommended for various ulcerative conditions (e.g. Diosc. *MM* 1.45.2; Orib. *CM* 43.36.47, *Syn.* 8.45.1; Marc. 11.1; Aët. 7.34; Paul. Aeg. 3.22.26, 3.66.3).

§10. *farina – imposita.*

Comparandum: Plin. 22.73.151

Bitter vetch was commonly used on spreading ulcers (Diosc. *MM* 2.108.2, *Eup.* 1.191.1, 1.193.1; Gal. K11.138; Orib. *CM* 44.22.16, *Syn.* 3.35.27, 7.11.22, *Eun.* 3.25.21; Paul. Aeg. 4.19.2). Its meal was considered cleansing (Cels. 5.5.2; *Cyran.* 1.1), and a suitable sarcotic (Gal. K10.163, 177; Orib. *EM* 98.8; Paul. Aeg. 4.40.1).

See Celsus (5.28.3D) for the use of medical instruments to apply medicaments.

§11. *lupini – siccat.*

Comparandum: Plin. 22.74.155.

Lupines were used, but not described as desiccants (e.g. Diosc. *Eup.* 1.193.2; Gal. K11.885; Ps-Gal. K14.397; Orib. *Eun.* 2.10.4; Marc. 4.62; Aët. 1.162; Paul. Aeg. 3.3.4; Paul. Nic. 91).

§11. *cinis – sanat.*

Comparandum: Plin. 23.3.6.

§11. *folia – medentur.*

Comparanda: Plin. 23.34.69 for ulcers generally; Marc. 4.48.

Olive leaves were used on *noma* and putrid ulcers (Diosc. *MM* 1.105.1–2; Aët. 7.32).

§12. *cauliculi – comprimunt.*

Comparanda: Plin. 23.38.78 for the head; Marc. 4.49.

Pliny's use of wild olive beyond this was limited (23.38.76, 23.38.78).

§12. *contra – adhibentur.*

Comparandum: Plin. 23.38.77 for abscesses.

§13. *ulcera – expurgat.*

This is a repeat of *Medicina Plinii* 1.3.3 (see that commentary for comparanda).

§13. *fici – vocant.*

Comparanda: Plin. 23.63.119; Diosc. *MM* 1.128.5, *Eup.* 1.163; Orib. *EM* 95.1; Paul. Aeg. 4.35.1.

§14.*carcinomati – est.*

Comparanda: Plin. 23.63.123 for *carcinoma* and *phagedaena*; Cels. 5.28.2E; Garg. 49.

The *Medicina Plinii* only recommends this for *carcinomata*; the omission of *phagedaena* is curious as the format of this chapter was justified as allowing the author to include treatments suitable for multiple ulcerative conditions (3.4.1).

§14.*nuces – impositae.*

Comparanda: Plin. 23.77.148 for gangrene; Marc. 4.51.

Walnuts and their oil were most commonly used to treat gangrene which was considered an ulcerative condition (Diosc. *MM* 1.125.2, *Eup.* 1.191.1; Gal. K12.14; Orib. *CM* 44.22.25; Aët. 1.185; Paul. Aeg. 4.19.2–3; Paul. Nic. 91).

§15. *glans – ilicina.*

Comparanda: Plin. 24.3.7; Diosc. *MM* 1.106.2, *Eup.* 1.193.1; Marc. 4.52.

Ilicina: a later spelling of *iligna*; *ilignus* is holm-oak, *Quercus ilex.*

§15. *ulceribus – inlinitur.*

Comparanda: Plin. 24.16.25 for shingles/creeping ulcers; Diosc. *MM* 3.76.2, *Eup.* 1.161.1.

§16. *pix – medetur.*

Comparanda: Plin. 24.23.38; Marc. 4.53.

Dioscorides (*MM* 1.72.2) recommended raw pitch with honey.

Dry or Bruttian pitch was variously used (Diosc. *MM* 1.72.5; Gal. K13.785; Aët. 15.14; Paul. Aeg. 4.39.1).

Raisins were commonly used with other medicaments (e.g. Diosc. *MM* 5.3.3; Ps-Gal. K14.397; Orib. *EM* 95.1; Aët. 15.7; Paul. Aeg. 4.35.1).

§16. *aqua – foventur.*

Comparanda: Plin. 24.28.42; Marc. 4.54.

Mastic decoctions were used to treat *noma* and *phagedaena* (Diosc. *MM* 1.70.2, *Eup.* 1.190.3; Paul. Aeg. 4.44.1) and mastic was used in other treatments (e.g. Orib. *Syn.* 1.19.18, *Eun* 3.18.3; Aët. 9.42).

§17. *pilulae – melle.*

Comparandum: Plin. 24.29.44.

The author either misread Pliny's text, mistaking *malandriasque* as a reference to apples and *veteres* for worms, or this passage is the victim of textual corruption. An early manuscript reads *Pilulae de platanis tusae emendant vermes tullunt. Malatusa ex melle* (*Cod. Sang. 752*, 56). Textual corruption would explain a lack of Latin comparanda for this. Rose (1875, 77) uses this as an excuse to rewrite the text to more closely follow Pliny, disregarding the use of sources other than Pliny.

Plane tree bark was more commonly used (Gal. K12.104; Orib. *Syn.* 3.35.32; Paul. Aeg. 4.44.6, 7.3.16).

§17. *hedera – ulcerum*.
Comparanda: Plin. 24.47.78; Diosc. *MM* 2.179.3; Seren. 62 l. 108; Ps-Apul.
99.5; Marc. 4.55.
Ivy was used more broadly (Diosc. *Eup.* 1.193.1; Gal. K12.30; Orib. *Eun.*
2.1κ.54; Aët. 1.205).

§17. *idem – melle*.
Comparandum: Plin. 29.9.31.
Like at 3.3.7, the author specified greasy wool when Pliny had not.
Burnt greasy wool was commonly applied to moist ulcers with honey (Diosc.
MM 2.73.1; *Cyran.* 2.33; Gal. K12.349; Orib. *CM* 43.57.20, *Syn.* 3.35.29,
7.11.11, *Eun.* 2.1ε.20, 3.25.11; Aët. 3.159; Paul. Aeg. 7.3.5).

§18. *cinis – exaequat*.
Comparanda: Plin. 30.39.113; Marc. 4.56–7.
The *Medicina Plinii* combines Pliny's dung ash and soda with the use of femur
ash.
The use of *pecus*, an imprecise term (see commentary on *Med. Plin.* 1.6.5), to
determine the type of dung suggests its source was not terribly important;
elsewhere specific directions relating to varieties of dung were given by the
author and Pliny; Pliny even described the different natures of sheep and
cattle dung (17.6.52).
Burnt sheep dung was included in some remedies (Gal. K12.302; Aët. 2.116),
and burnt, crushed bone was used as a desiccant (*Cyran.* 3.9).

§19. *ulcera – coercet*.
Comparanda: Plin. 32.44.126; Diosc. *MM* 2.28.1.
Pliny misread Dioscorides and attributed the use of *smaris* (*Spicara smaris*)
to *mena* which preceded it in Dioscorides' text; the *Medicina Plinii* repeats
this error. Aëtius (2.184) made a similar error, and late lexicographers and
scholiasts conflated these fish (e.g. Hesych. *Lex. Σ* 1229; Schol. in Opp.
1.108, 3.188).
Smaris is a member of the same genus as *mena*, and little damage likely
resulted as both were used to treat ulcers (Diosc. *Eup.* 1.179.1; *Cyran.* 4.46;
Orib. *CM* 14.58.2).

§19. *fistulae – auferunt*.
Comparandum: Plin. 32.44.127.
Burnt, pickled *menae* heads were recommended by some (Diosc. *MM* 2.29.1;
Gal. K12.333; Aët. 2.155; Paul. Aeg. 7.3.10). This use of linen pieces was
described as a "tent treatment" (Hippoc. *Fist.* 3, 4; Gal. K11.125).

§20. *serpentium – cicatricem*.
Comparanda: Plin. 36.57.180: Marc. 4.58.
Calx non lota: literally "unwashed lime"; an unusual form of the term *calx viva*
to denote quicklime. Quicklime was considered better than slaked lime for

medicinal use (Plin. 36.57.180), and was used to check ulcers (Diosc. *Eup.*
1.179; Orib. *CM* 14.58.2), and in eschar-creating medications for *noma*
(Gal. K10.325).

Pliny recommended quicklime alone, but the author mistakenly mixed quicklime with rose oil and vinegar. Adding oil was a way to remove quicklime's
caustic nature (Plin. 24.1.3, 33.30.94), and Dioscorides (*MM* 5.115.3) recommended its use with lipids to bring over scars unrelated to ulcers.

§20. *symphitum – sanat.*
Comparandum: Plin. 26.88.148 for bringing over a scar.
Galen recommended comfrey (Gal. K11.135; K13.767, 769).

§21. *plantaginis – mensura.*
Comparanda: Plin. 26.78.126, 28.74.241; Diosc. *MM* 2.126.3. Ps-Apul. 1.22.
Plantain was used for multiple ulcerative conditions (e.g. Diosc. *MM* 2.126.2;
Gal. K11.838; Orib. *Eun.* 2.1α.61, 3.25.12; Aët. 1.46; Paul. Aeg. 3.59.1,
7.3.1).
Bull's bile was used (Hippoc. *Ulc.* 12, 15; Gal. K13.807–8; Marc. 4.8); see
commentary on *Medicina Plinii* 3.4.6 for the use of leek.
Leek juice with bull's bile was rarely used for any complaint. Dioscorides
(*MM* 2.78.3) recommended them for "singing in the ears", but an eleventh-
century manuscript says it treated fistulas (Scorialensis III R 3 in Wellman
1907, 106). This perfectly matches this treatment, but bull bile and leek
juice were recommended for ear complaints (Celsus 6.7.6; Gal. K12.615,
616; Paul. Aeg. 3.25.1).

§21. *carcinomata – una.*
Comparanda: Plin. 28.74.242; Marc. 4.59.
Serenus (62 l.1084) recommended hare rennet with wine.
Caper was used on ulcers, but not *carcinomata* (Diosc. *MM.* 2.173.3; Gal.
K12.10; Orib. *CM* 14.58.1, *Eun.* 2.1κ.17; Aët. 1.180).

§22. *gangraenis – cinis.*
Comparanda: Plin. 28.74.242; Marc. 4.60.

§22. *caesus – purgat.*
Comparandum: Plin. 28.74.243.
As simples, crude pitch, sulphur, and grease were used to cleanse (Cels. 5.5.2); wax
and fat treated ulcers (Hippoc. *Ulc.* 21); goat lard treated *phagedaena* (Orib.
Syn. 3.25.6); and pitch and sulphur treated creeping ulcers (Diosc. *MM.* 1.72.2).

5. *panis quas paniculas nos dicimus*

This chapter begins the author's discussion of specific abscess varieties. The
logic for his chosen order is not obviously apparent, although treating them suc-
cessively from 3.5 to 3.8 was eminently sensible given the number of common

treatments, especially among *pani*, *strumae*, and boils, although there is also some commonality with parotid gland swellings.

Panus: a superficial abscess named after its resemblance to a bobbin; Greeks called it a φύγεθρον/φύγεθλον. Celsus (5.28.10) described *pani* as painful, occurring on the crown, armpits, or groin, slow maturing, and occasionally accompanied by a slight fever.

Panicula: the diminutive form of *panus*.

§1. *nasturcium – discutit.*
Comparanda: Plin. 20.50.128; Marc. 32.8. Cf. *Med. Plin.* 3.6.2.
Dioscorides (*MM* 1.72.5) recommended Bruttian and Lycian pitch.

§1. *maturis – discocta.*
Comparandum: Plin. 22.73.152. Cf. *Med. Plin.* 3.6.2.
Marcellus (32.8) recommended lentils prepared differently.

§1. *ervum – prohibet.*
Comparanda: Plin. 22.73.152; Marc. 32.9.

§2. *lupini – maturant.*
Comparanda: Plin. 22.74.156; Marc. 32.16. Cf. *Med. Plin.* 1.7.2, 3.6.2.
See commentary on *Medicina Plinii* 1.7.2.

§2. *ficum – imponunut.*
Comparanda: Plin. 23.63.122; Diosc. *MM.* 1.128.2; Garg. 49; Marc. 32.17. Cf.
    Med. Plin. 1.7.3, 3.7.4.
See commentary on *Medicina Plinii* 1.7.3.

§2. *viscum – imponunt.*
Comparandum: Plin. 24.6.11.
This combination was also used for parotid swellings and *strumae* (Diosc. *MM*
    3.89.2, *Eup.* 1.135.1, 1.138.2, 1.139.1, 1.140.2, 1.145.4; Paul. Aeg. 4.22.4).
Serenus (39 l. 746) recommended mistletoe in a poultice, and Scribonius (82)
    included it in a compound.

§2. *galbanum – prodest.*
Comparanda: Plin. 24.13.21; Marc. 32.12. Cf. *Med. Plin.* 3.6.3, 3.7.5.
Galbanum was a dispersive medicament (Diosc. *MM* 3.83.1) and was included
    in compounds for this reason (Scribon. 82, 263; Gal. K11.914, K13.787–8).

§3. *feniculi – dolorem.*
Comparanda: Plin. 24.120.188; Marc. 32.13.
Önnerfors (1964, 69) disagrees that the author sourced this from Pliny because
    he referred to the decoction of fenugreek meal; however this preparation is
    identical to Pliny's, and he misread Pliny's fenugreek for fennel elsewhere
    (see 2.4.3, 2.21.5).

§3. *aperit – impositus.*

Comparanda: Plin. 30.22.75; Marc. 32.3.

Pigeon dung preparations were also applied to *pani, strumi,* and parotid swellings (*Med. Plin.* 1.7.3, 3.6.6; Seren. 39 ll. 739–40).

§4. *echinorum – aperit.*

Comparanda: Plin. 32.34.106: Marc. 32.15.

The author added oil to Pliny's advice; Dioscorides (*MM* 2.4.1–2, 5.115.3) stated that calcined murex shells formed quicklime, and added lipids formed a dispersive medicament.

§5. *cancri – imposita.*

Comparandum: Plin. 32.34.107.

The author did not specify an Egyptian fish-pickle.

§5. *creta – cohibet.*

Comparanda: Plin. 35.57.195; Marc. 32.14. Cf. *Med. Plin.* 1.7.4.

See commentary on *Medicina Plinii* 1.7.4.

§5. *ursinus – tritus.*

Comparandum: Plin. 28.61.217.

§5. *ungulae – decoctum.*

Comparanda: Plin. 28.61.217–8; Marc. 32.40, 32.13.

The author significantly simplified Pliny's advice.

§6. *quidam – hemina.*

Comparandum: Plin. 32.34.106.

Litharge was known for its dispersive properties (Cels. 5.11.1).

6. strumis [id est scrofae quae nascuntur in gutture]

This chapter continues the author's exposition on the treatment of abscess varieties. Given that *strumae* most often arose on the neck, as the subheading "i.e. for the *scrofula* which rise in the throat" notes, the inclusion of this chapter in Book Three rather than Book One, indicates that the author considered this as not restricted to that part of the body. In addition to advising similar treatments to those for upper body inflammations, the author also provided similar ministrations to those recommended for *pani* in the previous chapter, and boils in the following one.

Struma, χοιράς: a swelling of the lymphatic glands frequently translated as scrofula, or scrofulous swellings or sores. Struma and scrofula are technical terms in modern medicine: a swelling of the thyroid gland, often referred to as goitre, or other thyroid complaints, and a *Mycobacterium tuberculosis* infection in the lymph nodes in the neck which causes an abscess respectively. *Strumae* were described as causing swelling and abscesses, so was likely used for both these conditions. Celsus (5.28.7) described *strumae* as especially difficult to treat by drugs or surgical intervention owing to recurrences.

§1. *caprifici – constat.*
Comparandum: Plin. 23.64.130.

§1. *echinorum – pulte.*
Puls: porridge made from any grain or legume.
Pounded sea-urchin shells were recommended with vinegar (Plin. 32.28.88; Marc. 15.54). Alum was likely used for its dispersive properties (Cels. 5.12).

§2. *nasturcium – hederae.*
Comparanda: Plin. 20.50.127 (covered with a cabbage leaf); Ps-Apul. 20.4; Marc. 15.78.
The use of cress was recommended by Paul. Aeg. (4.33.2).
A remarkably similar treatment for *strumae* in animals was recorded featuring bean meal, cress seed, and oil applied in a cabbage leaf (*Hippiatr. Cant.* 11.7; *Geopon.* 12.27.1). This suggests that Latin treatments influenced late Greek texts, but not those devoted to human care. Its inclusion of oil suggests this might have been a binding agent in *lomentum*.

§2. *marrubium – adipe.*
Comparanda: Plin. 20.89.242; Marc. 15.78.
Horehound was included in compounds (Orib. *EM* 90.4; Paul. Aeg. 4.33.5).

§2. *lens – discocta.*
Comparanda: Plin. 22.70.143; Diosc. *MM* 2.107.2, *Eup.* 1.145.4; Theod. 1.11.27.

§2. *lupinum – contritumque.*
Comparanda: Plin. 22.74.154; Marc. 15.37. Cf. *Med. Plin.* 1.7.2, 3.5.2.
See commentary on *Medicina Plinii* 1.7.2.
Lupine preparations with vinegar were commonly recommended (Diosc. *MM* 2.109.2, *Eup.* 1.145.4; Gal. K11.886; Ps-Gal. 14.408; Orib. *CM* 45.21.3, *Syn.* 7.29.1, *Eun.* 2.10.7, 3.44.1; Aët. 1.162; Paul. Aeg. 4.33.1).

§3. *folio – imponuntur.*
Comparanda: Plin. 23.63.118; Ps-Theod. *Ad.* I,10(26). Cf. *Med. Plin.* 1.21.2.
Unripe figs were a well-attested treatment (Diosc. *MM* 1.128.5, *Eup.* 1.145.3; Orib. *Syn.* 7.29.6, *Eun.* 3.44.6; Aët. 15.5; Paul. Aeg. 4.33.2; Paul. Nic. 116).

§3. *sucus – fermento.*
Comparandum: Plin. 24.10.16.

§3. *galbanum – imponitur.*
Comparanda: Plin. 24.13.21; Marc. 15.51; Ps-Theod. *Ad.* I,10(26). Cf. *Med. Plin.* 3.5.2, 3.7.5.
Galbanum was commonly included in topical compounds (e.g. Cels. 5.18.5; Scribon. 81; Gal. K13.807; Orib. *EM* 90.1; Aët. 12.49; Paul. Aeg. 4.33.3).

§3. *mustelae – imponitur.*
Comparanda: Plin. 30.12. 36; Marc. 15.79.
Weasel blood was used in other ways (Diosc. *MM* 2.5.1, *Eup.* 1.145.4; *Cyran.* 2.7; Ps- Gal. K14.401).

§4. *cochleae – imponitur.*
Comparanda: Plin. 30.12.37; Marc. 15.80; Ps-Theod. *Ad.* I,10(26).
Pliny stated snails should be sourced from shrubs.
Asp ash was noted for its dispersive properties, and thus included in compounds (Gal. K13.927; Aët. 15.16; Paul. Aeg. 4.33.2, 7.17.57).

§5. *adeps – bibere.*
Comparanda: Plin. 30.12.37; Diosc. *MM* 2.16.1, *Eup.* 1.145.3; Aët. 15.5.
Typically, Latin authors referred to snakes, whereas Greek writers referred to vipers. Their preparation was often identical: compare Pliny's directions to Dioscorides' (*MM* 2.16.2).
The measurements regarding how much to cut off snakes given in the *Medicina Plinii* precisely matches the advice Galen was taught by the Marsi for vipers (K11.143–4). The Marsi were an Italian tribe renowned for their snake lore, so this does not necessarily reflect a Greek influence.

§6. *fimum – acri.*
Comparanda: Plin. 30.12.38; Diosc. *MM* 2.80.4; Ps-Theod. *Ad.* I,10(26).
Darnel meal was sometimes used instead of barley (Diosc. *Eup.* 1.145.2).

§6. *talpae – abluunt.*
Comparanda: Plin. 30.12.38; Marc. 15.81; Ps-Theod. *Ad.* I,10(26).
The use of the patient's hands might have been magical; *Cyranides* (2.3) recommended holding a mole in the hands until it died.

§7. *talpae – sunt.*
Comparanda: Plin. 30.12.38; Marc. 15.58.

§8. *vermes – arescunt.*
Comparandum: Plin. 30.12.39.
Aëtius (2.168) included a similar magic-medical treatment matching the number of worms to swellings.

§8. *circumligantur – est.*
Comparanda: Plin. 30.12.40; Diosc. *Eup.* 1.145.2. Cf. *Med. Plin.* 1.7.5.

§8. *milipedae – apostemata.*
Comparandum: Plin. 30.12.40. Cf. *Med. Plin.* 1.7.4.

§9. *calx – auxiliatur.*
Comparanda: Plin. 36.57.180; Marc. 15.59; Ps-Theod. *Ad.* I,10(26).
Similar treatments were recommended elsewhere (Diosc. *Eup.* 1.145.1; Ps-Gal.
   K14.408; Orib. *EM* 94.3, *Syn.* 7.29.6, *Eun.* 3.44.6; Paul. Aeg. 4.33.1; Paul.
   Nic. 116).

§9. *fel – discutit.*
Comparandum: Plin. 28.51.190; cf. Marc. 15.53.

§10. *ungulae – inlinitur.*
Comparanda: Plin. 28.51.191; Diosc. *Eup.* 1.145.2; Marc. 15.60.
Ass hoof ash and oil was also recommended (Diosc. *MM* 2.42.1; Gal. K12.341;
   Orib. *CM* 45.21.5; Aët. 2.157).

§10. *fimum – inlinitur.*
Comparanda: Plin. 28.51.191; Diosc. *Eup.* 1.145.1; Ps-Gal. K14.408; Orib.
   EM 94.3; Paul. Aeg. 4.33.2; Paul. Nic. 116.
Pliny did not specify goat dung.

§10. *bubulum – imponitur.*
Comparandum: Plin. 28.52.192.

§10. *ebuli – alligantur.*
There is no further evidence for the use of dwarf elder.

7. furunculis

This chapter continued the author's discussion of abscesses from the previous chapters, for which it shared a treatment (the application of *galbanum*). This is the penultimate abscess chapter, followed by advice on the treatment of *carbunculi*.

Boils received limited attention in ancient texts. Referred to in Greek as δοθιήν, Hippocrates (*Aff.* 35) stated that they were caused by excessive phlegm and Celsus (5.28.8) only devoted one paragraph to their treatment.

§1. *fimi – inlinitur.*
Comparandum: Plin. 30.34.108.
Cyranides (3.3) recommended applying chicken dung. White chicken dung
   was specified by Serenus (37 ll. 714–5).

§1. *muscae – minimo.*
Comparandum: Plin. 30.34.108 (using the fourth "medical" finger).

§2. *sordes – portionibus.*

Comparanda: Plin. 30.34.108; Seren. 37 ll. 716–7.

Sordes ex auriculis: ear wax but has been translated literally.

§2. *nitrum – extrahit.*

Comparanda: Plin. 31.46.118; Diosc. *MM* 5.113.3, *Eup.* 1.135.2; Orib. *CM* 44.30.1.

Soda was recommended with leaven (Diosc. *Eup.* 1.135.2; Paul. Aeg. 4.23.1). Resin was used alone (Cels. 5.28.8), or with barley meal (Seren. 37 l. 710).

§3. *nasturcium – concoquitur.*

Comparanda: Plin. 20.50.130; Garg. 13; Ps-Apul. 20.5.

Leaven was recommended alone (Cels. 5.28.8), with soda (see above), or in plasters (Orib. *CM* 9.25.1, *Syn.* 3.77.1). Cress was used with brine (*MM* 2.155.2; *Eup.* 1.135.2).

§3. *novem – sanat.*

Comparandum: Plin. 22.65.135 (each grain drawn around three times).

§4. *ficus – imponuntur.*

Comparanda: Plin. 23.63.122; Garg. 49. Cf. *Med. Plin.* 1.7.3, 3.5.2.

Variously dried fig decoctions were recommended (Diosc. *MM* 1.128.2; Orib. *CM* 9.34.6, 44.30.8, *Syn.* 3.80.6; Paul. Aeg. 4.23.1).

§5. *galbanum – se.*

Comparanda: Plin. 24.13.21; Cels. 5.28.8; Diosc. *MM* 3.83.2; *Eup.* 1.135.1; cf. *Med. Plin.* 3.5.2, 3.6.3.

Galbanum was included in compounds (Gal. K13.812; Orib. *EM* 92.1; Aët. 15.13; Paul. Aeg. 4.34.2).

§5. *sevum – sevum.*

Comparandum: Plin. 28.70.234.

Dioscorides (*MM* 5.109.5; *Eup.* 1.135.1) and Oribasius (*CM* 44.30.5) recorded similar treatments.

§5. *limacis – purgat.*

There is no further evidence for the use of slug ash.

8. *carbunculis*

This chapter concluded the author's discussion of abscesses. While *carbunculus* is often translated as carbuncle, which today often describes a cluster of interconnected boils, this was not the description commonly given, perhaps as a result of the limited advice provided for the treatment of boils.

Carbunculus, ἄνθραξ: Celsus (5.28.1) described it as a skin lesion, primarily red in colour, with a few, often black, projecting pustules with blackened flesh between them. Ἄνθραξ was a malignant pustule, possibly small pox. This was not modern anthrax, although some symptoms are similar. Pliny (26.4.5) stated this was a recent disease to Rome from southern France.

§1. *fimus – imponitur.*
Comparanda: Plin. 30.33.107; Seren. 38, ll. 726–7.
Pigeon dung was variously used (Diosc. *MM* 2.80.4, *Eup.* 1.188.1; Theod. 1.20.62; Aët. 15.15; Ps-Theod. *Ad.* I,20(62)).

§1. *mullorum – prodest.*
Comparandum: Plin. 32.44.127.

§2. *ruta – trita.*
Comparanda: Plin. 20.51.141; Ps-Apul. 90.6; Theod. 1.20.61.
Soda was sometimes added (Orib. *EM* 105.1; Theod. 1.20.61).

§2. *ervi – rumpit.*
Comparanda: Plin. 22.73.152; Diosc. *MM* 2.108.2, *Eup.* 1.189.1; Theod. 1.20.61.
Bitter vetch meal preparations were recommended (Orib. *CM* 9.38.1; Paul. Aeg. 3.22.26).

§2. *idem – triti.*
Comparanda: Plin. 22.74.156; Seren. 38 l. 729.
Boiled lupines were used (Diosc. *MM* 2.109.2, *Eup.* 1.188.1; Theod. 1.20.62).

§2. *fimus – imponitur.*
Comparanda: Plin. 30.34.107; Theod. 1.20.61 specifying sheep dung.
Sheep dung with honey was recommended (Orib. *EM* 105.16; Paul. Aeg. 4.25.5).

§3. *ficus – extrahunt.*
Comparanda: Plin. 23.63.123; Orib. *Syn.* 7.12.8, *Eun.* 3.28.8; Theod. 1.20.61; Paul. Aeg. 4.25.3; Paul. Nic. 90.

§3. *nuces – impositae.*
Comparanda: Plin. 23.77.148; Diosc. *MM* 1.125.2, *Eup.* 1.189.1; Orib. *CM* 43.57.28, *EM* 105.17, *Syn.* 7.12.8, *Eun.* 3.28.8; Theod. 1.20.61; Paul. Aeg. 4.25.3; Paul. Nic. 90.

§3. *pix – purgat.*
Comparandum: Plin. 24.23.38.
Similar treatments were recommended (Diosc. *Eup.* 1.189.1; Plin. 20.82.217, 23.12.16; Garg. *Recensio altera* 78 (Rose 1875, 196); Orib. *EM* 105.17; Theod. 1.20.62; Paul. Aeg. 4.25.3).

§4. *herba – inlinitur.*
Comparanda: Plin. 24.61.102; Diosc. *MM* 1.76.1, *Eup.* 1.188.1; Gal. K11.853–4; Orib. *CM* 43.57.13–4; Ps-Apul. 86.3; Aët. 1.71.
Sabina: savin, *Juniperus sabina.*

§4. *cerebrum – imponitur.*
Comparandum: Plin. 28.74.243.
A plaster of baked piglet brain and honey was recommended (*Cyran.* 2.44), as were other cooked brains (Plin. 28.60.214; Plac. 7β.1; Marc. 33.37).

9. ambustis

While this chapter represents a shift away from abscesses by the author, its placement following *carbunculi* is curious; Celsus followed his burns advice (4.27.13) with a discussion of the treatment of *carbunculi* (4.28.1), likely owing to his use of cautery to treat *carbunculi*. While the author similarly positions these close, he did not recommend this. It is also strange that this chapter was separated from "burns caused by the cold" (frostbite) by chapters devoted to dog-bites and scarring. This only makes sense if, like Celsus' placement of *carbunculi* after burns, it was because of his recommendation to use cautery to treat rabid dog-bites (3.10.9).

Consistent with Celsus' (4.27.13B) advice that oily products be used, many of these remedies featured lipids (oil or wax), counter to modern first aid practice.

§1. *fimus – inlinitur.*
Comparanda: Plin. 30.35.109; Theod. 1.19.60.
Sheep dung was recommended with rose cerate (Diosc. *MM* 2.80.3, *Eup.* 1.170.1; Gal. K12.302; Aët. 2.116). Pigeon dung preparations were recommended (Diosc. *MM* 2.80.4; *Eup.* 1.170.1; Orib. *Syn.* 7.6.5; Paul. Aeg. 4.11.2).

§2. *garum – nominatur.*
Comparandum: Plin. 31.44.97.
The interdiction against mentioning *garum* suggests that this was at least semi-magical.

§2. *cancrorum – oleo.*
Comparanda: Plin. 32.40.119; Theod. 1.12.60.

§3. *hordei – inspargitur.*
Comparandum: Plin. 22.45.134.

§3. *lens – additur.*
Comparanda: Plin. 22.70.145; Cels. 5.27.13A; Theod. 1.19.60.
Oribasius (*Syn.* 7.6.4) recommended a lentil meal and honey plaster; other boiled lentil treatments omitted honey (Orib. *EM* 106.1, *Syn.* 7.6.2, *Eun.* 3.20.2; Paul. Aeg. 4.11.1).

§4. *vitis – reddit.*

Comparandum: Plin. 23.3.6 (vine bark ash).

Adding oil might have been an attempt to meet contemporary medical practice.

§4. *prodest – sapae.*

Comparandum: Plin. 23.33.68 (must).

Wine lees required less processing than must (Plin. 14.11.80), so was likely a cheaper option.

§§4–5. *olivarum – prohibet.*

Comparandum: Plin. 23.36.73.

Pickled olives were more often recommended (Diosc. *MM* 1.105.4, *Eup.* 1.169.2; Orib. *Syn.* 7.6.7, *Eun.* 3.20.5; Theod. 1.19.60; Paul. Aeg. 4.11.1).

§5. *myrti – spargitur.*

Comparanda: Plin. 23.81.163; Ps-Theod. *Ad.* I,19(60).

§5. *flos – imponitur.*

Comparanda: Plin. 24.47.79; Diosc. *MM* 2.179.1; Gal. K12.30; Orib. *Eun* 3.1κ.53; Aët. 1.205.

§5. *hordeum – prodest.*

Comparanda: Plin. 29.11.40; Seren. 59 l. 1047–8.

Barley preparations with lipids were recommended (Diosc. *Eup.* 1.170.1; Orib. *Syn.* 7.6.2, *EM* 106.1; Aët. 2.133; Paul. Aeg. 4.11.1).

§6. *ambusta – sequuntur.*

Comparandum: Plin. 29.11.40.

Serenus (59 l. 1043–4) recommended a similar use of egg white for a "flame burn", which might have been a poetic way to differentiate between burns and frostbite.

Eggs were commonly used to prevent blisters and treat burns (Diosc. *MM* 2.50.1, *Eup.* 1.169.3, *Cyran.* 2.47a, 3.55; Gal. K12.353; Orib. *Syn.* 7.6.2, *Eun.* 2.1ω.5; 3.20.2; Paul. Aeg. 4.11.1).

§6. *ova – inliniuntur.*

Comparandum: Plin. 29.11.45.

Egg yolks were used with other medicaments (Scribon. 221; Gal. K12.353; Orib. *Eun* 2.1ω.5).

§7. *oleum – reprimit.*

Comparanda: Plin. 31.45.103; Diosc. *MM* 5.109.6, *Eup.* 1.169.1.

§7. *eis – reddat.*

Comparanda: Plin. 32.40.119; Ps-Theod. *Ad.* I,19(60).

Cyranides (2.5) also recommended frog ash with vinegar.

§8. *efficax – inspargitur*.
Comparanda: Plin. 32.40.119, 36.25.130.

§8. *fimus – ponderibus*.
Comparanda: Plin. 28.71.235 (hare or goat dung); Ps-Theod. *Ad.* I,19(60).

§9. *gluten – applicare*.
Comparandum: Plin. 29.71.236.
The author mistakenly added *sordes* to Pliny's description.
The application of bull's glue was recommended (Diosc. *MM* 3.87.1, *Eup.*
    1.169.3; Orib. *Eun.* 3.20.5; Paul. Aeg. 7.3.19).

10. canis rabiosi morsui

Except for the use of cautery, placed at the end of this chapter, burns and their
treatment have nothing in common with rabid or non-rabid dog-bites (this topic
of the subsequent chapter). Rabid dog-bites were considered venomous, so their
inclusion outside the toxicology discussion at the end of this book is surprising.

There was confusion as to whether rabies could even be treated in antiquity:
Pliny stated that a remedy was only found in his lifetime (25.6.17), but then provided additional treatments; Aelian stated that bites could not be survived (*NA*
4.40, 9.15), and then gave a remedy (*NA* 14.20).

Writers often confused rabid and non-rabid dog-bites, and some treatments
were used for both human and animal victims (Veget. *Mulomed.* 2.148.1).

§1. *salsamentum imponitur*.
Comparanda: Plin. 32.17.47; Diosc. *MM* 2.28.1; Columella 6.31.1; Ps-Diosc.
    Ther. 2; Veget. *Mulomed.* 4.11; Cassius 67; Pall. *Agric.* 14.13.2; Paul. Aeg.
    5.3.3; *Hippiatr. Berol.* 87.10.
Fish-pickle was used for all dog-bites, and for venomous bites generally (Aët.
    13.12).

§1. *rutae – aceto*.
Comparanda: Plin. 20.51.133; Ps-Apul. 90.7.
Pliny and the author used different measurements but recommended the same
    dose (Plin. 21.109.185).
Rue was used to treat both rabid (Orib. *EM* 117.6; Ps-Apul 90.7; Paul. Aeg.
    5.3.3) and non-rabid dog-bites (Diosc. *Eup.* 2.120.3).

§2. *folia – medentur*.
Comparandum: Plin. 23.63.119.

§2. *rosae – pavorem*.
Comparanda: Plin. 25.6.17, 8.63.152; Veget. *Mulomed.* 2.148.2.

§2. *plantago – bestiarum.*
Comparandum: Plin. 25.77.125.

§3. *lana – soluta.*
Comparandum: Plin. 29.9.32.

§3. *cinis – devoratum.*
Comparandum: Plin. 29.32.98.

§4. *vermis – tollit.*
Comparandum: Plin. 29.32.98.

§4. *est – prohibet.*
Comparandum: Plin. 29.32.99.
When simplifying Pliny's text, the author dropped to word "saliva" which was
    used to describe what the slime was found in. Saliva was understood as the
    source of infection (Ael. *NA* 9.15).

§5. *omnia – coctum.*
Comparanda: Plin. 29.32.99; Diosc. *MM* 2.47.1, *Eup.* 2.120.1; Gal. K12.335;
    Ael. *NA* 14.20; Orib. *Syn.* 8.12.6; *Mulomed. Chiron.* 5.515.LV; Veget.
    Mulomed. 2.148.1; Aët. 6.24; Paul. Aeg. 5.3.3, 7.3.7.

§§5–6. *crista – melle.*
Comparandum: Plin. 29.32.100.

§6. *salliuntur – edantur.*
Comparandum: Plin. 29.32.100.
The preservation of rabid dogs for this purpose is recorded nowhere else; for
    a similar preservation of venomous creatures to treat bites see *Medicina
    Plinii* 3.35.2.

§7. *lactens – devoratur.*
Comparandum: Plin. 29.32.101.
This combined magic (drowning to combat hydrophobia and matching the
    sex), and a variation on a well-known treatment (eating dog liver).

§8. *fimus – imponitur.*
Comparandum: Plin. 29.32.101.
Cyranides (3.3) also recommended the application of chicken dung of unspeci-
    fied colour and vinegar.

§8. *glebulae – inlinuntur.*
Comparandum: Plin. 29.32.101.

§8. *catulus – umbilicum.*
Pup rennet was recommended (*Cyran.* 2.21; Theod. 2.8.27).

§9. *pavescentibus – marini.*
Comparandum: Plin. 32.20.57.
Seal grease was used to treat *scabies* instead of rabies (Columella 6.32.2; Pall. *Agric.* 14.24.3; *Antidot. Brux.* 204), but there was a Latin veterinary tradition that these were treated the same (Columella 6.31.1; Veget. *Mulomed.* 4.11.1; Pall. *Agric.* 14.13.2).

§9. *aquam – sanantur.*
Comparanda: Plin. 34.44.151, 32.17.47; Cels. 5.27.2A; Prom. *Ther.* 9; Gal. K14.280; Orib. *Syn.* 8.12.3; *Mulomed. Chiron.* 5.515.LV; Veget. *Mulomed.* 2.148.1; Cassius 67.
Paul. Aeg. (5.3.3) stated this should only be used after simple draughts had been tried.
Cauterisation was used well into the nineteenth century.

11. morsui canis non rabiosi

The discussion of non-rabid dog-bites immediately after rabid dog-bites was logical, although it would not have assisted the ongoing confusion between their treatments. The placement of this chapter immediately prior to the author's discussion of scarring might reflect an experience related to scarring from a dog attack given that he sought to address topics as they came to mind.

§1. *nitrum – imponuntur.*
Comparandum: Plin. 31.46.118.
The inclusion of axle-grease might have been the result of crasis, but axle-grease was used as a suspension agent for applying soda to dog-bites (Diosc. *MM.* 5.113.3, *Eup.* 2.120.4).
Soda and vinegar were recommended (Philum. 5.3; Aët. 13.2; Paul. Aeg. 5.4.1). Resin was included in plasters (Scribon. 201, 210).

§1. *allex – concerptis.*
Comparandum: Plin. 31.44.96.
Allex: sediment of *garum*; originally a waste product or lees, it became a specifically made product (Plin. 31.44.95).
Similar salted fish products were recommended: *garum* (Diosc. *MM* 2.32.1; Plin. 31.44.97); *liquamen* (Theod. 1.21.66); pickled tuna (Diosc. *MM* 2.31.1); fish-pickle (Diosc. *Eup.* 2.120.3; Philum. 5.5; Paul. Aeg. 7.3.19); and salted *mena* (*Cyran.* 4.41).

§1. *alium – tritum.*
Comparanda: Plin. 20.23.50; Diosc. *Eup.* 2.120.2; Garg. 18.

Garlic was recommended for both non-rabid (Philum. 5.6; Ps-Gal. K14.516–7, 573–4) and rabid dog-bites (Diosc. *MM* 2.152.2; Orib. *EM* 117.1; Paul. Aeg. 5.3.3).

§1. *menta – contrita.*

Dioscorides (*MM* 3.34.2) recommended mint with salt; Paulus Aegineta (5.3.3) recommended a mint plaster for rabid dog-bites.

§2. *marrubium – vetere.*
Comparandum: Plin. 20.89.244.

§2. *urtica – sale.*
Comparandum: Plin. 22.15.32.
This was also recommended for rabid dog-bites (Diosc. *MM* 4.93.1, *Eup.* 2.120.3; Orib. *EM* 117.6).

§3. *cinis – oleo.*
Comparanda: Plin. 23.3.6; Diosc. *Eup.* 2.120.3.
This was also recommended for rabid dog-bites (Orib. *EM* 117.6; Paul. Aeg. 5.3.3).

§3. *acetum – spongia.*
Comparanda: Plin. 23.27.55; Orib. *Eun.* 3.71.1. Cf. *Med. Plin.* 3.36.2.
The *Medicina Plinii* conflates Pliny's recommended use of vinegar for venomous bites with the use with sulphur on a sponge for anal conditions.
Theodorus (1.21.66) recommended cold water or *oxymel* in a sponge.

§3. *ramorum – triti.*
Comparandum: Plin. 23.63.119.

§3. *nuclei – triti.*
Comparanda: Plin. 23.75.144; Diosc. *MM* 1.123.1; Garg. 53; Orib. *CM* 11.α.44.
Dioscorides (*Eup.* 2.120.3) recommended bitter almonds and honey for rabid dog-bites.

§3. *nucum – contritae.*
Comparanda: Plin. 23.77.148; Diosc. *MM* 1.125.1.
This was also recommended for rabid dog-bites (Diosc. *Eup.* 2.120.4; Paul. Aeg. 5.3.3).

§4. *easdem – iubent.*
Comparandum: Plin. 23.77.149 for rabid dog-bites.

§5. *spongiae – melle.*
Comparandum: Plin. 31.47.129.

Sponges were also recommended wet with water, vinegar, *posca*, or vinegar
and soda (Philum. 5.3; Aët. 13.2; Paul. Aeg. 5.4.1).

§5. *faex – imponitur.*
Comparandum: Plin. 23.32.67.
Melanthium: either a transliteration of μελάνθιον, *Nigella sativa*, which has no
association with dog-bites, or chamomile. Chamomile was used to treat rabid
dog-bites, but not in this manner (Orib. *Syn.* 8.12.3; Aët. 6.24; Paul. Aeg. 5.3.3).

12. cicatricibus quibus color reddi debet

As suggested above, the author's placement of this advice after dog-bites might
imply some experience regarding scars resulting from mauling. That noted, there
is no apparent logic for placing this prior to frostbite. The inclusion of this advice
again illustrates the author's interest in "cosmetic medicine".

§1. *arietinus – est.*
Comparanda: Plin. 30.41.120; Plac. 6α.3, 6β.3.
Pliny did not specify ram's tallow.
Soda was included in compounds (Orib. *EM* 99.4; Cassius 9; Paul. Aeg. 4.47.1).

§1. *adeps – rosaceo.*
Comparandum: Plin. 28.25.89 for skin blemishes.

§1. *utuntur – decocta.*
Comparandum: Plin. 30.41.120.
The use of snake's slough might have been semi-magical.

§2. *fimus – melle.*
Comparandum: Plin. 30.41.120.
Oribasius (*EM* 99.5) recommended pigeon dung with water.

§2. *fel – marini.*
Comparandum: Plin. 32.44.127.

§2. *erucae – bubulo.*
Comparanda: Plin. 20.49.125; Garg. 14.
Rocket seed and bile were also used with litharge (Diosc. *Eup.* 1.108.1, 1.109.1;
Orib. *Syn.* 7.21.2, *Eun.* 3.37.2; Paul. Aeg. 4.47.1).

§2. *lupini – cocti.*
Comparandum: Plin. 22.74.156.

§2. *sevum – impositum.*
Comparanda: Plin. 28.74.245; Diosc. *MM* 2.76.18, *Eup.* 1.109.1; Orib. *Syn.*
7.21.2, *Eun.* 3.37.2; Ps-Theod. *Ad.* I,36(94); Paul. Aeg. 4.47.1.

§2. *fel – imponitur*.

Comparandum: Plin. 28.74.245.

Pliny described calf bile as the active ingredient and that doctors added myrrh, honey, and saffron. Yet despite the stated cynicism towards doctors' frauds by the author (Prol. 1), this discussion reflects none of Pliny's nuance. He replaced honey with oil, so it is possible that he sourced this elsewhere.

Cyranides (2.39) stated that bull's bile gave scars a uniform colour.

13. frigore exustis

Frostbite had no precise name in Greek, but in Latin it was literally "a burn caused by the cold", so it is strange the author separated this from burn treatments (3.9 above). He instead positioned this between chapters devoted to scarring and embedded matter, which have nothing in common with it. Frostbite was not subject to expansive medical discussion, but its dangers were described by medical and lay writers (e.g. Hippoc. *Liq.* 1; Lucian *Adversus indoctum*, 6; Tacitus *Annales*, 13.35).

§1. *ituri – excalefactoriam*.

Comparandum: Plin. 26.71.117 (*panax*).

Opopanax's warming properties were acknowledged (Diosc. *MM* 3.48.4; Gal. K12.94–5).

§1. *si – est*.

Comparandum: Plin. 22.57.119.

Pliny did not include wine.

§2. *rutae – imponuntur*.

Comparandum: Plin. 20.51.140.

Rue and oil had acknowledged warming properties (rue: Diosc. *MM* 3.45.1; Gal. K11.809, K12.100–1; oil: Cels. 2.33.5; Diosc. *MM* 1.30.2). Oil was even used to prevent frostbite (e.g. Polybius 3.72.6; Florus 1.22.12).

§2. *leporini   adalligatur*.

Comparandum: Plin. 28.62.221.

The inclusion of hare lung was the result of misreading Pliny's text.

§2. *aristolochiam – habet*.

Comparandum: Ps-Apul. 19.4.

Aristolochia had warming properties (Orib. *CM* 15.1.83; Paul. Aeg. 7.3.1), and Pliny (26.71.117) recommended rubbing with it.

§2. *axungia porcina*.

Comparanda: Plin. 28.37.137; Seren. 59 ll. 1051–2.

Dioscorides (*MM* 2.76.17) described all fats as warming. Pseudo-Apuleius (19.4) included axle-grease as an option with *aristolochia*.

14. extrahendis his quae corpori fixa sunt

Following on from frostbite, this chapter also does not relate to either that topic or the discussion of fevers which follows it. As a result, its positioning provides no insight into the author's approach.

§1. *Mus – coagulo.*
Comparanda: Plin. 30.42.122; Marc. 34.35, 32.32.
The attempt to simplify Pliny resulted in hare rennet being added to snails.
Lizard heads alone were recommended (Diosc. *MM* 2.64.1, *Eup.* 1.159.1; Gal. K12.334; Paul. Aeg. 7.3.10).
Ground snails with their shells were also plastered on (Diosc. *MM* 2.9.2, *Eup.* 1.159.1).

§2. *testarum – cinis.*
Comparanda: Plin. 32.43.125; Marc. 34.36.

§2. *alium – extrahit.*
Comparanda: Plin. 20.23.55; Marc. 34.37.

§2. *nasturcium – impositum.*
Comparandum: Plin. 20.50.128.

§2. *farina – trita.*
Comparanda: Plin. 20.92.250; Marc. 34.41.
Galen used wild cucumber root in a drawing compound (K13.343–4).

§2. *urticae – imposita.*
Comparanda: Plin. 22.15.38; Marc. 34.42.

§3. *harundinis – extrait.*
Comparanda: Plin. 24.50.85; Marc. 34.38.
Reed root was commonly recommended (Cels. 5.26.35C; Diosc. *MM* 1.85.1; Gal. K12.7; Orib. *Syn.* 7.17.2, *Eun.* 3.32.2; Paul. Aeg. 4.52.1, 7.3.10).
Reed splinters easily formed and were exceptionally sharp (Plin. 16.64.157).

§4. *radix – imponitur.*
Comparanda: Plin. 24.72.116; Marc. 34.39.

§4. *blattae – inlinuntur.*
Comparanda: Plin. 29.39.141–2; Marc. 34.40.

§5. *cancri – triti.*
Comparanda: Plin. 32.43.125; *Cyran.* 4.28; Gal. K14.242; Paul. Aeg. 7.3.10.

§5. *testarum – aceto.*

Comparandum: Plin. 32.43.125 (purple-fish ash with water).

§5. *fimus – visci.*

Comparanda: Plin. 28.76.245; Marc. 34.43.

The simplification of Pliny by the author resulted in erroneously combining rennet with frankincense and mistletoe.

Dung (Paul. Aeg. 7.17.1) and mistletoe (Diosc. *MM* 3.89.2) had drawing properties, and frankincense was included in drawing plasters (Gal. K13.344, 507).

15. Ad quartanis

This chapter started the author's discussion of fevers which encompassed three chapters. While it was perfectly logical to address quartan, tertian, and periodic fevers in successive chapters, the text gives no explanation for this order except that the final discussion might have addressed more than one kind of fever, and thus provided a potential segue to other conditions.

Quartan fever is the malarial infection of *Plasmodium malariae* parasites. Its 72-hour development cycle causes an equally cyclical recurrence of symptoms; a day of fever and chills, two days without, followed by a day of fever and chills. This was counted as four days and gave the disease its name.

Pliny (30.30.98) believed that normal medical practice could do little for this and as a result he described a number of "tied on" remedies, i.e. amulets, and remedies which he might have attributed to the Magi (LCL: *Pliny Natural History VIII*, 340). Amulets were a common treatment and prophylactic for quartan fever. Their identification as medical or magical changed over time; wearing amulets against quartan fever was made a capital crime by Constantius II in 359 CE because they were deemed *veneficia*, magic/poison (Ammianus Marcellinus 19.12.14).

§1. *caput – cruce.*

Comparandum: Plin. 28.12.46.

The decline in crucifixions in the fourth century (Cook 2014, 416) could explain its limited reception.

§2. *fimi – pedibus.*

Comparandum: Plin. 28.66.229 (ox dung ash sprinkled with children's urine on digits).

Pliny described this as a "Magian" treatment.

§2. *leporis – accessionem. . .*

Comparanda: Plin. 28.66.229; *Cyran.* 2.24; Seren. 48 1. 908; Plac. 3β.4.

§2. *. . . leonis – datur.*

Comparandum: Plin. 28.25.90.

Pliny described this as a "Magian" treatment.

§3. *viperae – dimittitur.*
Comparandum: Plin. 30.30.98–99.

§4. *ranae – unctionem.*
Comparanda: Plin. 32.88.113; Seren. 48 ll. 912–3; *Cod. Sang. 751,* 272.
Its preparation at a liminal location (crossroads) made this a magical act
(Johnstone 1991, 224).

§4. *alii – bibitur.*
Comparandum: Plin. 20.23.56.
Silphium products and garlic were recommended elsewhere, but not together
(Hippoc. *Morb.* 2.43; Cels. 3.16.2; Seren. 48 ll. 899–900; Aët. 3.110; Paul.
Aeg. 2.22.1, 2.45.1).

§5. *hirundinis – propinatur.*
Comparandum: Plin. 30.30.102.
Although not explicitly magical, Pliny placed this within his list of magical
treatments.

§5. *rubetae – leucopeo.*
Comparandum: Plin. 32.38.114.
This appears to be the result of the crasis of Pliny by the author.

§6. *semen – datur.*
Comparanda: Plin. 20.73.194; Seren. 48 ll. 904–6.
The author misread *anesum* (anise) as *anethum* (dill) as he did at 1.1.2. and
replaced "vinegar and a *cyathus* of honey" with a "*cyathus* of honeyed
vinegar".

§7. *in – sequitur.*"
Variations of this spell, demanding a disease's flight because it was chased
by a supernatural entity, were outlined in texts (Marc. 8.193; *Hippiatr.
Paris.* 22); written on paper amulets against malaria (*Pap. Oxy.* 8.1151;
Suppl. Mag. 25); and inscribed on gems (State Hermitage Museum, artefact
no. Ж. 1517 in Nagy 2011, 76; Medailles et Antiques de la Bibliotheque
nationale de France, inv. 58.2220bis), and metal amulets (Schlumberger
1892, 75–8, no. 2–3). One metal amulet even evoked Solomon as the
pursuer (Schlumberger 1892, 74–5, no. 1). This spell's inclusion likely
reflected contemporary magical treatment, except that all other examples
were written in Greek. The only other Latin example is an Anglo-Saxon
charm from a twelfth-century manuscript (Cotton MS Faustina A x, f. 116r;
Grattan & Singer 1952, 45).
The evocation of biblical figures to magically cure quartan appear multiple
times on surviving paper amulets (*Suppl. Mag.* 3, 10, 14, 19).
Misnaming quartan fever as tertian in an incantation also occurred in the
Physica Plinii (*Cod. Sang. 751,* 272).

The need for clean paper was a common requirement for paper amulets (e.g. Seren. 51 l. 935; Marc. 8.56, 8.57, 8.59, 10.34).

Gaius Seius was the later Latin magical equivalent to John Doe.

§8. *item – dicat.*

Heim (1892, 483) describes this as a transfer incantation.

The only other appearance of "by bread and salt" is on a first-century CE wooden tablet and assumed to be a social invitation as it also referred to guests (Tomlin 2016, 126: WT31).

16. tertainis

The author here followed his chapter on quartan fever with his discussion of tertian fever before continuing to provide advice for periodic fevers.

Tertian fever is the malarial infection of either *Plasmodium vivax* or *Plasmodium falciparum* parasites. Their 48-hour development cycle causes an equally cyclical recurrence of symptoms; a day of fever and chills, a day without, followed by a day of fever and chills. This was counted as three days and thus gave the disease its name.

The *P. vivax* infection was sometimes called "benign tertian fever", while *P. falciparum* was referred to as malignant, semi- or sub-tertian fever (Retief & Cilliers 2004, 128) and as an "illegitimate" tertian was treated differently. Celsus (3.3.2) and Galen (K11.26–7) said that this distinction was necessary for treatment, but was not addressed in this text.

§1. *spongiae – inlinitur.*
Comparanda: Plin. 31.47.129; *Cod. Sang.* 751, 271.

§1. *ante – remittitur.*
Comparanda: Plin. 32.28.115; *Cod. Sang.* 751, 271.

§2. *pulei – subditur.*
Comparanda: Plin. 20.54.155; Seren. 49 ll. 919–20; Ps-Apul. 93.6.

§3. *urticae – sit.*
Comparandum: Plin. 22.16.38.
Using patronymics to identify the subject of magical practices was common. Pliny provided the same directions for two other treatments attributed to the Magi (21.104.176, 22.24.50).

§4. *herba – videat.*
Comparandum: Plin. 24.107.170.

§5. *lacerta – capiat.*
Comparandum: Plin. 30.30.104. Cf. *Med. Plin.* 3.17.3.
This seems to have been an attempt to bind the fever and transfer it to the lizard.

§6. *aranei – bibuntur*.

Comparandum: Plin. 30.30.104.

The author seems to have deliberately used a different vocabulary to Pliny: *aluta* (patch) instead of *spleniolum anacollema* replacing the use of resin applied with wax. This might have been an attempt to simplify Pliny's instructions, but this led to the omission of a spider which was used by Pliny and Greek writers (Diosc. *MM*. 2.63.1, *Eup*. 2.25.1; *Cyran*. 2.16; Paul. Aeg. 7.3.1), and where on the body it was to be stuck.

There are two *anacollemata* prescriptions recorded which included wax and resin (Gal. K12.741, repeated by Orib. *EM* 84.3, *Syn*. 3.153.1).

17. febribus periodicis [id est febres quae de accessione nascuntur]

This chapter concluded the author's exposition relating to fevers. Periodic fever could refer to various conditions which shared the symptom of recurrence. The title's non-specific language reflected Pliny's description of the fevers treated by this advice: quotidian (daily), recurrent, and periodic fevers. This ambiguity might have influenced the decision to later add the subheading "that is fever which arise on occasion". Quotidian fevers are thought to relate to a number of different malarial and non-malarial infections, and its description in medical sources is extremely confused (Retief & Cilliers 2004, 134). Leaving this potentially miscellaneous chapter to the end of his fever discussions might have been a deliberate act.

§1. *iecur – linteolo*.

Comparandum: Plin. 32.38.113 for periodic fever.

Asellus piscus: literally "donkey fish", identified as hake.

Pliny and the author implied that these stones could only be found during the full moon; Aelian (*NA* 6.30) described it as the only having what resembled mill-stones in their brains with no reference to the moon, but this was the only fish described as having what resembled mill-stones in their brains. Perhaps catching them during the full moon was a magical requirement (cf. Plin. 30.8.22).

§1. *utile – sale*.

Comparandum: Plin. 31.46.104 for unspecified fever.

Celsus (3.9.2) also recommended this for fevers without remission.

§2. *cancris – oportet*.

Comparandum: Plin. 32.38.114 for a recurrent fever.

§3. *oculus – habet*.

Comparanda: Plin. 28.66.228 for quotidian fever; Plac. 8.4, 14.2.

§3. *recidivas – capiat*.

Comparandum: Plin. 30.30.104. Cf. *Med. Plin*. 3.16.5.

18. lethargicis

This chapter marks a change in the author's focus. *Lethargus* might have been the author's next topic because it was sometimes accompanied by a fever. It was followed by a chapter devoted to *phrenitis* because these two diseases were commonly paired together in medical texts.

Lethargus, λήθαργος: a form of extreme tiredness which at its most extreme was a coma (Cels. 3.20.2–3; Gal. K10.931). Lethargy should be understood by its pathological definition of morbid drowsiness or prolonged, unnatural sleep.

These remedies mostly sought to elicit a response from patients rather than address its cause.

§1. *cimices – quattuor.*
Comparanda: Plin. 29.17.63; Seren. 55 ll. 1003–5; Ps-Theod. *Ad.* II,2(15).
Pliny adapted this treatment from Dioscorides' treatment for asp-bites, a symptom of which was lethargy (Diosc. *MM* 2.34.1).

§2. *castoreum – inlinitur.*
Comparanda: Plin. 32.13.28; Cels. 3.20.1l; Diosc. *Eup.* 1.14.1; Aret. *CA* 1.2.2, 1.2.11; Gal. K10.932; Theod. 2.3.15; Alex. *Therap.* 1; Paul. Aeg. 7.3.10; Paul. Nic. 11; *DMAC* 2.3.
Castoreum acted as a stimulant, inducing sneezes to wake the patient. It was also used with other medicaments (e.g. Diosc. *MM* 2.24.1, *Eup.* 1.10.1; Aret. *CA* 1.2.12; Gal. K12.340–1; Orib. *Eun.* 2.1κ.33; Theod. 2.3.15; Cassius 63; Aët. 2.177; Alex. *Therap.* 1.529; Paul. Aeg. 3.9.3; *DMAC* 2.3).

§2. *ruta – olfacienda.*
Comparanda: Plin. 20.51.138; Diosc. *Eup.* 1.10.1; Seren. 55 ll. 1001–2; Ps-Apul. 90.9; Ps-Theod. *Ad.* II,2(15).
Rue treatments were widely recommended (Celsus 3.20.4; Diosc. *Eup.* 1.14.1; Plin. 20.20.43; Aret. *CA* 1.2.8; Theod. 2.3.15; Cassius 63; Aët. 1.32; *DMAC* 2.3).

§2. *sisymbrium – aceto.*
Comparanda: Plin. 20.90.246; Ps-Theod. *Ad.* II,2(15).
Sisymbrium, σισύμβριον: water mint, *Mentha aquatica*, or less likely bergamot-mint or water cress.

§2. *urtica – frons.*
Comparanda: Plin. 22.15.31; Diosc. *Eup.* 1.14.1; Cassius 63; cf. Aret. *CA* 1.2.13.

§3. *spondilium – instillatur.*
Comparanda: Plin. 24.16.25; Diosc. *MM* 3.76.2, *Eup.* 1.14.1.

§3. *mustelae – adalligatur.*
Comparanda: Plin. 30.29.97; Ps-Theod. *Ad.* II,2(15).

Presumably burnt weasel liver smelled pungent.

Despite the use of *adalligo*, a verb used to describe tying on amulets, this use of lung does not appear to be magical.

§4. *palumbi – odore.*
This likely sought to elicit a response through a terrible smell.

§4. *euphorbio – tanguntur.*
Comparanda: Plin. 26.72.118; Seren. 55 ll. 1001–2; Ps-Theod. *Ad.* II,2(15).
Cassius (63) said that *euphorbea* promoted sneezing. Various *euphorbea* preparations were recommended (Aret. *CA* 1.2.11, 1.2.13; Aët. 3.114; Alex. *Therap.* 1.531).

§4. *capri – patitur.*
Comparanda: Plin. 28.67.230; Seren. 55 ll. 997–8; Ps-Theod. *Ad.* II,2(15).
This sought to work via smell; burning other keratin-rich parts of goat, hair or hide, was recommended (*Cyran.* 2.4; Plac. 5α.4, 5β.8), as was burning other horns (Cels. 3.20.2; Aët. 6.3).

§5. *vulturis – fricabis.*
Hand-tying might have been a binding ritual, but the application of *aristolochia* to the hands makes no clinical sense as lethargy treatments were normally applied to the head.

19. phreneticis [qui sensum perdunt] et qui somnum non capiunt

The placement of *phrenitis* next to *lethargus* here and in all classical medical texts facilitated the contrast of its sleeplessness (its predominant symptom), with lethargy's drowsiness. As a result, those treatments which were not soporific were similar to those for lethargy. Celsus (3.18.15) warned that if a *phrenetic* patient were forced to sleep, it could cause lethargy.

Phrenitis, φρενίτις: commonly defined as a brain inflammation, but this fails to consider the variously identified sites of φρήν (the seat of mental faculties): heart, diaphragm, and brain. The placement of treatments depended on this (Sakai 1991, 193–205). Latin medical writers more consistently attributed it to the brain (Murphy 2013, 44).

§1. *rosaceo – accedit.*
Comparandum: Plin. 32.13.28.
Castoreum and sulphurwort were normally used separately (Marc. 1.25 is an exception), often accompanied by rose oil and other medicaments (Diosc. *MM* 3.78.2, *Eup.* 1.10.1; Aret. *CA* 1.1.11; Aët. 5.121; Paul. Nic. 10; *DMAC* 1.3).

§1. *alium – datur.*
Comparanda: Plin. 20.23.52; Garg. 18.

§2. *sucus – tempora.*
Comparanda: Plin. 20.51.138; Cels. 3.18.8; Seren. 7 l. 99. Cf. *Med. Plin.* 3.18.2.
Other rue preparations were used (Plin. 20.51.138; Diosc. *Eup.* 1.10.1; Paul.
Aeg. 3.2.2; Paul. Nic. 10; *DMAC* 1.3).

§2. *spondilium – capiti.*
Comparandum: Plin. 24.16.25. Cf. *Med. Plin.* 3.18.3.
Spondylium, normally applied to the head, was used with other medicaments
(Diosc. *MM* 3.76.2, *Eup.* 1.10.1; Aret. *CA* 1.1.11; Marc. 1.25; Cassius 62;
Paul. Nic. 10).

§2. *suffitus – prodest.*
Comparanda: Plin. 29.9.31; Seren. 7 ll. 93–4.
Pliny did not specify greasy wool.

§2. *pulmo – alligatur.*
Comparanda: Plin. 30.29.95; Seren. 7 ll. 91–2. Cf. *Med. Plin.* 3.18.3.

§3. *adipe – dormit.*
Placitus (19.4) recommended this to promote sleep.

§3. *pellem – pone.*
The ignorance of the patient suggests this was a magical treatment, perhaps
of Greek origin. Greek literature described hares as sleepy (Xenophon
Cynegeticus, 5.27), especially after escaping hunters (Ael. *NA* 13.14;
Anthologia Palatina 9.94), so this might have been a form of sympathetic
magic to calm the patient like a hare after a chase.
White hares were not Italian (Varro *Rustica*, 3.12.6; Plin. 8.81.217; Pausanias
8.17.4), so this might not have been an easily sourced treatment.

§4. *lauri – dormit.*
Pseudo-Theodorus (*Ad.* II, 2(12)) described multiple uses of laurel leaves, but
with spells written on them; one directed that three leaves be placed without
the patient's knowledge under the pillow. These tap into a strong Greek
tradition of using laurel leaves with spells or magic words written on them
to treat insomnia (Ps-Gal. K14.489, 526–7; *Suppl. Mag.* 74 ll. 1–7, 96 ll.
51–2; Legrand 1881, 11; Delatte 1927, 90, 550–1).
In addition to showing the influence of Greek magic, it also illustrates the
understanding of disease's symptoms by the author; he did not just choose
treatments by simply matching diseases' names.

§4. *semen – dormit.*
Dactylus: might refer to finger-shaped dates (Plin. 13.9.46), grapes (Columella
3.2.1; Plin. 14.3.15), mussels (Plin. 9.87.184), or grass (Plin. 24.119.182).
Poppies and lettuce were both regarded as soporifics (Diosc. *MM* 2.136.1; Plin.
10.38.126, 20.26.64). Poppy decoctions were recommended despite the risk

of lethargy (Cels. 3.18.12; Plin. 20.76.202; Aët. 6.2; Ps-Theod. *Ad.* II,2(12); Paul. Aeg. 3.2.2; Paul. Nic. 10).

§5. *seminis – dormit.*

Theodorus (2.2.11) recommended applying lettuce seed boiled in oil to the head, or boiled in water and used to foment the face.

20. cardiacis

The author's decision to follow *phrenitis* with *cardiacus* might reflect his understanding that φρήν could refer to the heart, but the text includes nothing to support this. Its placement prior to his discussion of epilepsy might have been because both could lead to a loss of consciousness and death.

Cardiacus, καρδιακός: while this could refer to various conditions including heartburn and heart disease (LCL: *Celsus I*, 302), Celsus (3.19.1) used the phrase *cardiacus morbus* whose symptoms included excessive weakness when the stomach was languid, and wasting from extreme sweating on the chest, neck, head, feet, and legs. This has been interpreted as heart syncopation which could result in a loss of consciousness and lead to death (Aret. *CA* 2.3.1; *DMAC* 10.3; LCL: *Celsus I*, 302).

Celsus recommended treatment in three parts: repressive plasters applied to the breast; arrest sweating; and reverse weakness through diet. The treatments given in the *Medicina Plinii* addressed the first two.

§1. *aqua – sale.*
Comparanda: Plin. 20.34.87; Ps-Theod. *Ad.* II,29(91).

§1. *ruta – imponitur.*
Comparanda: Plin. 20.51.139; Ps-Theod. *Ad.* II,29(91).
This matches Celsus' description of a repressive plaster (2.33.3).

§2. *rutae – sistit.*
Comparanda: Plin. 20.51.142 (rue, rose oil, and aloe); Ps-Apul. 90.8; Ps-Theod. *Ad.* II,29(91).
Rose oil was recommended for *cardiacus* sweats (Cels. 3.19.2; Diosc. *Eup.* 2.27.1; Aët. 9.1).
Aloe was included in compounds (Aret. *CA* 2.3.13; Aët. 9.1; Alex. *Therap.* 2.281).

§3. *radix – inhibet.*
Comparanda: Plin. 20.98.260; Ps-Theod. *Ad.* II,29(91).
Giant fennel juice was thought to promote perspiration (*Cyran.* 5.13); this might account for the treatment's limited reception.

§3. *vinum – imponitur.*
Comparanda: Plin. 23.23.44; Ps-Theod. *Ad.* II,29(91).

Wine in sponges was cooling and repressive (Cels. 2.33.3). Wine was used to address sweating alone (Plin. 23.25.50), and to treat *cardiacus* (Paul. Nic. 56). Sponges addressed the sweating directly (Aret. *CA* 2.3.16; *DMAC* 10.3).

§4. *myrti – sinistrae.*
Comparandum: Plin. 23.81.160 (white myrtle seed and *polenta*); cf. Ps-Theod. *Ad.* II,29(91).
Barley groat-based plasters were variously recommended (Aret. *CA* 2.3.13, 2.3.16; Cassius 64; Aët. 9.1).

§4. *folia – mammae.*
Comparanda: Plin. 24.73.118; Ps-Apul. 88.4; Theod. 2.12.36; Ps-Theod. *Ad.* II,29(91).
Bramble was a cooling represent (Cels. 2.33.4), and its leaves were used in plasters (Diosc. *MM* 4.37.1, *Eup.* 2.28.1; Orib. *Eun.* 3.9.1; Aët. 9.1; Paul. Nic. 56).

§5. *sucus – datur.*
Comparanda: Plin. 24.73.120; Ps-Theod. *Ad.* II,29(91).

§5. *cornus – perunguntur.*
Comparanda: Plin. 28.79.260 (goat horn ash and myrtle oil); Ps-Theod. *Ad.* II,29(91).
Myrtle oil, unguent, and cerate were also recommended (Cels. 3.19.2; Diosc. *Eup.* 2.27.1; Aët. 9.1).

§5. *pulvis – statuit.*
Comparanda: Plin. 15.37.123, 23.81.161; Cels. 3.19.2; Diosc. *MM* 1.112.3; Theod. 2.12.36; Aët. 9.1.
Myrtle leaves were not always used dried (Orib. *EM* 37.4; *DMAC* 10.3), and they were not always specifically used to check sweats (Diosc. *Eup.* 2.28.1; Orib. *Eun.* 3.9.1; Aët. 9.1).

21. comitialibus

Like *cardiacus*, epilepsy could attack a sufferer with little chance to prepare. This chapter appears to have been the last disease of that kind the author devoted a chapter to prior to starting his long exposition on mostly skin-related conditions.

In Latin epilepsy was called *morbus comitialis*, "comitial disease", owing to epileptic seizures being bad omens necessitating the cancellations of *comitia* meetings (Isid. *Etym.* 4.7.7); *morbus maior*, "greater disease" (Cels. 3.23.1); *caduca* or *caducus morbus*, "falling sickness" because seizures caused sufferers to fall (Isid. *Etym.* 4.7.5); and *epilepsia*, the transliteration of ἐπιληψία. In addition to that name, Greeks called it the "sacred disease" owing to the tradition that it was caused by supernatural beings. Despite being judged as irrational (e.g. Hippoc. *Morb. sacr.* 1), this belief seems to have continued throughout antiquity, and epilepsy was described as the result of demonic possession in Late Antiquity (Isid. *Etym*. 4.7.6). The ongoing supernatural element could explain the inclusion of so many magical treatments.

Multiple forms of the disease were noted by doctors (Hippoc. *Morb. sacr.* 1; Cels. 3.23.1; Aret. *SA* 1.4.1; Gal. K8.180–194; Alex. *Therap.* 1.567; Clark & Rose 2013, 65–6), but the author of the *Medicina Plinii* made no reference to varieties. He also seemed to be unaware that patients did not need to be roused following a seizure (Cels. 3.23.2).

§1. *testiculi – bibuntur*.
Comparandum: Plin. 28.63.224.

§1. *cum – repetit*.
Comparandum: Plin. 28.17.63.
A similar use of nails occurred even during the late nineteenth century in rural Sussex (Museum of Witchcraft and Magic, artefact no. 1218).

§2. *dantur – est*.
Comparandum: Plin. 28.6.34.
Drinking human blood was a famous treatment (*Med. Plin* 3.21.5 and commentary). This is a magical variation: the power of human blood was transferred to the animal via the weapon.

§2. *lapillus – gestatur*.
Comparanda: Plin. 30.27.91; Diosc. *MM* 2.56.1, *Eup.* 1.21.1; *Cyran.* 3.50; Cassius 71; Alex. *Therap.* 1.561.
The simplification of Pliny by the author resulted in a failure to state that the stones came from chicks. Scientific study of some swallows indicates that swallow-stones (gastroliths) are only found in chick's gizzards (Chişamera & Traian 2007, 473).
Details of how swallow-stones were gathered and worn varied between writers. This was also recommended for "lunacy" (Damig. 10), a term used for epilepsy in Late Antiquity (Isid. *Etym*. 4.7.6).
The use of swallow-stones continued into later folk medicine (Duffin 2013).

§3. *hirundinis – praestat*.
Comparanda: Plin. 30.27.91; Seren. 56 ll. 1014, 2021–2; Theod. *Physicorum* 2.7.
Gastroliths are thought to have been consumed by chicks from the nest (Chişamera & Traian 2007, 473); this might have been the result of this being observed.

§4. *alium – sumitur*.
Comparandum: Plin. 20.23.56.

Serenus (56 l. 1015) recommended *apium elixum* "well-boiled *apium*" which might have been a copyist's error.

§4. *tenentes – appetuntur.*
Comparandum: Plin. 20.73.192.
The author misread *anesum* (anise) as *anethum* (dill) as he did at 1.1.2.

§§4–5. *testiculi – postea.*
Comparandum: Plin. 30.27.87; cf. Plin. 30.27.92.
The forbidding of wine days in advance of a seizure is odd because they cannot be foretold days in advance. Celsus (3.23.3) recommended complete abstinence from wine.

§5. *sanguis – bibitur.*
Comparandum: Plin. 30.27.88.
A variety of different animal's blood was recommended (Plin. 32.14.35; Diosc. *MM* 2.79.2; *Eup.* 1.20.2; *Cyran.* 2.7).

§5. *sed – liberat.*
Comparanda: Plin. 28.2.4, 28.10.43; Cels. 3.23.7; Aret. *CD* 1.4.7–8.
The bland description of this within the *Medicina Plinii* is extremely odd; all other medical texts strongly criticised its use.
This continued to be recommended in early modern Europe (Stuart 1998, 359–60).

§6. *fel – editur.*
Comparandum: Plin. 30.27.88.
Cochleari vel ligula: As liquid measures, these were the same (11.375 millilitres), but the description of *cochlear* as half a *drachma* by the author is significantly smaller (*Med. Plin.* Prol. 9; Isid. *Etym.* 16.26.3).
Lamb bile was recommended with its blood (*Cyran.* 2.33), and other biles were used in treatments (Diosc. *MM* 2.78.4, *Eup.* 1.19.1; Cassius 71).

§7. *viverra – abigat.*
Comparandum: Plin. 30.27.90.
While Latin has a specific word for ferret (*viverra*), Greek does not differentiate between ferrets, weasels, and similar animals, referring to γαλῆ for all. The consumption of γαλῆ was commonly recommended (Diosc. *MM* 2.25.1, *Eup.* 1.20.3; Ps-Gal. K14.401; Aët. 2.167; Paul. Aeg. 7.3.3); Aretaeus (*CD* 1.4.8) stated that he had not tested this.

§8. *cochlearum – sale.*
Comparandum: Plin. 30.27.90.
Nettles were recommended by Dioscorides (*Eup.* 1.20.3) and Aretaeus (*CD* 1.4.13).

§§8–9. *iecur – cadavere.*

Comparandum: Plin. 30.27.92.

Pliny recommended eating either a vulture liver or the vulture if it had eaten human remains.

Human flesh, typically the liver, was another taboo treatment (Scribon. 17; Aret. *CD* 1.4.8); this recommendation is similar to the "consumption" of human blood magically via a third party at *Medicina Plinii* 3.21.2, except that it is the consumption of flesh (cf. *Med. Plin.* 3.21.12).

The consumption of vulture was recommended elsewhere (Theod. *Physicorum Codex B*, 2.7; *Vulture Epistles*, (Mackinney 1943, 495)).

§9. *fel – erigit.*

Comparanda: Plin. 32.14.37; Diosc. *Eup.* 1.20.3.

§10. *coagulum – aceto.*

Comparandum: Plin. 32.37.112.

Drinking seal's rennet with other medicaments was recommended (Theophr. 9.11.3; Diosc. *MM* 2.75.2, *Eup.* 1.20.2, 1.19.1).

§10. *castoreum – datur.*

Comparandum: Plin. 32.37.112.

Drinking *castoreum* in different honeyed draughts was recommended (Aret. *CD* 1.4.6; Orib. *EM* 2.2; Cassius 71; Aët. 6.16).

§11. *his – I.*

Comparandum: Plin. 32.37.112.

§12. *mustelae – sumitur.*

Comparandum: Plin. 32.37.112.

Mustela marina: "sea-weasel"; a name given to various fish including rockling, burbot, and lamprey. Sheat-fish liver was recommended by *Cyranides* (4.13).

§12. *carnes – depellunt.*

Comparandum: Plin. 28.63.226.

This Magian treatment seems to have used human remains magically via the funeral pyre (cf. *Med. Plin.* 3.21.9). Given Roman laws regarding burial practices, this was likely considered "unclean".

§12. *caprini – adhibetur.*

Comparanda: Plin. 28.63.226; Diosc. *Eup.* 1.23.1; Orib. *EM* 2.3; Aët. 6.14; Alex. *Therap.* 1.559.

Strong smells were used to detect epilepsy; Pliny recommended burnt sulphur (35.50.175) and bitumen (35.51.182) too.

Modern anecdotal evidence suggests that strong, unpleasant smells can induce a seizure.

22. *hydropicis*

This commences a collection of chapters, with the exception of broken bones (3.25), which provide treatments for complaints associated with skin. While dropsy might not seem skin-related, the retention of fluid was considered as being under the skin, as indicated by those treatments which sought to draw the fluid out via the skin directly.

Hydrops, ὕδρωψ: today clinically defined as subcutaneous fluid retention or oedema, but translated as "dropsy" and its sufferers, *hydropicus*, as "dropsical". Varieties of dropsy were described by doctors (e.g. Cels. 3.21.1–2), but the author only addressed the disease as a whole. Latin medical texts also treated what was called οἴδημα by Greek doctors, a painless, spongy swelling of the feet and legs as a result of dropsy (Gal. K10.953–4, K11.101), under that heading.

A number of the treatments within the *Medicina Plinii* were devoted to controlling thirst, a major symptom of the disease (e.g. Hippoc. *Int.* 26; Polybius 13.2.2; Ovid *Fasti*, 1 ll. 215–6; Cels. 3.21.2, 3.21.4) and an essential treatment (Cels. 3.21.2), but these treatments were not all sourced from dropsy treatments.

§1. *lapidem – liberabitur.*
Önnerfors (1964, 84) identifies Pliny 37.54.141 as the source for this, but Pliny recommended placing an Indian agate in the mouth to allay thirst. If the author did acquire this from Pliny, he appears to have analysed the text and adapted a treatment to reduce thirst to a disease with that symptom, and thus recommended agates to treat dropsy. However, there was a strong tradition of carrying agates as described by the author to treat dropsy.

The Orphic *Lithica* (42) described how "jasper-agate" helped dropsy and checked thirst, but Pliny separated "jasper-agates" (37.54.139) from "Indian agates". Aëtius recommended green "jasper-agate" to check thirst and assist dropsy (2.37), but also referred to "agates" in another treatment (15.5). Pseudo-Dioscorides (*Lapid.* 13) described "jasper-agate" identically to Aëtius, but only referred to its usefulness for dropsy. None of these described how it was used or how it helped, but *Physiologus Graecus* (*redactio prima* 46) described the use of a "green Indian stone" to treat dropsy: it was bound to the patient and "with accompanying rituals, prayers, and drinking, the stone cleansed patients of putrid fluids". *Physiologus* called it "Indian stone", matching Pliny; described it as "frog green" rather than the "emerald green" as described by Pseudo-Dioscorides and Aëtius (compare also how Pliny 37.54.141 implied that green was a common agate colour); and said it cured dropsy. It seems probable that "agate", "green agate", "Indian agate", "jasper-agate", and "Indian stone" referred to the same stone.

§1. *vomitus – inlinuntur.*
Comparanda: Plin. 30.31.105; Plac. 9.28.

§2. *sablone – obruuntur.*
Comparanda: Plin. 31.38.72; Cels. 3.21.6; Diosc. *MM* 5.148.1; Aulus Gellius 19.8.3; Seren. 27 l. 502; Orib. *CM* 10.8.1–16; Theod. 2.32.107; Aët. 3.9; *DMAC* 45.3).

Sablo/sabulo: typically referred to course sand or gravel, but *marinum sablo* suggests it was used here interchangeably with *harena*, "fine sand".

§2. *spongiae – apponuntur.*
Comparandum: Plin. 31.47.128.
Wet rather than dry sponges were used for οἴδημα like this (Gal. K10.953–4, K11.101–2; Orib. *CM* 44.28.2, 46.21.41, *Syn.* 7.35.2, *Eun.* 3.51.2; Aët. 15.1; Paul. Aeg. 4.27.1; Paul. Nic. 121; Leo 7.5).

§2. *adeps – tactis.*
Comparandum: Plin. 32.39.117.

§3. *cancri – iure.*
Crabs were diuretics (Hippoc. *Reg.* 2.48; Diocl. *Fr.* 224; Plin. 32.31.101), and excessive fluid was typically drained from the body through urination.
Pseudo-Theodorus (*Ad.* II,32(108)) recommended eating baked crabs.

§3. *alium – evacuat.*
Comparanda: Plin. 20.23.52 (garlic and centaury for dropsy, garlic and split fig to empty bowels); Ps-Theod. *Ad.* II,32(108).
Clearing the bowels was occasionally recommended (Cels. 3.21.9; Plin. 21.78.134, 24.20.30). Garlic was used as a diuretic for dropsy (Diosc. *MM* 2.152.3, *Eup.* 2.65.5).

§4. *scilla – compescit.*
Comparanda: Plin. 20.39.99; Diosc. *MM* 2.171.1; cf. Ps-Apul. 42.4.
Celsus (3.21.10) recommended sucking a cooked squill, but not for thirst.

§4. *scillae – urinam.*
Comparanda: Plin. 20.39.100; Ps-Apul. 42.1; Ps-Theod. *Ad.* II,32(108); *Antidot. Brux.* 34.
Baked squill, often in *oxymel* was recommended (Diosc. *MM* 2.171.3, *Eup.* 2.66.5, 2.119.5; Orib. *EM* 51.3; Paul. Aeg. 3.48.2).
Squills are scientifically proven diuretics (Attard *et al.* 2015, 5–7) used for centuries to treat dropsy (Stannard 1974, 684–713).

§5. *sinapem – imponuntur.*
Comparanda: Plin. 20.87.237; Ps-Theod. *Ad.* II,32(108).
Mustard applications were used (Cels. 3.21.10; Garg. 29); cumin and fig were recommended together (Gal. K13.257); and cumin was included in compounds (Orib. *EM* 51.1; Paul. Aeg. 3.48.3).

§5. *ficus – imponuntur.*
Comparanda: Plin. 23.63.123 (wine-boiled figs, wormwood, and barley meal); Ps-Theod. *Ad.* II,32(108).

Soda's inclusion might have been because the author misread Pliny (cf. Diosc. *MM* 1.128.3; Garg. 49), but soda was recommended with figs (Diosc. *MM* 5.113.3), so the addition might have been deliberate.

Fig-based plasters were used (e.g. Diosc. *MM* 3.23.3, *Eup.* 2.66.1–2; Gal. K13.257; Orib. *CM* 9.34.4, *Syn.* 3.80.4; Aët. 3.179).

§6. *folia – dantur.*
Comparandum: Plin. 23.81.162.
A myrtle potion with other medicaments was recommended (*Pap. Oxy.* 8.1088, ll. 63–5).

§6. *radices – exinaniunt.*
Comparanda: Plin. 24.35.52; Seren. 26 ll. 498–9; Ps-Theod. *Ad.* II,32(108).
Elder root juice was a diuretic (Theod. 2.32.108; Cassius 76). Elder was included in other treatments (Diosc. *MM* 4.173.3, *Eup.* 2.65.1; Aët. 1.19; Paul. Aeg. 7.4.11).

§7. *est – exinaniunt.*
Comparanda: Plin. 24.47.77; Ps-Apul. 120.1; Ps-Theod. *Ad.* II,32(108).
Chrysocarpus, χρυσόκαρπος: "with golden fruit"; the golden-berried variety of ivy known as "poet's ivy" (e.g. Vergil *Eclogues*, 3, ll. 38–39; Plin. 16.62.147) or black or Dionysian ivy (Diosc. *MM* 2.179.1). It has been identified as a variant of English ivy (*Hedera helix*) or *H. nepalensis* instead.
Ivy berries were diuretic (Plin. 24.47.75).

§8. *testudo – possit.*
Comparanda: Plin. 32.39.118; Ps-Theod *Ad.* II,32(108).

§9. *fimus – inlinitur.*
Comparandum: Plin. 28.68.232.
Applied cattle manure was thought to extract the fluid (*Cyran.* 2.6; Orib. *EM* 51.3; Paul. Aeg. 3.48.2), but its use was attributed to the death of the philosopher Heraclitus (Tatian. *Ad Gr.* 3; Diogenes Laertius 9.1.3; *Suda* H 472).

§9. *vincae – sanitatem.*
Comparanda: Plin. 21.99.172; *Cyran.* 5.22.
Periwinkle was a diuretic (Diosc. *Eup.* 2.119.3; Orib. *Eun.* 2.16.1).

§10. *elleborum – adalligamentum.*
Önnerfors (1964, 85) identifies Pliny 25.22.55 (cf. Diosc. *MM* 4.162.3, *Eup.* 2.66.2) as the source for this, but this is an extraordinarily different treatment.
All other references to the use of hellebore related to its purgative qualities (e.g. Hippoc. *Reg.* 3.76; Seren. 26 l. 506; *DMAC* 45.3).
Adalligamentum: a noun derived from the verb *adalligo*; this could relate to an amulet, but its use here seems more akin to a medical dressing.

23. morbo regio

This chapter continued the author's discussion of diseases related to the skin, especially those thought to feature fluids under the skin like dropsy, his previous topic of discussion; skin tone change associated with jaundice was often considered the result of bile settling under the skin (Hippoc. *Int.* 35, *Aff.* 32; Gal. K11.74). This chapter is followed by the author's discussion of erysipelas, so this might also constitute a focus on diseases whose symptoms changed the skin's colour.

Morbus regius: "royal disease", the most common name for jaundice, though etymological explanations for it differed (Cels. 3.24.5; Plin. 22.53.114). Other names were *arquatus morbus*, "rainbow disease" (Cels. 3.24.1; Lucilius 30.1007), and *aurugo/aurigo* derived from *aurium* "gold", relating to the symptomatic skin colour (Isid. *Etym.* 4.8.13). A Greek name was ἴκτερος, perhaps relating to the *icterus* bird used in treatment (Plin. 30.28.94), or named for the yellow-breasted marten, ἴκτις (Aret. *SD* 1.15.7). Jaundice was addressed as its own disease and as a symptom of liver and splenic diseases (Hippoc. *Epid.* 2.10; Gal. K2.114, 133), or other internal organ complaints (Aret. *SD* 1.15.2–4).

§1. *sordis – hauriuntur.*
Comparandum: Plin. 30.28.93.

§2. *vermes – propinantur.*
Comparandum: Plin. 30.28.93.
Earthworms prepared in potions were described as curing via urination (*Cyran.* 2.8; Gal. K14.242; Ps-Gal. K14.457; Aët. 2.168).

§2. *cerebrum – bibitur.*
Comparanda: Plin. 30.28.94; Plac. 26.1.

§3. *cineres – mulso.*
Comparandum: Plin. 30.28.94.

§3. *salsamentum – abstinentia.*
Comparandum: Plin. 32.31.101.

§4. *alium – propinatur.*
Comparanda: Plin. 20.23.52; Garg. 18; Seren. 57 l. 1027.
Oribasius (*EM* 50.12) recommended drinking a head of garlic with wine.

§4. *erucae – bibuntur.*
Comparandum: *Geopon.* 12.26.3 (wild rocket).
Önnerfors (1964, 85) attributes Pliny 20.49.126 as the source owing to the similarity in the gathering of rocket and how it was taken, but this was an aphrodisiac.
Geoponica provided no details about how or if it was to be taken.

§5. *cicer – cibo.*

Comparandum: Plin. 22.72.150.

Chickpea decoctions were commonly recommended (Hippoc. *Int.* 45, *Morb.*
3.17.v; Diosc. *MM* 2.104.1, *Eup.* 2.58.2–3; Plin. 26.76.124; Gal. K13.231–3;
Ps-Gal. K14.376; Orib. *EM* 50.4, 50.9–10, *Eun.* 4.98.6; Theod. 2.27.77).

§5. *nuces – eduntur.*

Comparandum: Plin. 23.76.146 (without forming pills).

Celsus (3.24.2–3) and Gargilius (53) recommended almond and wormwood
together with other medicaments, as did others who described the creation
of pills (Gal. K13.233; Orib. *EM* 50.5; Alex. *Therap.* 2.393).

Simple decoctions of wormwood were recommended (Diosc. *MM* 3.23.1; Orib.
CM 7.26.142, *EM* 50.3; Theod. 2.27.77; Paul. Aeg. 3.50.2; *DMAC* 33.3).

Almonds were always used with other medicaments (e.g. Diosc. *Eup.* 2.60.1;
Orib. *CM* 7.26.125; Aët. 3.41; Leo 5.24).

§6. *rubia – bibitur.*

Comparanda: Plin. 24.56.94; Diosc. *MM* 3.143.2, *Eup.* 2.119.4; Seren. 571. 1026.

Madder was taken in other ways (Diosc. *Eup.* 2.58.1; Gal. K13.234; Ps-Gal.
K14.456; Orib. *EM* 50.1, 50.3; Paul. Aeg. 3.50.2; *DMAC* 33.3).

§6. *herba – datur.*

Comparanda: Plin. 24.61.102; Ps-Apul. 86.1.

Savin was taken with honeyed (Ps-Gal. K14.455, 457; Ps-Apul. 86.1) or
peppered wine (Ps-Theod. *Ad.* II,27(77)).

§7. *canini – datur.*

Comparandum: Plin. 30.28.93.

This used *similia similibus* to form a magical link between the patient's and
hen's yellow skin.

§7. *folia – imponuntur.*

Dispersive plasters had a limited use (Cels. 3.24.5; Paul. Aeg. 3.50.2; Paul.
Nic. 62).

§8. *spondilium – bibitur.*

Comparanda: Plin. 24.16.25; Diosc. *MM* 3.76.2, *Eup.* 2.58.1, 2.60.1; Gal.
K12.135; Orib. *Eun.* 2.1σ.25; Paul. Acg. 7.3.19.

§§8–9. *fimus – ratione.*

Comparandum: Plin. 28.64.227.

§9. *cyminum – datur.*

Comparandum: Plin. 20.57.161.

Hippocrates (*Int.* 35) recommended a draught containing Egyptian cumin. Elsewhere it was utilised in compounds (Gal. K13.203, K14.164; Alex. *Therap.* 2.355).

24. igni sacro

Like the previous chapter devoted to jaundice, this discussion is devoted to a disease whose symptoms include a change in skin colour: erysipelas. Unlike the treatments for dropsy and jaundice, every treatment included here was applied. The application of treatments seems to be the only common element between this and the author's subsequent discussion of broken bones which seems to be completely out of place within this section of Book Three.

Ignis sacer: "holy fire"; erysipelas, the Streptococcal (most commonly *Streptococcus pyogenes*) skin infection which first appears in a small area with a burning sensation. It slowly spreads with a clear demarcation between red, swollen skin and normal, healthy skin.

This was also called *erysipelas*/ἐρυσίπελας but this did not always refer to erysipelas; some early Greek writers used this term to refer to any redness of the skin caused by eruption or ulceration. In addition to this, Celsus used the terms *ignis sacer* and *erysipelas* interchangeably but then described them as two distinct conditions (5.26.33, 5.28.4C-E; LCL: *Celsus III*, 590–1).

§1. *vermes – inlinuntur.*
Comparanda: Plin. 30.32.106; *Cyran.* 2.8; Seren. 40 l. 759; Aët. 1.113.

§1. *serpentium – balneo.*
Comparandum: Plin. 30.32.106.
Pig's bile was applied in the bath (Ps-Theod *Ad.* 1, 23(73)).

§2. *alii – inlinitur.*
Comparanda: Plin. 20.23.55; Seren. 40 ll. 762–3.

§2. *ruta – inlinitur.*
Comparanda: Plin. 20.51.141; Seren. 40 l. 760; Ps-Apul. 90.10.
Rue was recommended with other medicaments (Scribon. 245; Diosc. *MM* 3.45.4, *Eup.* 1.160.1–2; Gal. K13.836; Garg. 3; Marc. 4.64; Paul. Aeg. 4.21.2; Paul. Nic. 88).

§2. *lens – imponitur.*
Comparanda: Plin. 22.70.144; Diosc. *MM* 2.107.3.
Other lentil preparations were used (Cels. 5.26.33A; Diosc. *Eup.* 1.160.3; Orib. *CM* 44.24.10, *Syn.* 7.32.4, *Eun.* 3.47.4; Paul. Aeg. 4.21.1).

§3. *amurca – infunditur.*
Comparandum: Plin. 23.37.74.
Pliny did not specify the kind of *amurca* (see *Med. Plin.* 1.12.8).

§3. *herba – inlinitur.*
Comparanda: Plin. 24.61.102; Ps-Apul. 86.4.

§4. *ova – imponitur.*
Comparanda: Plin. 29.11.40, 29.11.41; Plac. 29.4; Theod. 1.23.73.
Various egg preparations were used (*Cyran.* 3.55; Seren. 40 ll. 756–8, 764–5;
    Plac. 29.9; Ps-Theod. *Ad.* I,23(73); Paul. Aeg. 3.59.5).
Celsus (5.36.33B) recommended beet leaves with other medicaments.

§4. *hyssopum – inlinitur.*
Comparandum: Plin. 30.32.106.
The author misread *oesypum* (wool grease) as *hyssopum.*
Pompholyx, πομφόλυξ: a zinc oxide sublimate named for its bubbly appear-
    ance when forming on the upper part of furnaces which processed copper
    using calamine (Diosc. *MM* 5.75.2; Riddle 1985, 149–52).
Sometimes lesser quality zinc oxide, σποδός, was used in treatments (Diosc.
    Eup. 1.160.4).
Hyssop was used, but with salt (Plin. 31.45.103).

§5. *grillus – terra.*
Comparandum: Plin. 30.32.106.

§6. *anseris – superlinitur.*
Comparandum: Plin. 30.32.106.

§7. *spongia – tegat.*
Comparandum: Plin. 31.47.128.
Elsewhere these were not used together (vinegar: Diosc. *MM* 5.13.1; Gal.
    K11.439; sponges: Orib. *EM* 103.3; Paul. Aeg. 4.21.1).

§7. *ursinus – imponuntur.*
Comparanda: Plin. 28.69.233: Seren. 40 l. 756; Ps-Theod. *Ad.* I,23(73).

§8. *est – Cimolia.*
Comparandum: Plin. 26.74.121.
Zoster, ζωστήρ: this was not discussed elsewhere. Jones (LCL: *Pliny
    Natural History VII,* 357) identifies it as a form of shingles; ἕρπης,
    "shingles"/"creeping ulcer", was discussed with *erysipelas* by Dioscorides
    (*Eup.* 1.161) and Oribasius (*CM* 44.26.8; *Syn.* 3.53.1).
Plantain juice and Cimolian chalk were recommended (Diosc. *MM* 2.126.3;
    Paul. Nic. 88).

§9. *aqua – inlinitur.*
Feathers were recommended to apply medicament elsewhere (Ps-Apul. 121.1;
    Ps-Theod. *Ad.* I,23(73)).

Pliny considered cistern-sourced water inappropriate because of potential contaminants (31.21.31–4).

See *Medicina Plinii* 3.24.4 for the use of egg.

25. *ossibus fractis*

The author's placement of this between chapters devoted to skin complaints, erysipelas and *scabies*, is bewildering. Logically it would have been better placed near the beginning of Book Three given that one of these treatments is identical to that relating to fractured joints in the first chapter (cf. *Med. Plin* 3.1.5 to 3.25.3).

§§1–2. *caninum – extrahit.*
Comparanda: Plin. 30.40.119; Iul. Afr. fr. 3.16, (D41); Seren. 52 ll. 949–53; *Hippiatr. Cant.* 62.2.
Pliny described these as equally effective.
Knitting bones normally took longer: small bone (ribs, cheeks) took 14 to 21 days; the humerus and femur took 27 to 40 days (Cels. 8.7.5).
Bandages and wool were commonly used (e.g. Hippoc. *Art.* 49; Cels. 8.8.1C; Diosc. *MM* 2.73.1), and wetting the wool was also recommended (Cels. 8.10.1E-G; Diosc. *MM* 2.73.1).
The need to extract bone fragments to assist healing was recommended (Cels. 8.8.1C), and ground earthworms and honey were used for this (Ps-Theod. *Ad.* I,38(97)).

§2. *laridum – solidat.*
Comparanda: Plin. 28.65.227; Ps-Theod. *Ad.* I,38(97).
Galen recommended lard in plasters (K13.544, 546).

§3. *articulorum – cera. . .*
Comparanda: Plin. 30.40.119; Marc. 34.66; cf. *Med. Plin.* 3.1.5.
Cerates were variously recommended (e.g. Hippoc. *Art.* 49; Gal. K13.536–7, 537–8, 539–40, 544, 546, 578), but Celsus used wax and cerates to hold bandages in place (8.10.1F).

§3. . . . *costis – sanat.*
Comparanda: Plin. 28.65.227; Seren. 52 ll. 954–5; Ps-Theod. *Ad.* I,38(97).
Bandaging was (and is) customary for ribs.

26. *scabei*

The author here returned to skin conditions. Its placement in close proximity to the following chapter devoted to *papulae* and itching complaints was logical, especially given the reference to a *scabies* treatment at 3.27. 2.

Scabies: any itching skin condition or associated roughness of skin, commonly translated as itch, mange, scab, roughness, scurf, or scabies. Although modern scabies is named after the Latin disease, they are not necessarily the same.

Identifying which skin complaints were meant by *scabies* is almost impossible. Cassius (15) said it was called *lepra* by Greeks (probably a form of leprosy), but he, Celsus (5.28.16, 6.6.31), and Pliny (20.69.178, 23.63.117) also combined *psora* (ψώρα) with *scabies*-related conditions. Pliny (20.2.4) also stated that *scabies* was *lichen*, which the *Medicina Plinii* addresses at 1.18.

§1. *plurimum – sedat.*
Comparanda: Plin. 28.75.244; Seren. 6 ll. 73–4; Ps-Theod. *Ad.* I,35(93).
Urine was used (Diosc. *MM* 2.81.1; Gal. K12.285; Aët. 2.108) but the only
    urine mud-pack prescribed for this in Greek treated horses (*Hippiatr. Cant.*
    57.5).

§2. *fimus – impositus.*
Comparandum: Plin. 28.75.244 for *bova*, a skin condition not dissimilar to
    scabies.
Heiffer dung was recommended by Serenus (6 l. 75).

§2. *sanguis – lixivo.*
Comparandum: Plin. 28.75.244 for canine *scabies.*
Lye is strongly alkali and can cause chemical burns. Hair might have made this
    safe for canine use, but human use was potentially problematic.
Lye was made from ashes by throwing fresh water on them and collecting it
    (Plutarch *Causes of Natural Phenomena*, 1 (911E)).

§3. *sanguis – inlinitur.*
Comparanda: Plin. 30.41.121; Ps-Theod. *Ad.* I,35(93).

§3. *alumen – melanthio.*
Comparandum: Plin. 35.52.185.
Soda and alum were used together elsewhere with other medicaments (Celsus
    5.28.16C; Columella, 6.31.2; Gal. K13.347; Garg. 30; Aët. 12.1; *Hippiatr.*
    Berol. 69.20).
Melanthium was little used for skin complaints (Ps-Theod. *Simp.* 84).

§3. *ocustarum – medentur.*
Comparandum: Plin. 30.10.30.
The first letter has been dropped from *locustarum.*

27. papulis et pruritui

The placement of this immediately following a chapter which addressed *scabies* was logical given their inherent nature; the fact that one treatment was used for both itch and *scabies* (3.27.2) illustrates just how appropriate this was. The author's exposition on skin conditions continued into the following chapter devoted to another similar conditions: pimples.

Papula: pustule or pimple. As an individual complaint, Celsus (5.28.18A-B) described two varieties of *papulae*, and numerous kinds of *pusulae* (5.28.15); *pusula/pustula* can relate to a pustule, inflamed sore, small prominence, or blister.

Pruritus: itching.

These terms appear to have been deliberately vague, giving the chapter a generic quality. This text contains no nuanced approach to these varieties of dermatological complaints.

The use of the baths in treatments by the author matches their usage for other similarly named conditions (Cels. 5.28.15D; Diosc. *Eup.* 1.118.1; Ps-Gal. K14.468; Marc. 16.25; Theod. 1.35.92; Cassius 16; Paul. Nic. 110).

§1. *lupinorum – inlinitur*.

Comparanda: Plin. 22.74.155; Seren. 6 ll. 82–3; Ps-Theod. *Ad.* I,35(93).

Celsus recommended lupine meal for large *pusulae* (5.28.15D). Lupine decoctions were recommended (Diosc. *MM* 2.109.1; Gal. K11.885, K12.496–7; Ps-Gal. K14.468; Orib. *Eun* 2.10.4; Aët. 1.162).

§1. *pruritus – impositae*.

Comparandum: Plin. 30.41.121.

Serenus (6 ll. 85–6), recommended these with sea foam.

§2. *nitrum – aspergitur*.

Comparandum: Plin. 31.46.116 for *papulae* and *pusulae*.

Soda was recommended for pimples or pustules with other medicaments (Cels. 5.28.15D; Diosc. *Eup.* 1.99.1, 1.119.1; Gal. K12.496–7; Orib. *EM* 105.1–4; Aët. 5.133, 6.68).

§2. *pruritum – sint*.

Comparanda: Plin. 32.40.191; Ps-Theod. *Ad.* I,35(93).

The *Medicina Plinii* fails to include *iecur* (liver) from Pliny's text; this transformed the treatment from decocted liver to multiple boiled down stingrays.

§3. *aluminis – inlinuntur*.

Comparanda: Plin. 35.52.185; Ps-Theod. *Ad.* I,35(93); cf. Diosc. *MM* 5.106.5, *Eup.* 1.119.1.

Honey and alum were used with other medicaments for various dermatological conditions (Diosc. *Eup.* 1.117.1; Aët. 16.129; Paul. Aeg. 3.3.2).

§3. *aeque – balneo*.

Comparandum: Ps-Theod. *Ad.* I,35(93).

This might have been an attempt by the author to adapt Pliny's advice (35.57.196) to the standard topical application of Cimolian chalk; it was variously prepared for this (Diosc. *MM* 2.80.3; Ps-Gal. K14.469; Orib. *CM* 10.27.16; Aët. 5.133, 6.68).

§4. *pustulis – inlinitur*.
Comparanda: Plin. 28.69.233; Seren. 6 l. 76.
Pseudo-Theodorus (*Ad.* I,35(93)) recommended burnt sow dung and vinegar.

§4. *sulphur – inlinitur*.
Liquamen: sauce made from whole fermented fish and salt.
Sulphur was used for various similar dermatological conditions (Cels. 5.28.18C; Diosc. *MM* 5.107.2, *Eup.* 1.100.1, 1.119.2; Gal. K12.482, 827; Ps-Gal. K14.395–7, 520; Orib. *EM* 77, 102.1, *Eun.* 3.21.6; Marc. 16.25; Theod. 1.35.93; Cassius 16; Paul. Aeg. 4.8.1).

28. varis

The author's continued exposition of inflamed skin blemishes used more precise terminology here. Pimples have more in common with the previous chapter's *papulae* and itches, than the following discussion of warts.

Varus: an inflamed spot on the skin or pimple. There are few references to pimples in Latin texts because treating them was considered a waste of time (Cels. 6.5.1). The inclusion of this again indicates the author's cosmetic interests.

§1. *folia – varos*.
Comparandum: Plin. 20.21.44.

§1. *farina – emendat*.
Comparandum: Plin. 22.73.151 for pimples and *macula*.
Macula: a disfiguring skin mark, spot, blemish, or mole.
Bitter vetch was used to address skin imperfections (Ovid *Medicamina faciei*, ll. 56–66; Cels. 6.5.3; Diosc. *MM* 2.108.2, *Eup.* 1.115.2; *Cyran.* 1.1, 2.6; Orib. *EM* 78.7; Aët. 8.11, 8.12, 8.14; Paul. Aeg. 3.25.3, 4.6.2).

§1. *oleum – inlinitur*.
Comparandum: Plin. 23.42.85.
Almond oil was recommended with other medicaments (Diosc. *MM* 1.33.2, *Eup.* 1.114.1; Aët. 8.11). Honey was used with other medicaments for pimples (Diosc. *Eup.* 1.116.1; Gal. K12.825; Ps-Gal. K14.352; Orib. *Syn.* 8.36.3, *Eun.* 4.51.2).

§2. *adeps – imponitur*.
Comparandum: Plin. 30.10.30.
Dioscorides recommended onion and salt (*MM* 2.151.2), or onion juice with zinc oxide (*Eup.* 1.116.1).

§2. *naevos – imposita*.
Comparanda: Plin. 22.67.137; Ps-Theod. *Ad.* I,36(94) for *macula*.
Naevus: a discoloured mark on skin, mole, or birthmark.

29. verrucis

This chapter concluded the author's discussion of spontaneous skin complaints; he moved next to bruising and swelling. While warts do not present as a blister or pustule, they did create a disfiguration, and thus suitably followed his previous chapters.

Varruca: a wart or skin excrescence. The term *clavus* can also refer to warts, but was mostly reserved for calluses by Pliny and the author (see introductory commentary to 2.27). This attempt at clarity was undermined by the similarity between many treatments for *verrucae* and *clavi*.

Greek generic terminology included ἧλος, which could mean callus; and θύμος, a wart-like excrescence. Specialised Greek terminology for what Celsus outlined as "wart-like blemishes" was used: *acrochordon* (ἀκροχορδών), thin-necked wart; *thymion* (θύμιον), large wart the colour of thyme; *myrmecia* (μυρμηκία) "ant-hill" wart which spread under the skin whose creeping sensation was compared to ants crawling on skin and was considered the opposite to *acrochordon*, (*Med. Plin.* 2.20.1 described it as a genital wart).

> §1. *verrucae – inlita*. . .
> Comparanda: Plin. 30.23.81; Seren. 63 l. 1096; Plac. 9α.18; Marc. 19.65; Ps-Theod. *Ad.* I,35(93). Cf. *Med. Plin.* 2.26.7.
> This was recommended for *acrochordona* (Diosc. *Eup.* 1.168.1), possibly for *myrmecia* (Iul. Afr. 3.17 (D42); Wallraff et al. 2012, 137, describe it as a dog urine mud-pack, but the text does specify), and for both (Paul. Nic. 113).

> §1. . . . *fimi – imposito*. . .
> Comparanda: Plin. 30.23.81; Ps-Theod. *Ad.* I,35(93).
> Marcellus (19.65) recommended burnt dog dung alone.

> §1. . . . *fimo – inlito*. . .
> Comparanda: Plin. 30.23.81; Marc. 19.67. Cf. *Med. Plin.* 2.26.2.
> See commentary on *Medicina Plinii* 2.26.2.

> §1. . . . *sanguine – recenti*. . .
> Comparanda: Plin. 30.23.81;.Marc. 19.66; Ps-Theod. *Ad.* I,35(93).
> Galen (K12.263) recommended this for *acrochordona*.

> §1. . . . *erinacei felle*. . .
> Comparandum: Plin. 30.23.81.

> §1. . . . *sanguine lacertae*. . .
> Comparanda: Plin. 30.23.81; Diosc. *Eup.* 1.166.1; Seren. 63 l. 1095. Cf. *Med. Plin.* 2.26.3.

> §1. . . . *fimo – nitro*.
> Comparandum: Plin. 30.23.81.

§2. *efficaciter – sutoricio. . .*

Comparanda: Plin. 20.48.123; Garg. 22.

Atramentum sutoricius: "cobbler's blacking", a solution of copper sulphate (blue vitriol).

This mix was also used to treat various types of warts (Diosc. *Eup.* 1.167.3; Orib. *EM* 114.8; Paul. Aeg. 3.59.2, 5.15.1).

§2. *. . . inmaturarum – mixto. . .*

Comparanda: Plin. 23.63.118 (unspecified fig latex and axle-grease); Ps-Theod. *Ad.* I,35(93).

Fig latex alone was recommended to treat various warts (Diosc. *MM* 1.128.4, *Eup.* 1.167.2, 1.116.1; Gal. K12.88; Orib. *EM* 114.8; Paul. Aeg. 3.59.2, 4.15.1, 7.3.18).

A small clinical trial using immature *Ficus caria* latex reported a 44 per cent success rate (Bohlooli *et al.* 2007, 524–6).

§2. *. . . capitum – trito. . .*

Comparanda: Plin. 32.45.128; Aët. 2.184.

Burnt pickled *smaris*, with which *mena* was confused (see commentary on *Med. Plin.* 3.3.18) was more frequently recommended (Diosc. *MM* 2.64.1, *Eup.* 1.166.1, 1.167.2; *Cyran.* 4.46; Orib. *EM* 113; Paul. Aeg. 3.59.2, 4.15.1).

§2. *. . . cinere – luto.*

Comparanda: Plin. 28.62.223; Marc. 34.49; Ps-Theod. *Ad.* I,35(93). Cf. *Med. Plin.* 2.26.2.

The urine mud-pack described by Iulius Africanus (see commentary on *Med. Plin.* 3.29.1) could be this one as the text did specify the source of the urine.

30. *livoribus et tumoribus*

While this chapter would have fitted well within the author's discussion of injuries at the beginning of Book Three, discussing bruises, swelling, dislocations, ruptures, sprains, and abrasions, he instead used it as a conclusion for skin conditions. This might suggest that the author was more concerned with the cosmetic implications of bruising rather than the actual injurious nature of some the problems outlined in his text. The *Medicina Plinii* does not differentiate between bruise varieties, as was common elsewhere, like Pliny's use of *suggilatio* "black and blue marks" in the treatments recommended by this author. This is the last chapter devoted to skin conditions, as the following chapter discusses *paralysis*.

§1. *recenti – imponitur.*

Comparanda: Plin. 20.13.24; Diosc. *MM* 2.112.1, *Eup.* 1.53.1; Gal. K12.809, 815, 817; Ps-Gal. K14.350–1; Marc. 19.53; Aët. 8.2; Paul. Aeg. 3.25.4.

§1. *alium – melle.*

Comparanda: Plin. 20.23.55; Diosc. *MM* 2.152.3, *Eup.* 1.53.1; *Geopon.* 12.30.2.

§1. *holus – se.*

Comparanda: Plin. 20.34.88; Cato *De agricultura*, 157.4.

This was likely also used in Greek medicine, but radish, ῥαφανίς, was often used interchangeably with ῥάφανος, which like *holus*, referred to both cabbage and vegetable generally. *Cyranides* (5.17), for example, used both words in its treatment of black eyes and livid spots.

§1. *apium – ovi.*

Comparandum: Marc. 19.49.

This might have been the result of crasis between Pliny's use of *apium* to treat bruises and its use with egg white to treat kidneys (20.44.115).

§2. *sinapis – remediat.*

Comparandum: Plin. 20.87.240.

While Pliny recommended mustard, honey, and goose grease, only the author outlined the mustard type, amounts, and application specifics; perhaps he formulated them from experience.

Alexandrian mustard: an uncommon term. The *Medicina Plinii* only specifies it here, but recommends mustard four times elsewhere. Pliny referred to it once in passing (12.14.28); Marcellus once (25.6), but recommended mustard ten other times; Galen used the term twice (K13.247, 252); Oribasius once (*Syn.* 3.162.1). This use of both "mustard" and "Alexandrian mustard" throughout individual texts implies a differentiation between them, perhaps relating to efficacy. The late Latin *Alphabet of Galen* (261) described Alexandrian mustard as the most effective. The name was likely because mustard's purportedly originated from Canopus, an old town outside Alexandria (Herod. *De prosodia catholica*, 3.1).

Mustard and honey was recommended by Dioscorides (*MM* 2.154.2, *Eup.* 1.53.1), and mustard and animal fats were also recommended (Gal. K12.811–2, 815; Ps-Gal. 14.351).

§3. *percussa – sanantur.*

Comparandum: Plin. 22.68.139.

The author simplified Pliny's advice.

Variously prepared bread was applied to abrasions (Diosc. *Eup.* 1.165.1; Orib. *Syn.* 7.5.3, *Eun.* 3.18.3; Paul. Aeg. 4.14.2; Paul. Nic. 100).

§3. *acrifolii – tumori.*

Comparandum: Plin. 24.72.116 for dislocations and swellings.

§4. *pulmones – imponuntur.*

Comparanda: Plin. 30.10.28 for bruises; Plac. 6β.3; Marc. 19.59.

§5. *columbine – utuntur.*
Comparanda: Plin. 30.10.28 for bruises; Plac. 30.14.

§5. *aqua – calido.*
Comparandum: Plin. 31.33.65 for bruises.

§5. *plantagine – canceromata.*
This advice might be the result of misreading Pliny 26.75.122, where plantain and salt were recommended for glandular swellings rather than injury-related swellings.
This cross-reference to *cancer* does not correlate with the use of plantain at *Medicina Plinii* 3.4.21.

§6. *sal – imponitur.*
Comparandum: Plin. 31.45.100.

§6. *livorem – tollit.*
Comparanda: Plin. 31.47.129; Gal. K12.808, 814–5, 817; Ps-Gal. K14.351; Marc. 19.47.

§7. *mirifice – oleo.*
Comparandum: Plin. 28.70.234, cf. *Med. Plin.* 2.22.3.

§§7–8. *vitiatis – pressi.*
Comparanda: Plin. 28.72.237–8; Diosc. *MM* 2.80.3.
The author simplified Pliny's advice. Pliny and this author alone addressed chariot-associated injuries.

§9. *proximam – inesse.*
Comparandum: Plin. 28.72.238.

§9. *luxatis – imponitur.*
Comparanda: Plin. 28.70.234; Ps-Theod. *Ad.* I,31(86).
Applications of hot cattle or swine dung preparations were recommended by Dioscorides (*Eup.* 1.218.3).

§10. *verris – trita.*
Comparanda: Plin. 28.70.234; Plac. 5α.24; Ps-Theod. *Ad.* I,31(86).

§10. *ruptis – mulieris.*
Comparandum: Plin. 30.22.71.

§10. *cancri – asinino.*
Comparandum: Plin. 32.32.103.

§11. *ponimus – medetur.*

Sagares cannot be further identified. The name appears in multiple inscriptions in Latin and Greek, but with no connection to pancration.

§§12–13. *in – tangatur.*

Tudicula: an instrument for crushing olives.

Another pancrationist's compound for burns and scarring contained litharge, white lead, possibly the plant *Plumbago europa*, wax, turpentine resin, and oil (Gal. K12.844–5).

Similar compounds were recorded (Scribon. 214: Orib. *EM* 87.6).

§14. *Nero – praebebat.*

Comparanda: Plin. 13.43.126; Diosc. *MM* 4.153.4.

The ability of *thapsia* to remove bruises had been known for centuries prior to Pliny (Arist. *[Pr.]* 9.9–10; Theophr. 9.20.3). It was often used with other medicaments (Cels. 5.18.24; Diosc. *Eup.* 1.53.1; Gal. K12.813–4, 818–9; Orib. *CM* 10.27.14; Marc.19.55; Paul. Aeg. 3.25.4).

Nero's nocturnal behaviour and subsequent beatings were recorded elsewhere (Tacitus *Annales*, 13.25; Suetonius *Nero*, 26).

§15. *si – fascias.*

Comparanda: Plin. 22.60.127; Gal. K12.576.

31. paralyticis

This short chapter reads as if its inclusion were an afterthought, which it might well have been given the author's intent to address complaints as they came to mind. All it has in common with the previous chapter is that it too might have better thematically fit earlier in Book Three, perhaps incorporated into its first chapter.

Paralysis: the relaxation of tendons resulting in weakened limbs; if this affected the whole body it was called *apoplexia* which quickly resulted in death (Cels. 3.27.1A).

§1. *nullus – holera.*

Comparandum: Plin. 20.34.85 (cabbage).

Oribasius (*EM* 73.18) recommended cabbage among other vegetables.

§1. *rubia – balnei.*

Comparandum: Plin. 24.56.94.

Drinking madder outside the bath was recommended (Diosc. *MM* 3.143.2; Aët. 1.148).

Bathing as a treatment was recommended (Cels. 3.27.1E; Paul. Aeg. 3.18.2–3; *DMAC* 21.3).

§2. *aliqui – euphorbio.*
Euphorbea was used topically with other medicaments (Gal. K13.1046–7; Orib. *EM* 73.4–5, *Syn.* 3.83.1; Theod. 2.19.54–5; Aët. 6.28, 12.1, 12.63; Alex. *Therap.* 1.585; Paul. Aeg. 3.18.3; Paul. Nic. 124; *DMAC* 21.3).

§2. *pingue – edendum.*
Comparanda: Plin. 30.26.86 as a prophylactic; Plac. 19.1.

32. psilotrum

This last chapter prior to the final discussion of toxicology also has nothing in common with the *paralysis*, though its focus on the cosmetic fits well within author's discussions of pimples, warts and bruises prior to that.

Psilothrum/psilotrum, ψίλωθρον: usually translated as "depilatory". Rather than remove hair, these applications sought to prevent hair regrowth. The focus on removed hair regrowth by the author is similar to his logic related to hair dyes (1.5).

§1. *sunt – renascantur.*
The author contextualised this use of depilatories as purely cosmetic, but some treatments related to the prevention of ingrown eye-lash regrowth. This might account for the lack of invective which usually accompanied hair removal in Roman culture (Olsen 2014, 182–205).

§2. *nam – auferantur.*
Comparandum: Plin. 32.47.136, cf. 14.25.123.
The removal of hair prior to the application of depilatories was commonly, but not always, described; it may have been a presumed practice.
Martial (*Epigrams*, 3.74, 12.21–2) and Juvenal (8 1. 114) referred to this use of resin.

§3. *sanguisugae – abluuntur.*
Comparanda: Plin. 32.47.136; *Cyran.* 4.8 for eye-lashes and body; Seren. 34 ll. 670–3.
The length of application was recorded only in the *Medicina Plinii.*
Other uses of leech ash were recommended address eye-lashes (Marc. 8.184; Theod. 1.12.41) and hair generally (Gal. K12.742; Aët. 7.69).

§3. *lacte – inlinitur.*
Comparanda: Plin. 30.46.133; Diosc *MM* 2.70.6 to thin hair.
Placitus (9α.14, 9β.18) recommended any dog's milk, and it was recommended for eye-lashes (Gal. K12.269; Marc. 8.181).

§4. *Amerinae – balneo.*
Comparandum: Plin. 24.37.58.
Ameria was an ancient town in Umbria.

§4. *sanguis vespertilionis.*

Comparanda: Plin. 30.56.132; Seren. 34 ll. 663–4; Aët. 2.85.

This was specifically recommended for eye-lashes by *Cyranides* (2.28) and Marcellus (8.181).

Bat blood used with additional medicaments was recommended for nearly two millennia prior to this to prevent eye-lash regrowth (*Ebers Papyrus* 424, in Nunn 2002, 201; Bryan 1974, 102; Gal. K12.740–1, 800; Aët. 7.69).

§4. *vipera – psilotrantur.*

Comparandum: Plin. 30.46.133.

This constitutes the only use of the verb *psilotro* in the entire Latin corpus.

Pliny stated that this was used instead of a depilatory, and the author turned Pliny's *psilotrum* into a verb to describe its action. As result, the sense of substitution was lost.

§5. *fel – inlinitur.*

Comparandum: Plin. 30.46.133.

Hedgehog bile was only recommended with other materials (Gal. K12.742, 800; Aët. 7.69).

§5. *et – frequenter. . .*

Comparandum: Plin. 26.93.164.

Pliny used this to kill hair still attached and as a depilatory following plucking; used with oil in the sun, it removed hair and promoted the regrowth of fine, blond hair until its continual use killed it completely at the root (Diosc. *MM* 4.164.3; Ps-Apul. *Interpol. ex Diosc.* II 309, 13 sqq).

Spurge juice's effect when mixed with oil was described as "more violent" (Gal. K12.141; Aët. 1.391).

The continual use of spurge juice alone would also kill hair (Gal. K12.141; Ps-Theod. *Simp.* 125). Its varied use was recommended (Diosc. *Eup.* 1.97.1; Gal. K6.627; Aët. 6.63).

§5. *. . . . et – quoque.*

The author mistook hyena bile for blood; hyena bile was a recognised depilatory (Plin. 28.27.97; Gal. K12.800; Marc. 8.175; Theod. 1.12.41).

33. Praef. venenis et venetatis morsibus

Like the chapter devoted to the breast (1.23), this preface acts as an introduction to the final topic of this text: toxicology. Why the author decided to discuss this after a chapter devoted to depilatories cannot be stated with any certainty, but venomous animals were used as depilatories, for example viper (described at *Med. Plin.* 3.32.4), and sea-hare which the author did not recommend. Perhaps this led him to this final topic, as he made no prior mention to toxicology.

34. antidotum contra venena

The author started his toxicological exposition with this highly simplified discussion of poisons. He provided here advice to prevent and address the ingestion of all poisons barring sea-hare, which was a topic in the following chapter.

§§1–2. *antidotum – noceant.*

Antidotum Mithridaticum/Mithridatum/Mithridatium: the name given to universal poison prophylactics after Mithridates VI Eupator of Pontus who researched toxicology. Six different *Mithridatica* recipes are extant (Cels. 5.23.3; Scribon. 170; Gal. K14.107–9, 115–7, 152–3). Pliny (29.8.24–5) was highly critical of these and similar compounds called *theriaci*. The *riacus* originated as a compound which specifically addressed venomous bites, but over time became similar to *Mithridaticum* and was used to treat multiple conditions. Over centuries, *theriacus* became known as "treacle" in English, and was offered for sale in European apothecaries as late as the nineteenth century (Watson 1966, 150).

This expense cannot be analysed comparatively owing to third century CE inflation. The concept of the psychological correlation between cost and effectiveness was noted by Galen (K14.216), and profiteering through the use of exotic *materia medica* and complicated compounds was described by Pliny (24.1.4–5). Many ingredients included in extant *Mithridatica* and *theriaci* were either imported from the east, difficult to obtain in large quantities (e.g. *castoreum*), or were labour intensive (e.g. saffron, opium).

§3. *alia – venenum.*

The author's safety concerns were likely based on Pliny's discussion of the inclusion of Indian cinnabar (29.8.25); it was confused with highly toxic *cinnabaris nativa*, also called *minium*, "red lead" (33.38.115–6), mercury sulphide.

Pliny did not provide the description of *Mithridaticum* poisoning recorded here.

§4. *Pompeius – ieiuno.*

Comparanda: Plin. 23.77.149; Garg. 3.

§§5–6. *electrum – naturale.*

Comparanda: Plin. 33.23.80–1; Serv. *Ad Aen.* 8.402; Isid. *Etym.* 16.24.1.

Poison-detecting cups, or cups which rendered poisons safe, were described elsewhere in classical literature (e.g. Ael. *NA* 3.41) and have survived to the present (Science Museum London, artefact no. A634419).

The description given by the author that manufactured *electrum* shared the poison-detection property of naturally occurring *electrum* was in direct opposition with Pliny, but consistent with his desire to provide cheaper alternatives.

§8. *centaurion – alvum.*

Comparandum: Plin. 25.79.127.

Fine centaury was more often described (Plin. 25.31.68; Diosc. *MM* 3.7.2; Gal. K12.21; Ps-Apul. 35.5).

§8. *aristolochiae – bibitur*.
Comparanda: Plin. 25.79.128, 25.55.101; Diosc. *MM* 3.4.4; Ps-Apul. 19.1.
All varieties of *aristolochia* were commonly used (e.g. Nic. *Ther*. l. 937; Gal. K14.82).

§8. *sanguis – toxica*.
Comparanda: Plin. 29.14.58; Diosc. *MM* 2.79.1; Seren. 45 ll. 853–5.
Toxicum, τοξικόν: poison applied to arrows or poisonous materials generally.

§9. *coagulum – datur*.
Comparandum: Plin. 29.33.104–5.
The author appears to have misread Pliny's text.

§9. *mustela – potatur*.
Comparanda: Plin. 29.33.105; Diosc. *MM* 2.25.1.
Weasels were commonly used in antidotes (Gal. K12.362), and preserved for medical use (Nic. *Ther*. ll. 689–99; Diosc. *MM* 2.25.1; Plin. 29.16.60).

§10. *sanguis – vino*.
Comparandum: Plin. 29.33.104.
Pontic ducks: the use of these was based on Mithridates' toxicological research; his theory stated that these ducks did not die from eating poisonous plants, therefore their blood could help its consumer to do the same (Plin. 25.3.6; Aulus Gellius 17.16).
Despite the availability of Mithridates' research (Plin. 25.3.5), duck's blood (not Pontic) was only occasionally recommended (Scribon. 177; Diosc. *MM* 2.79.1; Marc. 22.18).

§10. *asini – rest[r]ing<u>it*.
The author's vocabulary here mirrors Pliny's (28.45.158) except he replaced milk with blood. The use of ass blood was not described elsewhere, whereas milk was common (e.g. Cels. 5.27.12B; Scribon. 179; Diosc. *MM* 2.70.5; Gal. K14.138–9).

§10. *haedi – bibitur*.
Comparandum: Plin. 28.45.161.
Dioscorides (*MM* 2.79.1) described kid's blood as a beneficial antidote ingredient.

35. *contra leporem marinum et pastinacam*

Despite its heading, this chapter made no explicit reference to stingrays, and the only connection between sea-hare and stingrays apart from both being marine creatures is extraordinarily tenuous (Philostrotus *Vita Apollonii*, 6.32). Sea-hare is poisonous when ingested and stingrays have a venomous strike. Stingray-strike treatment was discussed by numerous writers, but there was also a tradition that they were incurable (Ael. *NA* 1.56, 2.50). By devoting a chapter to marine toxicology, the author created a segue from poisons to venomous bites or strikes which were the focus for the rest of his text.

§1. *saeviunt – lepore.*
Madness was commonly considered a potential outcome from administered poisons (Rives 2003, 321).

§1. *qui – vixit.*
Comparandum: Plin. 32.3.9.

§2. *atque – piscis.*
Comparandum: Plin. 32.3.9.

§2. *hoc – sumpta.*
Comparandum: Plin. 32.20.58–32.21.59.
Similarly prepared riverine crabs were recommended, likely following Nicander's advice (Nic. *Ther.* ll. 949–50; Diosc. *Eup.* 2.160; Ps-Diosc. *Ther.* 30; *Cyran.* 4.28).

§3. *malva – datur.*
Comparanda: Plin. 20.84.223; Diosc. *MM* 2.118.2 for all deadly poisons.
Mallow preparations were recommended (Nic. *Alex.* ll.486–7; Diosc. *Eup.* 2.160; Ps-Diosc. *Alex.* 30; Prom. *Ther.* 79; Gal. K14.139).

§3. *sanguis – bibitur.*
Comparandum: Plin. 29.33.104.
Goose blood was variously recommended (Diosc. *Eup.* 2.160.2; Ps-Diosc. *Ther.* 30; *Cyran.* 4.40; Prom. *Ther.* 79).

§3. *ad – tribus.*
Comparandum: Plin. 28.45.162 for stingrays and all marine creatures' strikes.
Pliny recommended a *drachma* of rennet in an unspecified amount of wine. Hare rennet was similarly recommended for stingray strikes (Prom. *Ther.* 16; Philum. 15.16).

36. contra murem araneum

It is difficult to determine why the author moved from his discussion of marine creatures to a mammal. Despite the sincerely held belief in antiquity that shrew-mice were venomous (Arist. *Hist. an.* 7(8).24; Nic. *Ther.* ll. 815–6; Plin. 8.83.227), they actually are not (Woodman 2004, 266–70). Their Latin name, literally "spider-mouse", focused on their supposed venomous nature, and likely explains why this chapter was followed by a discussion of spiders.

§1. *mus – obtusa*. . .

This is the earliest extant Latin description of the shrew-mouse. Its Greek name, μυγαλῆ, literally "mouse-weasel", was given for its appearance (Prom. *Ther*. 30; Philum. 33.1). Aristophanes of Byzantium (*Epit*. 2.373) described it as having small eyes and dim sight, but others described it as blind (Nic. *Ther*. l. 815; Ps-Garg. 21).

§1. . . . *et – occurritur*.

Comparanda: Plin. 29.27.89, cf. 8.83.227; Nic. *Ther*. ll. 815–6; Ael. *NA* 2.37; Marc. 15.47.

§2. *coagulum – imponitur*.
Comparanda: Plin. 29.27.88; Ps-Theod. *Ad*. I,21(68).

§2. *ipse – imponitur*.
Comparandum: Plin. 29.27.89.

If the shrew-mouse responsible for the bite was unavailable, another would suffice (Plin. 29.27.89; Gal. K14.246). Preserved shrew-mice were recommended in veterinary texts (Columella 6.17.5; Veget. *Mulomed*. 2.146; Pall. *Agric*. 14.18.7).

§2. *terra – imponitur*.
Comparanda: Plin. 29.27.89; Ael. *NA* 2.37.

This was based on the theory that something that would kill the animal would also "kill" the effect of its bite.

§2. *talpa – imponitur*.
Comparandum: Plin. 30.7.20.

This treatment was completely stripped of its context by the author, making Pliny appear to have written positively of this. When Pliny's advice is properly contextualised (30.6.16–30.8.22 among Magian treatments) he did not recommend this.

37. contra phalangium

The move from the "spider-mouse" to spiders was a logical progression. This chapter is not terribly long, and is followed by a significantly longer chapter devoted to snakes. Given that spiders and snakes are the most commonly recognised potentially venomous animals, it is not surprising that this was the author's chosen order of chapters.

Phalangium, φαλάγγιον: Aristotle (*Hist. an.* 8(9).39), Nicander (*Ther*. ll. 715–51), and Pliny (29.27.84–7) used this generically for all venomous spiders. Given this and the lack of further descriptions of spiders akin to those provided by Nicander and Pliny, it appears that the author sought to provide universal spider-bite remedies.

Pliny stated that *phalangia* were not found in Italy (29.27.84).

§1. *phalangium – intelleguntur.*

Comparandum: Plin. 22.81.163 for *solipuga*-bites.

Solipuga was a type of spider (Solin. 4.3), and spiders were commonly described as living in various leguminous crops, and thus posed a danger (Arist. *Hist. an.* 8(9).39; Theophr. 8.10.1; Nic. *Ther.* ll. 752–5; Plin. 18.44.156; Ael. *NA* 9.39).

Alia genera bestiolarum mortifera: this could refer to more than spiders. The provision of treatments and prophylactics which addressed multiple venomous bites and stings was common (e.g. Nic. *Ther.* ll. 652–5; Diosc. *MM* 3.24.3, *Eup.* 2.126.1; Plin. 20.67.175, 21.92.162, 23.31.63; *Cyran.* 4.28; Gal. K14.2, 175–6; Orib. *EM* 119.1–7); the creation of universal treatments was a popular goal (Totelin 2004, 15) and this fits that trend.

There are only four extant references to itching as a symptom of *phalangia*-bites, and it was considered a minor symptom (Prom. *Ther.* 6; Philum. 15.6; Aët. 13.20; Paul. Aeg. 5.6.1). It is impossible to determine why the author chose to focus on a minor symptom.

§2. *adversus – bibutur.*

Comparandum: Plin. 23.23.43.

§2. *acetum – sulphuris.*

Comparandum: Plin. 23.27.55. Cf. *Med. Plin.* 3.11.3.

Serenus (46 ll. 875–6, l. 862) recommended vinegar and sulphur, but not together, on spider- bites.

Variously prepared vinegar was recommended in sponges (Prom. *Ther.* 15.11; Philum. 15.11; Aët. 13.20). Galen recommended the use of sulphur on venomous strikes, but not explicitly for *phalangia* (K12.217).

§2. *radicis – bibitur.*

Comparanda: Plin. 24.47.79 (ivy juice with vinegar); Diosc. *MM* 2.179.3, *Eup.* 2.126.2; Ps-Apul. 99.4.

This was thought to have developed from witnessing deer eating wild ivy to counteract spider-bites (Ael. *VH* 1.8).

§3. *sucus – rubo.*

Comparandum: Plin. 24.73.120 for *araneus*-bite.

§3. *gallinacei – potione.*

Comparanda: Plin. 29.27.88; Cassius 68.

§3. *fimi – inponuntur.*

Comparandum: Plin. 29.27.88.

The source of the dung might not have been important (see commentaries on *Med. Plin.* 1.6.5 and 3.4.18).

38. contra serpentis et hominis morsum

The penultimate chapter of this text, this discussion of snake-bites is the longest within this exposition on toxicology. By addressing preventions and treatment, the author used a similar format here to that used for poisons. While it is entitled "Against snake's and human's bites", the specialised treatment of human-bites at the very end read like they were an afterthought prior to addressing asp-bites.

Greek writers usually referred to vipers rather than snakes (see commentary on *Med. Plin.* 3.6.5), in relation to bites as well as medicaments.

1. *serpentes – suffitu. . .*
Comparanda: Plin. 29.24.77; Ael. *NA* 1.45; Seren. 45 l. 838; Plac. 23.1.
Apart from releasing foul-smelling smoke, vultures and snakes were thought to
    enjoy a specific antipathy (Arist. *Hist. an.* 8(9).1), so this might have been
    semi-magical.

§1. . . . *ebuli – fumo. . .*
Comparanda: Plin. 25.71.119; Lucan ll. 9.915–21.

§1. . . . *nidore – cervini.*
Comparanda: Plin. 28.41.149, cf. 8.50.118, 10.90.195; Nic. *Ther.* ll. 35–6;
    Diosc. *MM* 2.59.1; Lucan ll. 9.915–21; Columella 7.4.6, 8.5.18; Cassius 70.

§2. *viperae – feriri.*
Comparandum: Plin. 29.22.71.
Nicander (*Ther.* l. 622) recommended drinking snake liver in wine.

§2. *erucis – mordent.*
Comparandum: Seren. 45 ll. 849–50.
Rocket was more commonly used to treat scorpion-strikes (e.g. Plin. 20.49.125;
    Cyran. 5.5; Orib. *EM* 119.7; Paul. Aeg. 5.8.3).

§2. *habentem – appetunt.*
Comparanda: Plin. 29.24.77; *Cyran.* 3.9; Plac. 23.6; *Vulture Epistles*, (Cumont
    1926, 30).
Vulture Epistles, *Cyranides*, and Placitus all described this as worn in hide.
    Again, this was likely owing to the perceived antipathy between vultures
    and snakes (see commentary on *Med. Plin.* 3.37.1).

§3. *raphanus – imponitur.*
Comparanda: Plin. 20.13.23 (radish cooked in *posca*); Seren. 45 l. 832.
Radish was recommended both topically and eaten (e.g. Diosc. *MM* 2.112.1;
    Prom. *Ther.* 21; Aët. 13.23; Paul. Aeg. 5.13.5).

§3. *alium – adicitur.*
Comparanda: Plin. 20.23.51; Garg. 18.

Garlic was variously recommended topically (Diosc. *MM* 2.152.2; *Cyran.* 5.18; Philum. 7.6, 21.4; Orib. *EM* 117.6).

§4. *radix – imposita.*
Comparandum: Plin. 20.98.260.
Giant fennel was more commonly drunk (e.g. Nic. *Ther.* ll. 594–8; Diosc. *MM* 3.77.1; Plin. 20.98.260; Seren. 45 l. 840).

§4. *farina – facit.*
Comparandum: Plin. 22.62.130.
Liquid pitch was often used with salt (Diosc. *MM* 1.72.1; Ps-Diosc. *Ther.* 19; Orib. *EM* 118.2; Paul. Aeg. 5.2.2, 5.13.5).

§4. *ervum – medetur.*
Comparandum: Plin. 22.73.151.
Human-bites were considered the most venomous (e.g. Plin. 28.8.40; Ael. *NA* 9.15), and combining their treatment with that of other venomous bites was not unusual (e.g. Prom. *Ther.* 10; Gal. K14.43, 189; Orib. *EM* 126.1).
Bitter vetch was commonly used for viper-bites (Ps-Diosc. *Ther.* 27; Philum. 17.3) in addition to human-bites (*MM* 2.108.2), and its meal was commonly included in *theriaci* devoted to all venomous bites.

§5. *vinum – imponitur.*
This remedy appears to be an erroneous crasis of Pliny's test (23.23.43–4) where the author took the use of unmixed wine as a remedy for venomous bites and placed it with the use of unmixed wine to treat *cardiacus* on a sponge, correctly recorded at 3.20.3.

§5. *mori – imponuntur.*
Comparandum: Plin. 23.71.138.
The topical use of mulberry leaves was very uncommon; Aëtius (13.23) included them once in a plaster.

§5. *hyssopi – bibitur.*
Hyssop, not specifically its seeds, was included in some treatments (Plin. 25.87.136, 31.45.98; Gal. K14.292; Paul. Aeg. 5.16.3). It was especially recommended for chilling bites (Plin. 23.23.43; Diosc. *Eup.* 2.124.1) because of its warming properties (Diosc. *MM* 3.25.1).

§6. *eius – est.*
Comparanda: Plin. 25.38.78, cf. 5.1.16; Diosc. *MM* 3.82.3.
This treatment was also specified for *pelias* snake-bites (Prom. *Ther.* 23; Philum. 28.2).

§7. *centauriae – bibitur.*

Comparanda: Plin. 25.55.100 (large centaury); Nic. *Ther.* ll. 500–7; Cels. 5.27.10.

Whether the failure by the author to specify the variety of centaury might have caused problems for his readers cannot be determined; Celsus also did this, and Pseudo-Apuleius (35.1) recommended small centaury in old wine.

§7. *vettonica – imponitur.*

Comparanda: Plin. 25.55.101; Diosc. *MM* 4.1.2; Gal. K12.24; Ps-Musa 43.

Celsus (5.27.10) might have recommended betony's application to Italian and colder climate snake-bites.

§7. *agarici – propinantur.*

Comparanda: Plin. 25.57.103; Diosc. *MM* 3.1.5.

Tree fungus was included in a variety of snake-bite antidotes and *theriaci* (e.g. Gal. K14.39, 259; Ps-Gal. K14.308; Orib. *EM* 118.1; Paul. Aeg. 5.13.2).

§8. *aristolochiae – bibitur.*

Comparanda: Plin. 25.55.101; Ps-Apul. 19.5.

Pliny elsewhere wrote that the long variety of *aristolochia* was more suitable (25.54.97). Dioscorides (*MM* 3.4.4) recommended the same dosage outlined by the author, but of round *aristolochia*; and Crateuas (*Fr.* 1, 2) referred to both large and round varieties being drunk in wine.

Different preparations of *aristolochia* were recommended for various snake-bites (Theophr. *Hist. pl.* 9.13.3, 9.20.4; Nic. *Ther.* ll. 509–19; Ps-Diosc. *Ther.* 29; Philum. 25.3, Paul. Aeg. 5.15.1, 5.17.1, 5.18.1). Such was *aristolochia*'s use that it was described outside of medical literature (e.g. Cicero *De divinatione*, 1.10.16, 2.21.47).

§8. *et – plagae.*

Comparandum: Plin. 25.55.101.

Aristolochia's topical application without vinegar was described elsewhere (Theophr. 9.13.3, 9.20.4; Crateuas *Fr.* 1, 2; Diosc. *MM* 3.4.4).

§8. *fimus – imponitur.*

Comparanda: Plin. 20.15.59; Diosc. *MM* 2.80.2.

When the variety of dung was specified, goat was most common, though not necessarily decocted in wine (Cels. 5.27.8; Ps-Diosc. *Ther.* 27; Gal. K12.299; Philum. 17.3, 17.10; Aët. 13.23; Paul. Aeg. 5.13.5).

§9. *mus – adicitur.*

Comparandum: Plin. 29.15.59.

This was also used for scorpion-strikes (Diosc. *MM* 2.69.1; Gal. K12.365).

§9. *viperae – prodest.*

Comparanda: Plin. 29.21.69; Ps-Gal. K14.490; Seren. 45 ll. 828–30.

Viper flesh rendered into *theriaci* or pastilles was common (e.g. Diosc. *MM* 2.16.1; Plin. 29.21.70; Gal. K14.262–7, 290–2).

§9. *carnibus – venenum*.
Comparanda: Plin. 29.25.78; Diosc. *MM* 2.49.1, *Eup.* 2.123.1; Orib. *EM* 118.2.
Variations of this treatment were recorded elsewhere (Plin. 29.26.81; Ps-Gal. K14.489; Aët. 13.23; Paul. Aeg. 5.13.5).

§10. *item – imponitur*.
Comparandum: Plin. 29.25.78 (hen's brain).
It is impossible to determine precisely where the author found his reference to pigeon brains.

§10. *sal – melle*.
Comparanda: Plin. 31.45.98; Diosc. *MM* 5.109.4.
Origanum ὀρίγανος: oregano or marjoram; various types were described, especially by Nicander (*Ther.* ll. 575, 559, 617, 626–8).
Pliny and Dioscorides recommended all four ingredients together, whereas the text of the *Medicina Plinii* is ambiguous and could be read as "salt with *origanum*" distinct from "hyssop in honey", or all together. The use of these ingredients was recommended by Philumenus (17.4) who transposed the combination from that possibly provided here.
The use of *origanum* likely originated with the theory that tortoises were able to eat viper flesh because they ate ὀρίγανος (Arist. *Hist. an.* 8(9).6, *Mirabilibus auscultationibus*, 11).
Pliny (25.87.136) described a similar remedy of salt, hyssop, honey, and cumin; the author perhaps chose this remedy over it because cumin was an exotic spice.

§10. *fraxini – adiciuntur*.
Comparanda: Plin. 16.24.64; Diosc. *MM* 1.80.1; Gal. K14.203; Theod. 1.24.74.

§§11–3. *non – tribus*.
Comparanda: Plin. 20.100.264; Gal. K14.185–6, 201–3; Garg. 39.
There are some notable differences between the *Medicina Plinii's* and Pliny's records of this compound: the author switched from *drachmae* to *denarii* mid-prescription; wrote *amuli* (starch) instead of *ami*; and misread *anesum* (anise) as *anethum* (dill) as he did at 1.1.2. All three Latin renderings stated that pastilles weigh the same as a *victoriatus* were made and that this was inscribed at the temple of Asclepius on Cos.
Galen referred to Pliny's text, calling the compound "*theriacus* of Antiochus for viper-bites" that Pliny said was engraved beside the doors of Asclepius (K14.183). Galen later recorded a *theriacus* ascribed to Antiochus Philometor that was recorded by Eudemus in its original poetic form along with a prose rendering of it (K14.185–6); he did this without any reference to Pliny or Asclepius. These were repeated with no additional information later in his work (K14.201–3).

Watson (1966, 13) argues that the Antiochus Philometor *theriacus* differs from Pliny's, but a close reading of the poem indicates that this is erroneous. The ingredients are the same: Pliny used a transliteration of ἄμι (Diosc. *MM* 3.62.1), *ami*, "ajwain"; σέλινον "celery" corresponds with *apium*; and Jones (LCL: *Pliny Natural History VI*, 156) points out that the *seminis* associated with fennel in Pliny might also refer to *apium*, ajwain, and anise, therefore matching the poem's recipe using seeds from all four plants. The amounts of *opopanax*, thyme, spignel and trefoil seeds also match if the potential difference between the weight of Hellenistic *drachmae* and Roman *denarii* is ignored. The use of the liquid measure ὀξύβαφον, likely used to fit the poetic metre, for the amounts of anise, fennel, ajwain, celery seeds, and bitter vetch meal was interpreted by Pliny and the author as equalling six *denarii*, whereas one of Galen's prose renderings (K14.202–3) made it equal four *drachmae*. Galen included multiple errors in this prose rendition, so this section of his text is suspicious, and this is the basis of Watson's argument. The poem described that this compound was then made into pastilles weighing half a *drachma* (compare this to a *victoriatus* equalling half a *denarius*), and the more accurate prose rendering (K14.185–6) recommended that it be mixed in three *cyathi* of wine, matching Pliny and the *Medicina Plinii*.

King Antiochus: determining which Antiochus is difficult. The name "Antiochus the Great", ascribed by Pliny, makes Antiochus III of Syria (223–187 BCE) tempting (Watson 1966, 13), but it only fits with Gargilius' "Antiochus of Syria". Galen's "Philometor" only correlates with Antiochus VIII Grypus (Josephus *Antiquitates Judaicae*, 13.325). The conflicting titles make it impossible to identify Antiochus with certainty.

Storing pastilles in a glass container was not recorded elsewhere; it might have been influenced by the other references in the *Medicina Plinii* to glass vessels to store compounds (2.4.12, 2.4.14, 2.17.15), or the use of specialist containers for antidotes recorded elsewhere (e.g. Scribon. 170, 173; Gal. K14.268, 293).

§14.*hominis – solvuntur*.
Comparandum: Plin. 28.43.156.

§14.*sordes – plagae*.
Comparandum: Plin. 28.4.40.

39. contra aspidem

This is the final chapter of the *Medicina Plinii*, and likely addressed asp-bites separate from and immediately following the treatment of snake-bites because of the author's inclusion of Antiochus' *theriacus* which explicitly made the point that asp-bites required different treatment. This had been understood for centuries prior to this. Analysis of Nicander's descriptions of symptoms identifies two families of snakes: *Viperidae* whose venom usually causes respiratory failure;

and *Elapidae*, to which asps belong, whose venom contains neurotoxins causing unconsciousness, swallowing difficulties, and respiration paralysis (Scarborough 1977, 6–9). Like modern clinical practice, it was recognised in antiquity that these required different treatments.

There was confusion regarding whether asp-bites were treatable: Aelian stated that victims recovered when treated by excision, cauterisation, or dangerous drugs (*NA* 2.5), but later wrote that no one survived (*NA* 6.38); Pliny stated that the only remedy was immediate amputation (8.35.85), but again provided treatments.

§1. *adversus – biberet.*
Comparandum: Plin. 29.18.65.

§§2–3. *intra – efficacissimam.*
Comparanda: Plin. 23.27.56; Cels. 5.27.4.
Vinegar was occasionally included in treatments (e.g. Diosc. *MM* 4.7.1, *Eup.* 2.125; Philum. 16.7) but not on its own like this.

§4. *si – superest.*
Comparandum: Plin. 29.18.65.
Aelian (*NA* 9.16) described in great detail how asp venom could gain entry into the body via broken skin.

Bibliography

Anon. (2018). "Red threads & amulets: Roman and late antique artefacts from Egypt (13 December 2018)." https://blogs.kent.ac.uk/egypt-artefacts/2018/12/13/red-threads-amulets/, accessed 15/3/2019.

Attard, E. *et al.* (2015). "The phytochemical constitution of Maltese medicinal plants – Propagation, isolation and pharmacological testing." Rao, V. & Rao, L. (eds.) *Phytochemicals – Isolation, characterisation and role in human health.* Intech: 3–44. www.intechopen.com/books/phytochemicals-isolation-characterisation-and-role-in-human-health/the-phytochemical-constitution-of-maltese-medicinal-plants-propagation-isolation-and-pharmacological (DOI: 10.5772/60094), accessed 20/3/2017.

Biraben, J.-N. (1998). "Disease in Europe: Equilibrium and breakdown of the pathocenosis." Grmek, M. (ed.) & Shugaar, A. (tr.) *Western medical thought from antiquity to the middle ages.* Cambridge, MA, Harvard University Press: 319–54.

Bohlooli, S. *et al.* (2007). "Comparative study of fig tree efficacy in the treatment of common warts (*Verruca vulgaris*) vs. Cryotherapy." *International Journal of Dermatology* 46: 524–6. (DOI: 10.1111/j.1365–4632.2007.03159.x), accessed 27/4/2017.

Bondeson, J. (1998). "*Phthiriasis*: The riddle of the lousy disease." *Journal of the Royal Society of Medicine* 91: 238–334. (DOI: 10.1177/014107689809100617), accessed 24/10/2018.

Brodersen, K. (2016). "Antike Reiseapotheke." *Damals* 48(8): 45–6.

Bryan, C. (1974). *Ancient Egyptian medicine, the papyrus ebers.* Chicago, IL, Ares Publishers.

Buffa Giolito, M. F. (2000). "'Topoi' della tradizione letteraria in tre prefazioni di testi medici latini." Pigeaud, A. & Pigeaud, J. (eds.) *Les textes medicaux Latins comme littérature.* Nantes, Université de Nantes: 13–31.

Butcher, K. & Ponting, M. (2012). "The beginning of the end? The Denarius in the second century." *The Numismatic Chronicle* 172: 63–83.

Castiglioni, A. (1964). "Pseudo-Plinian medicine." *Bulletin of History of Medicine* 20: 201–6.

Chişamera, G. & Traian, M. (2007). "Contributions to the knowledge of the food structure of red-rumped swallows (*Hirundo daurica rufula* temm. 1835) (Passeriformes: Hirundinidae) in Romania and Turkey [Partial results of "Focida" 2006 expedition in Turkey]." *Travaux du Muséum National d'Histoire Naturelle "Grigore Antipa"* 50: 463–77.

Clark, P. & Rose, M. (2013). "Psychiatric disability and the Galenic medical matrix." Laes, C., Goodey, C. F. & Rose, M. L. (eds.) *Disabilities in Roman antiquity, disparate bodies a Capite ad Calcem.* Leiden, Brill: 45–72. (DOI: 10.1163/9789004251250_004).

Cook, J. (2014). *Crucifixion in the Mediterranean world.* Tübingen, Mohr Siebeck. (DOI: 10.1628/978-3-16-153125-5).

Coromines, J. (1939). "Catalan rolder 'sumac'." *Romania* 65: 218–21.

Corsini, A. R. & Segoloni, M. P. (1989). *Medicinae Plinii concordantiae (Alpha – Omega A 101)*. Hildesheim, Olms.

Cumont, F. (1926). "Le sage Bothros ou le phylarque Arétas?" *Revue de Philologie* 50: 13–33.

Dalby, A. (2003). *Food in the ancient world from A-Z*. London, Routledge.

Daremberg, C., Saglio, E. & Pottier, E. (1904). *Dictionaire des Antiquités Grecques et Romaines, Tome Troisième Deuxième partie (L-M)*. Paris, Librairie Hachette.

De Grandsagne, M. (1832). *Histoire Naturelle de Pline, Tome Quatorzième*. Paris, Panckoucke.

Delatte, A. (1927–39). *Anecdota Atheniensia I: Textes grecs inédits relatifs à l'histoire des religions; II: Textes grecs relatifs à l'histoire des sciences*. Liege, H. Vaillant-Carmanne.

Dey, D. *et al.* (2015). "Antimicrobial activity of pomegranate fruit constituents against drug-resistant *Mycobacterium tuberculosis* and β-lactamase producing *Klebsiella pneumoniae*." *Pharmaceutical Biology* 53(10): 1471–80. (DOI: 10.3109/13880209.2014.986687), accessed 4/3/2018.

Doody, A. (2009). "Authority and authorship in the *Medicina Plinii*." Doody, A. & Taub, L. (eds.) *Authorial voices in Greco-Roman technical writing*. Trier, WVT: 93–158.

Doody, A. (2010). "Specialist readings: Art and medicine from the natural history." Doody, A. (ed.) *Pliny's encyclopedia: The reception of the natural history*. Cambridge: Cambridge University Press: 132–72. (DOI: 10.1017/CBO9780511676222.006), accessed 15/3/2019.

Duffin, C. (2013). "Chelidonius: The Swallow stone." *Folklore* 124(1): 81–103. (DOI: 10.1080/0015587X.2012.747479), accessed 9/5/2017.

Estel, C. (1968). *Über die volksmedizinischen Anteile der "Medicina Plinii Secundi Junioris"*. Diss. med. Erfurt (unpublished).

Ferraces Rodríguez, A. (2008). "Un extracto de la Medicina Plinii y una fuente ignorada de la Physica Plinii." *Mittellateinisches Jahrbuch* 43: 165–76.

Fischer, K.-D. (1988). "Anweisungen zur Selbstmedikation von Laien in der Spätantike." *Actes XXX: Congrès international d'histoire de la médicine*. Düsseldorf Vicom: 867–74.

Fischer, K.-D. (2012). "Wenn kein Arzt erreichbar ist: Medizinische Literatur für Laien in der Spätantike." *Medicina nei secoli – arte e scienza* 24(1): 379–401.

Fischer, K.-D. & Kudlien, F. (1989). "Die sogenannte Medicina Plinii." Herzog, R. (ed.) *Restauration und Erneuerung: Handbuch der lateinischen Literatur der Antike 5*. Munich, Beck: 75–7.

Formisano, M. (2004). "The "natural" medicine of Theodorus Priscianus." *Philologus* 148(1): 126–42. (DOI: 10.1524/phil.2004.148.1.126), accessed 3/4/2019.

Gertler, H. (1966). *Über die Bedeutung der "Medicina Plinii Secundi Junioris"*. Habil. med. Erfurt (unpublished).

Gibson, A. (1983). "A group of roman surgical and medical instruments from Cramond, Scotland." *Medizinhistorisches Journal* 19(4): 384–93.

Gowling, E. (2017). "Aëtius' Extraction of Galenic Essence." Lehmhaus, M. & Mattelli, M. (eds.) *Collecting recipes: Byzantine and Jewish pharmacy in dialogue*. Berlin, De Gruyter: 83–102. (DOI: 10.1515/9781501502538–005), accessed 4/4/19.

Grattan, J. & Singer, C. (1952). *Anglo-Saxon magic and medicine*. Oxford, Oxford University Press.

Groag, E. *et al.* (eds.) (1933–). PIR – *Prosopographia Imperii Romani Saeculi I, II, III*, 2nd edn. Berlin, De Gruyter.

Heim, R. (1892). "De usu incantamentorum." *Incantamenta Magica Graeca Latina*. Leipzig, Teubner: 465–576.

Horden, P. (2013). "Prefatory note: The uses of medical manuscripts." Zipser, B. (ed.) *Medical books in the Byzantine world*. Bologna, Eikasmós Online: 1–6.

Johnstone, S. (1991). "Crossroads." *Zeitscrift für Papyrologie und Epigraphik* 88: 217–24.

Koch, W. (1939). *Medicina Plinii, Übersetzung 2: Teil*. Diss. med. München (unpublished, 16 p. translating only 1.16–2.6).

Kudlien, F. (1988). "Heilkunde." *Reallexikon für Antike und Christentum 14*. Stuttgart, Hiersemann: 223–49.

Langslow, D. (1991). *The formation and development of Latin medical vocabulary: A. Cornelius Celsus and Cassius Felix*. Ph.D. dissertation, University of Oxford.

Legrand, E. (1881). *Bibliotheque grecque vulgaire*. Paris, Maisonneuve.

Linder, G. (1969). *Die magischen Mittel und die Mittel der Dreckapotheke in der "Medicina Plinii Secundi Junioris"*. Diss. med. Erfurt (unpublished).

Luck, G. (2006). *Arcana Mundi: Magic and the occult in the Greek and Roman worlds*. Baltimore, MD, Johns Hopkins Press.

Mackinney, L. (1943). "An unpublished treatise on medicine and magic from the age of Charlemagne." *Speculum* 18(4): 494–6.

Murphy, K. (2013). *The conceptualization and treatments for Phrenitis, mania and melancholia in Aretaeus of Cappadocia and Caelius Aurelianus*. MA Thesis, University of Calgary.

Nagy, A. (2011). "Magical gems and classical archaeology." Entwistle, C. & Adams, N. (eds.) *Recent research on engraved gemstones in late antiquity c. AD 200–600*. London, The British Museum.

Nunn, J. (2002). *Ancient Egyptian medicine*. Norman, OK, University of Oklahoma Press.

Nutton, V. (1995). "Medicine in late antiquity and the early middle ages." Conrad, L. I. et al. (eds.) *The Western medical tradition 800 BC to AD 1800*. Cambridge, Cambridge University Press: 71–83.

Nutton, V. (2013). "Byzantine medicine, genres, and the ravages of time." Zipser, B. (ed.) *Medical books in the Byzantine world*. Bologna, Eikasmós Online: 7–18.

Olsen, K. (2014). "Masculinity, appearance, and sexuality: Dandies in Roman antiquity." *Journal of the History of Sexuality* 23(2): 182–205. (DOI: 10.7560/JHS23202), accessed 29/4/2017.

Oman, C. (1916). "The decline and fall of the Denarius in the third century A.D." *The Numismatic Chronicle and Journal of the Royal Numismatic Society* 16: 37–60.

Önnerfors, A. (1963). *In Medicinam Plinii Studia Philologica*. Lunds Universitets Årsskrift N. F. 1.55.5. Lund, Gleerum.

Önnerfors, A. (1965). "Die mittelalterlichen Fassungen der Medicina Plinii." *Berliner Medizin* 16: 652–5.

Önnerfors, A. (1993). "Magische Formeln im Dienste römischer medizin." *Aufstieg und Niedergang der römischen Welt* II 37.1. Berlin and New York, De Gruyter: 157–224.

Photos-Jones, E. et al. (2015). "Testing Dioscorides' medicinal clays for their antibacterial properties: The case of Samian Earth." *Journal of Archaeological Science* 57: 257–67. (DOI: 10.1016/j.jas.2015.01.020), accessed 20/10/2018.

Pittinger, J. (1975). "The mineral products of Melos in antiquity and their identification." *The Annual of the British School at Athens* 70: 191–7.

Rehren, T. et al. (1999). "Litharge from Laurion. A medical and metallurgical commodity from South Attika." *L'Antiquité Classique* 68: 299–308. (DOI: 10.3406/antiq.1999.1348), accessed 28/12/2018.

Retief, F. & Cilliers, L. (2004). "Malaria in Graeco-Roman times." *Acta Classica* 47: 127–37.

Riddle, J. (1985). *Dioscorides on pharmacy and medicine*. Austin, TX, University of Texas Press.

Rider, J. (1589). *Bibliotheca scholastica*. Oxford, Joseph Barnes.

Rives, J. (2003). "Magic in Roman Law: The reconstruction of a crime." *Classical Antiquity* 22: 313–39. (DOI: 10.1525/ca.2003.22.2.313), accessed 12/11/2015.

Rose, V. (1874). "Über die Medicina Plinii." *Hermes* 8: 18–66.

Sakai, A. (1991). "Phrenitis: Inflammation of the mind and the body." *History of Psychiatry* 2: 193–205. (DOI: 10.1177/0957154X9100200606), accessed 17/2/2017.

Scarborough, J. (1977). "Nicander's toxicology I: Snakes." *Pharmacy in History* 19: 3–23.

Scarborough, J. & Fernandes, A. (2011). "Ancient medical use of Aristolochia: Birthwort's tradition and toxicity." *Pharmacy in History* 53: 3–21.Schäfer, J. (1939). *Medicina Plinii, übersetzt und in Hinsicht auf unsere Volksmedizin untersucht*. Diss. med. Munich (unpublished; 30 p. translating only 1.1–15).

Scheidel, W. (2011). "The Roman slave supply." Bradley, K. & Cartledge, P. (eds.) *The Cambridge world history of slavery, Volume 1: The ancient Mediterranean world*. Cambridge, Cambridge University Press: 287–310. (DOI: 10.1017/CHOL9780521840668.016), accessed 3/1/2019.

Schlumberger, G. (1892). "Amulettes Byzantins Anciens Destinés a Combatrre les Maléfices & Maladies." *Revue des Études Grecques* 5: 299–308.

Segoloni, M. P. (1990). "Il prologus della Medicina Plinii." Santini, C. & Scivoletto, N. (eds.) *Prefazioni, prologhi, proemi di opere tecnico-scientifiche latine*. Rome, Herder: 361–6.

Sigerist, H. E. (1958). "The Latin medical literature of the early middle ages." *Journal of History of Medicine and Allied Sciences* 13: 127–46.

Sparkes, B. (1982). "Production and exchange in the classical and Roman periods." Renfrew, C. & Wagstaff, M. (eds.) *An island polity: The archaeology of exploitation in Melos*. Cambridge, Cambridge University Press: 228–35.

Stannard, J. (1974). "Squill in ancient and medieval materia medica, with special reference to its employment for dropsy." *Bulletin of the New York Academy of Medicine* 50(6): 684–713.

Steier, A. (1931). "Medicina Plinii." *Realencyclopädie der classischen Altertumswissenschaft XV* 1: 81–5.

Stoll, U. (1992). *Das 'Lorscher Arzneibuch', ein medizinisches Kompendium des 8. Jahrhunderts (Codex Bambergensis medicinalis 1): Text, Übersetzung und Fachglossar*. Stuttgart, Steiner.

Stuart, K. (1998). "The executioner's healing touch: Health and honor in early modern German medical practice." Reinhart, M. (ed.) *Infinite boundaries: Order, disorder, and reorder in early modern German culture*. Kirksville, Sixteenth Century Journal Publishers: 349–80.

Taylor, W. *et al.* (2018). "Origins of equine dentistry." *Proceedings of the National Academy of the Sciences of the United States of America* 115(29): E6707–15. (DOI: 10.1073/pnas.1721189115), accessed 11/1/2019.

Tomlin, R. (2016). *Roman London's first voices: Writing tablets from the Bloomberg excavations, 2010–14*. London, Museum of London Archaeology Monographs.

Totelin, L. (2004). "Mithridates' antidote – a pharmacological ghost." *Early Science and Medicine* 9: 1–19. (DOI: 10.1163/1573382041153179), accessed 18/12/2016.

Verma, R. *et al.* (2014). "Rubus fruticosus (blackberry) use as an herbal medicine." *Pharmacognosy Reviews* 8: 101–4. (DOI: 10.4103/0973-7847.134239), accessed 14/5/2018.

Watson, G. (1966). *Theriac and Mithridatium: A study in therapeutics*. London, Wellcome Historical Medical Library.

Whitehouse, D. (2001). *Roman glass at the Corning Museum of glass*. New York, NY, Hudson Hills.

Williams, F. *et al.* (2017). "Internal parasites from the 2nd-5th century AD latrine in the Roman Baths at Sagalassos (Turkey)." *International Journal of Paleopathology* 19: 37–42. (DOI: 10.1016/j.ijpp.2017.09.002), accessed 13/5/2018.

Woodman, N. (2004). "Designation of the type species of Musaraneus Pomel, 1848 (Mammalia: Soricomorpha: Soricidae)." *Proceedings of the Biological Society of Washington* 117(2): 266–70.

Index